Clinical Voice Pathology:
Theory and Management

Third Edition

Clinical Voice Pathology
Theory and Management
Third Edition

Joseph C. Stemple, PhD
Director
Blaine Block Institute for Voice Analysis and Rehabilitation
Dayton, Ohio

Leslie Glaze, PhD
Director of Clinical Programs
Department of Communication Disorders
University of Minnesota, Minneapolis, Minnesota

Bernice Gerdeman Klaben, PhD
Director of Clinical Practice
Blaine Block Institute for Voice Analysis and Rehabilitation
Dayton, Ohio

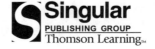

Singular
PUBLISHING GROUP
Thomson Learning

COPYRIGHT © 2000 Delmar. Singular Publishing Group is an imprint of Delmar, a division of Thomson Learning. Thomson Learning™ is a trademark used herein under license.

Printed in Canada
5 6 7 8 9 10 XXX 05 04 03

For more information, contact Singular Publishing Group, 401 West "A" Street, Suite 325 San Diego, CA 92101-7904; or find us on the World Wide Web at http://www.singpub.com

Library of Congress Cataloging-in-Publication Data
Stemple, Joseph C.
    Clinical voice pathology: theory and management / Joseph C. Stemple, Leslie E. Glaze, Bernice K. Gerdeman.—3rd ed.
        p.   cm.
    Includes bibliographical references and index.
    ISBN 0-7693-0005-7 (softcover: alk. paper)
    1. Voice disorders. I. Glaze, Leslie E. II. Gerdeman, Bernice K. III. Title.
    [DNLM: I. Voice Disorders. WV 500 S824c 2000]
RF510.S74 2000
616.85'5—dc21   99-057053

Contents

9   Rehabilitation of the Laryngectomized Patient

Preface

Through our many years of clinical work, we have discovered the enjoyment and the challenge of working with the voice-disordered population. Each patient provides us with questions that must be answered to return the voice to an improved condition. To answer these questions, voice pathologists must draw on many areas of knowledge, including anatomy, physiology, etiologic correlates, and laryngeal pathologies. Diagnostic skills must be honed, which include developing an effective patient interview style, techniques for the perceptual analysis of voice, and, more recently, an understanding of voice acoustics, aerodynamics, and evaluation of vocal fold movement patterns. Finally, the voice pathologist must understand and be able to initiate a wide range of therapy techniques that, through the diagnostic procedure, have been determined to be the treatments most likely to effect positive vocal change.

This text was developed as an aid to speech-language pathology students in their study of clinical voice pathology and to clinicians currently working with individuals with voice disorders. The ordering of the chapters was designed to slowly build the areas of knowledge necessary to manage the patient. Chapter 1 presents a history of voice disorders and describes the manner in which speech-language pathologists became involved with evaluation and treatment of these disorders. The importance and advantages of the "team approach" are emphasized. Chapter 2 describes the anatomy and physiology of the laryngeal mechanism, including recent information that expands our traditional knowledge of the cellular-layered micro-structure of the vocal fold. Recent advances in our understanding of the self-oscillating mechanism that governs vocal fold vibration are also described.

Chapter 3 offers a presentation of common etiologies associated with the development of voice disorders, whereas Chapter 4 presents a discussion of laryngeal pathologies categorized as structural changes in the vocal fold, neurogenic voice disorders, systemic contributions to laryngeal pathology, disorders of voice use, and idiopathic voice disorders. With the knowledge of anatomy and physiology, common etiologies, and laryngeal pathologies, the reader is then prepared to learn how to conduct the diagnostic voice evaluation. Chapter 5 details the voice evaluation, including the patient interview and various methods of perceptually analyzing voice production. Chapter 6, which has been greatly expanded in this edition, presents information on instrumental assessment of vocal function, providing the reader with an introduction to the basic science principles of acoustics, aerodynamics, and laryngeal videostroboscopy. This foundation is then bridged to the practical tasks of clinical analysis of vocal function in the voice laboratory.

Following the diagnostic voice evaluation, the voice pathologist is prepared to initiate a treatment plan. Chapter 7 provides the reader with a large sampling of treatment suggestions and therapy techniques. This chapter, also greatly expanded in this edition of the text, introduces the philosophies related to voice treatment, including hygienic, symptomatic, psychogenic, physiologic, and eclectic voice therapy orientations. The reader will find detailed descriptions of management approaches to be used with the wide variety of voice disorders.

Chapter 8 presents some comments on the professional voice. Salespeople, teachers, ministers, actors, singers, and others who are dependent on a healthy vocal system for their livelihoods are considered professional voice users. Because of their dependence on the vocal mechanism, professional voice users with voice disorders often require special considerations regarding the physical and emotional well-being and their courses of treatment. This chapter discusses these treatment considerations.

The final chapter, Chapter 9, deals with the total rehabilitation of the laryngectomized patient and the patient's family. From preoperative counseling to the reestablishment of oral communication, the rehabilitative processes are discussed from the perspective of the rehabilitation team. Oral communication methods, including artificial larynges, esophageal voice, and the use of surgical prostheses are described and illustrated in detail.

Clinical voice pathology has rapidly become a specialty within the field of communication disorders. It is our hope that this text will help to prepare students and clinicians who are interested in treating voice disorders by providing the appropriate science foundation, which permits the development of the artistic nature of voice care.

Numerous individuals have contributed to the development of this text. We are deeply indebted to Sadanand Singh, who strongly encouraged and supported the development of this expanded third edition. In addition, the guidance of our editor, Marie Linvill, was instrumental in bringing this text to print. We also wish to acknowledge the invaluable assistance of Sandy Doyle, Brad Bielawski, and Kristin Banach at Singular Thomson Learning. We are grateful for the efforts of Barbara Weinrich, Karen Kelly, and Richard Glaze in helping us completing the final draft. Finally, it is with sincere gratitude that we acknowledge Nancy Pinter, Administrative Assistant for the Blaine Block Institute for Voice Analysis and Rehabilitation, for her technical support and computer skills during the manuscript preparation.

Acknowledgments

A writing project of this kind may occur only with the support of those closest to us, through the teachings and works of those who came before us, and by the experience gained through working with those around us. With deep gratitude we acknowledge our families who have supported our goals and projects with love, patience, and endurance, and our teachers and colleagues, who inspired, encouraged, and challenged our learning and our patients, whose strength and perseverance make the entire process meaningful, productive, and ultimately worth our every professional effort.

Medical Illustrations Based on Original Artwork by John Barrord, MD, and Computer-generated Illustrations by Loralee McAuliffe

Dr Barrord is an otolaryngologist and head and neck surgeon in private practice in Middletown, Ohio who enjoys a longstanding avocation as an artist and illustrator. He created the original artwork for the 2nd edition (1994) of this text. His artistic talent, combined with his knowledge of the surgical anatomy of the larynx, made Dr Barrord an ideal illustrator for that text. We remain indebted to his efforts and have based figures in this 3rd edition on his original drawings.

Ms McAuliffe has worked as a freelance illustrator for more than 20 years. In the past 10 years, she has come to specialize in computer-generated medical illustrations. Through her unique talents, the original pencil drawings were transformed to cleaner, brighter line drawings to illustrate our 3rd edition. We extend our sincerest appreciation to Ms McAuliffe for her state-of-the-art talents, her ingenuity, and her creativity.

Laryngeal Photography by Jean Abitbol, M.D.

We are also indebted to the extraordinary generosity of Dr Jean Abitbol, who allowed us to reprint images of various laryngeal pathologies from his remarkable collection. Dr Abitbol is a practicing otorhinolaryngologist and head and neck surgeon at Hospitaux à la Faculté de Medecine in Paris, France. He is an internationally recognized clinician and scholar in laryngology. Dr Abitbol is the author of numerous publications related to laryngeal anatomy, pathology, and phonosurgery. He is also a frequent lecturer at interdisciplinary voice conferences worldwide. It is a privilege to incorporate some of his images in this text.

1

Voice: A Historical Perspective

Voice, articulation, and language are the major elements of human speech production. When a disorder related to any of these elements is present, the ability to communicate may be impaired. Voice is the element of speech that provides the speaker with the vibratory signal upon which speech is carried. Regarded as magical and mystical in ancient times, today the production of voice is viewed as both a powerful communication tool and an artistic medium. It serves as the melody of our speech and provides expression, feeling, intent, and mood to our articulated thoughts. It provides great expression and joy for both the listener and the performer as it is expressed artistically through the many varieties of vocal performance.

This text is concerned with the study of both normal and abnormal voice production. It is meant to introduce the reader to the science of voice production, the causes of voice disorders, and the pathologies of vocal function. You will explore methods of evaluation of voice disorders and delve into the wide array of management techniques; all are designed to return the

1

pathological voice to an improved state of equilibrium. Treating voice disorders is extremely rewarding. The vast majority of the time, patients with vocal difficulties who follow the prescribed treatment plans significantly improve their voice quality in a relatively short period of time.

A voice disorder exists when a person's quality, pitch, and loudness differ from those of similar age, gender, cultural background, and geographic location.[1-4] In other words, when the perceptual properties of voice are so deviant that they draw attention to the speaker, a voice disorder may be present. A voice disorder may also exist when either the structure, the function, or both of the laryngeal mechanism no longer meet the voicing requirements established for the mechanism by the speaker. These requirements include vocal difficulties that others do not readily recognize, such as the negative effects of vocal fatigue, but are reported to be present by the speaker. Successful management of a voice disorder is dependent on the individual recognizing the problem and accepting the need for improvement.

The effects of a voice disorder depend on the voicing needs of the individual. Those with a great need for normal voice production, such as professional voice users, may be unusually concerned with the presence of even minor vocal difficulties. Those with low vocal needs may not be greatly concerned with even more severe vocal problems. Identifying the vocal needs of each patient is extremely important in successfully treating voice disorders.[5]

The voice pathologist plays a major role in the evaluation and management of voice disorders. This role focuses on three major goals: (a) evaluation of laryngeal function using perceptual, acoustic, aerodynamic, and visual imaging techniques; (b) identification and modification or elimination of the functional causes that have led to the development of the voice disorder; and (c) developing a therapy plan that will remediate the voice disorder and return the voice to improved function. To accomplish these goals, voice pathologists must have an extensive understanding and knowledge of the normal anatomy and physiology of the laryngeal mechanism, as well as knowledge of common laryngeal pathologies. They also must understand etiologic factors that lead to the development of voice disorders, as well as appropriate diagnostic techniques and skills for discovering the causes. Finally, based on the previous knowledge, voice pathologists must develop a bank of clinical management approaches for remediating the voice disorder.

Only in the recent history of voice disorders have speech-language pathologists played this evaluation and management role. Indeed, the first persons in the profession who became interested in the remedial aspects of voice did so only about 70 years ago.[6,7] The advent of voice therapy was a unique blend of the knowledge that speech correctionists, as speech-language pathologists were then called, gained from training in the areas of public speaking, oral interpretation, and theater arts. This training was combined with understanding in the areas of anatomy, physiology, psychology, and pathologies of the laryngeal mechanism. In more recent history, voice pathologists have been required to also gain knowledge in vocal fold histology, biomechanics of laryngeal tissue, voice acoustics, aerodynamics of voice production, and visual imaging and interpretation of vocal function.[8-13] These years during which speech-language pathologists have dealt with the remediation of voice disorders represent only a small component of time when compared with the total history of the evaluation and treatment of voice disorders. Let us begin by looking to the past as a means of gaining an understanding and appreciation of the current knowledge of clinical voice pathology.

Ancient History

The earliest accounts of voice disorders, as with other medical information, were handed down orally. These accounts were mainly represented by folk remedies for various recognized disorders. Folklore remedies for disorders of the throat included the gargling of liniment derived from centipedes, the juice of crabs, and an owl's brain, as well as inhaling the ashes of a burned swallow. Plant remedies included gargles made from cabbage, garlic, nettles, pennyroyal, and sorrel. Wearing beads of various kinds or a black silk cord around the throat was also recommended, as was the excommunication of sore throats in the name of God.[14]

One of the earliest written histories of a voice disorder was presented about 1600 BC in the Edwin Smith Papyrus. One of many Egyptian papyri discovered in burial tombs, the Edwin Smith Papyrus contained early medical writings. It described 50 traumatic surgical cases, beginning with injuries to the head and continuing down the body to the thorax. One of these cases was a detailed description of a crushing injury to the neck, which caused the loss of speech. The Egyptian writings contained a hieroglyph portraying the lungs and trachea (Figure 1-1). The larynx was not pictured because no organ for voice had yet been identified.[15]

The ancient Hindu civilization presented much medical information including mention of diseases of the throat. The most notable information was presented in the Sanskrit-Atharva-Veda (700 BC). Among the Hindus, surgical achievements were tonsillectomy and rhinoplasty. Nose flaps became a necessity in this civilization, for cutting off the nose was the corporal punishment for adultery. Hindu gargles for throat disorders included oils, vinegar, honey, the juices of fruit, and the urine of sacred cows.[16]

In the fifth century BC, Hippocrates, the "Father of Medicine," was responsible for finally separating medicine from magic. One of Hippocrates' greatest contributions to medicine was his insistence on the value of observation. Observation

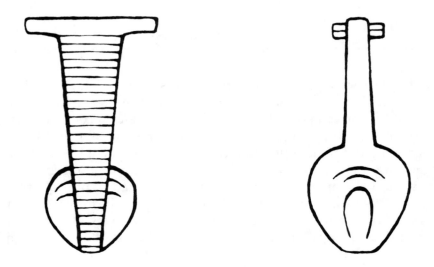

Figure 1-1. Egyptian hieroglyphs of the trachea and lungs.

remains one of the voice pathologist's most powerful diagnostic tools. Hippocrates made many observations regarding diseases associated with the throat and voice, although he, too, failed to identify the source of voice. Several of these observations, as translated by Chadwick and Mann,[17] include:

Aphorism 58:	Commotion of the brain, from any cause, is inevitably followed by loss of voice.
Coan Prognosis 240:	Aphonia is of the most serious significance if accompanied by weakness.
Coan Prognosis 243:	Aphonia during fever in the manner of that seen in seizure, associated with a quiet delirium, is fatal.
Coan Prognosis 252:	A shrill whining voice and dimness of the eyes denote a spasm.

These examples demonstrate that Hippocrates studied symptoms more than treatments of diseases. Hippocrates was the first person to write that observation of voice quality, whether it be clear or hoarse, is one means by which a physical diagnosis may be reached.[17] Observation of voice quality remains a powerful diagnostic tool to this day.

Aristotle was the first writer to refer to the larynx as the organ from which the voice emanates. In his *Historia Animalium*,[18] written in the late fourth century BC, he stated that the neck was the part of the body between the face and the trunk, with the front being the larynx and the back, the gullet. He further stated that phonation and respiration took place through the larynx and the windpipe.[15]

This information lay dormant until five centuries later when the first true anatomist, Claudius Galenus, was born in Asia Minor in AD 131. Galen (Figure 1-2) derived his knowledge of anatomy from the dissection of animals. He greatly advanced the knowledge of the upper air passages and the larynx and described the warming and filtering functions of the nose. He also distinguished six pairs of intralaryngeal muscles and divided them into abductor and adductor muscles. The thyroid, cricoid, and arytenoid cartilages were described, as was the activity of the recurrent laryngeal nerves.

In experiments with pigs, Galen demonstrated that pigs would always cease squealing when the recurrent laryngeal nerve was severed. This led him to conclude that muscles move

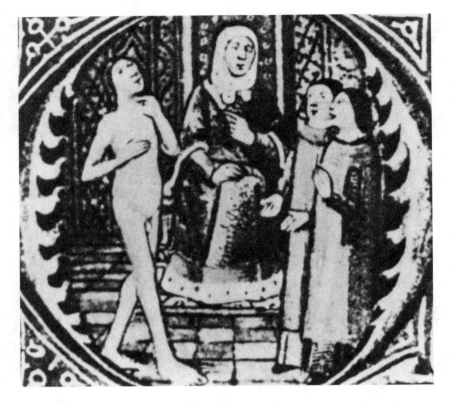

Figure 1-2. Claudius Galenus (Galen).

certain parts of the body on which breathing and voice depend and that these muscle movements are dependent on nerves from the brain. Galen, therefore, proved that the larynx was the organ of voice, thus disproving that the "voice was sent forth by the heart,"[14] which was still a popular belief.

The Renaissance

Galen did much to further medical progress, but his theories and views, which were by no means totally accurate, were blindly accepted for 1500 years as the world went through the Dark Ages. This historical period of intellectual and artistic stagnation was finally broken in the late 14th and early 15th centuries AD with the invention of the printing press, the astronomical discoveries of Copernicus and Galileo, and the discovery and exploration of the western hemisphere. With these and other discoveries, the world began the great growth period known as the Renaissance.

A genius of the renaissance, the bold artist Leonardo da Vinci (1452-1519) did not hesitate to exchange his painting brush for a dissection scalpel to explore the human anatomy. Andreas Vesalius (1514-1564) reformed the knowledge of anatomy (Figure 1-3). In his 1542 publication, *De Humani Corporis Fabrica*,[19] this 29-year-old anatomist and artist corrected many of

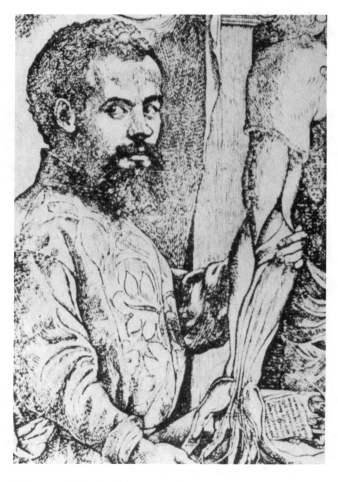

Figure 1-3. Andreas Vesalius, 1514-1564.

the age-old errors of Galen. He clarified the laryngeal anatomy and presented the function of the epiglottis. Vesalius' work is considered to be the anatomic classic of all time.[14]

During this time period, Bartolomeus Eustachius (1520-1574; Figure 1-4) was one of the first anatomists to accurately describe the structure, course, and relations of the eustachian tube. More interesting were his descriptions and carvings of the anatomy of the larynx, which were not discovered until the 18th

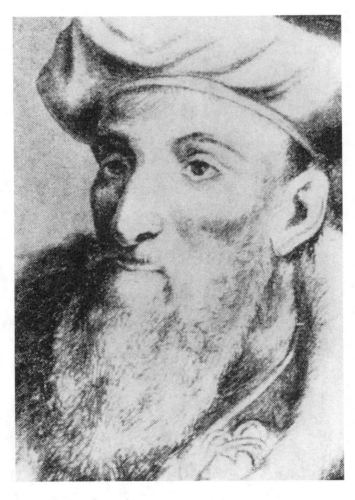

Figure 1-4. Bartolomeus Eustachius, 1520-1574.

century in the Vatican Library and are even more detailed and accurate than those of Vesalius. Fabricius, of Padua, authored the first monograph of the larynx (1600) entitled, *De Visione Auditu*.[20] In his monograph, Fabricius named the posterior cricoarytenoid muscles and described the action of the other laryngeal muscles.

The 17th to 19th Centuries

The discoveries of anatomy, physiology, and pathology of the laryngeal mechanism continued, highlighted by descriptions of the laryngeal ventricles by the Italian anatomist Giovanni Morgagni (1682-1771); further clarification of the purpose of the epiglottis by Francois Magendie (1783-1855) of Paris; the functions of the laryngeal cartilages and muscles in the production of voice by Robert Willis in Cambridge in 1829; and, finally, in Frederick Ryland's (1837) publication called *Treatise on the Disease and Injuries of the Larynx and Trachea*.[21] This important publication clearly described the diseases of the larynx (Figure 1-5) as they were understood before the use of the laryngeal mirror.

The Laryngeal Mirror

Since the time of Aristotle, many minds had considered the idea of examining the larynx in living humans. It was not until 1854, however, that a Parisian singing teacher named Manuel Garcia (1804-1906; Figure 1-6) made the discovery that ushered in the modern era of laryngology.

Strolling through the gardens of Palais-Royal on a bright September day, Garcia observed the flashing sun in the window-panes of the quadrangle buildings:

> Suddenly I saw the two mirrors of the laryngoscope in their respective positions, as if actually present before my eyes. I went straight to Charriere, the surgical instrument maker, and asking if he happened to possess a small mirror with a long handle, was informed that he had a little dentist's mirror, which had been one of the failures of the London exhibition of 1851. I bought it for six francs. Having also obtained a hand mirror, I returned home at once, very impatient to begin my

experiments. I placed against the uvula the little mirror (which I heated in warm water and carefully dried), then flashing upon its surface with the hand mirror a ray of sunshine, I saw at once, to my great joy, the glottis, wide and open before me, and so fully exposed that I could perceive a portion of the trachea. When my excitement had somewhat subsided, I began to examine what was passing before my eyes. The manner in which the glottis silently opened and shut and moved in the act of phonation, filled me with wonder.[22]

Further Advancements

The use of the laryngeal mirror (Figure 1-7) was taken up quickly in the major medical centers of the world, with the major improvement of artificial illumination made in Budapest by

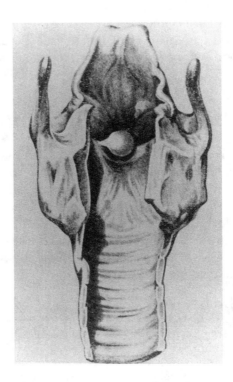

Figure 1-5. Polyps of the larynx from Ryland.[21]

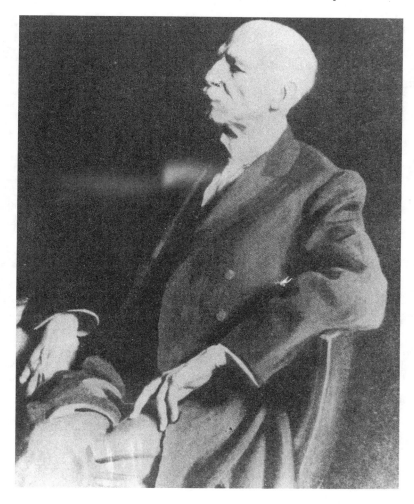

Figure 1-6. Manuel Garcia at the age of 100.

Johann Czermak in 1861.[23] The laryngeal mirror was first introduced in the United States in 1858 by Ernst Krakowizer, but credit for the development of laryngology as a specialty in the United States was given to Louis Elsberg of New York, and J. Dobs Cohen of Philadelphia. Elsberg taught laryngoscopy in the University Medical School of New York in the 1860s, and Cohen published the first American textbook on diseases of the throat in 1872. Cohen also performed the first total laryngectomy in the United States.

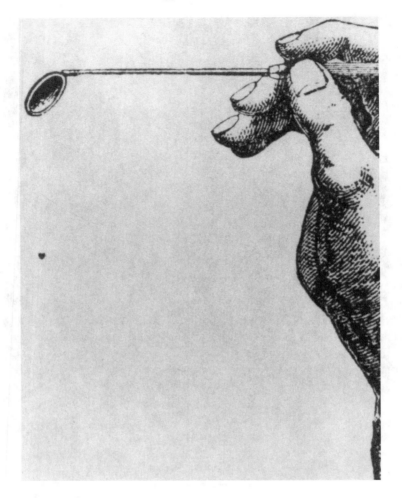

Figure 1-7. The position of the hand and the laryngeal mirror.

Other laryngeal examination techniques followed including stroboscopy (1878), direct laryngoscopy (1895), and ultra-high speed photography developed at the Bell Telephone Laboratories in 1937. These techniques are further described in Chapters 5 and 6. Medical treatment of laryngeal pathologies has advanced greatly just in the past 20 years. The philosophy of surgical intervention has changed from one of lesion excision to a philosophy of vocal conservation. Indeed, a new subspecialty in otolaryngology has developed known as phonosurgery, which is defined as surgery to improve voice quality. Special microsurgical instruments have been designed specifically for the purpose of permitting phonosurgeons to excise laryngeal lesions while maintaining the integrity of the vocal fold mucosa and thus voice quality. Perhaps the most remarkable recent achievement in voice treatment was the laryngeal transplant performed at the Cleveland Clinic in January 1998.[24] The success of the transplant for both voice and swallowing has been quite remarkable. The future of this procedure will evolve over the next several years.

Voice Therapy

The evaluation and treatment of voice disorders remained the province of the medical profession until about 1930. It was at this time that a few laryngologists, as well as singing teachers, instructors in the speech arts, and a fledgling group of speech correctionists became interested in retraining individuals with vocal disorders.[25] Using drills and exercises borrowed from training manuals designed to enhance the normal voice, these specialists attempted to modify the production of the disordered voice. Enterprising teachers created many of these rehabilitation techniques and tailored them to individual students' needs. The techniques, however, were not based on scientific principles of laryngeal, respiratory, and resonatory physiology. Nonetheless, it is particularly interesting how many of these techniques remain with us today, as testimony to the insight and creativity of early speech pathologists.

In the 1930s, the study and practice of voice therapy were greatly advanced with the publication of two books, *The Rehabilitation of Speech* by West, Kennedy, and Carr,[26] and Charles Van Riper's *Speech Correction Principles and Methods*.[27] In their chapter related to voice disorders, West, Kennedy, and Carr concentrated on the organic problems of voice and diseases related to laryngeal dysfunction. These authors understood that when the voice is disordered, there is always a reason, and if properly studied, the reason will be discovered. Causes of the disorder may be neuropathological, emotional, or the result of improper vocal habits and structural pathology. To rehabilitate voice, the authors suggested techniques including (a) ear training, (b) breathing exercises, (c) relaxation training, (d) articulatory compensations, (e) emotional retraining, and (f) special drills and exercises to be used with cleft palate and velopharyngeal insufficiency.

Van Riper stressed remedial measures to be used specifically by speech correctionists. He was the first author to suggest that voice disorders could be classified under the major headings of disorders of pitch, intensity, and quality. Van Riper advocated that voice therapy should follow a medical examination, to rule out organic pathology, and a detailed evaluation of pitch, intensity, and quality. His description of therapy techniques was the most elaborate of the time, and included several therapy approaches:

- recognition of the problem by the patient
- production of a new, more appropriate sound
- stabilization of the new vocal behavior in many contexts
- habituation of the new voicing behavior in all situations

These early foundations of voice rehabilitation have evolved into several general voice management orientations. These orientations may be classified as:

- hygienic voice therapy
- symptomatic voice therapy
- psychogenic voice therapy
- physiologic voice therapy
- eclectic voice therapy

In short, hygienic voice therapy concentrates on discovering the behavioral causes of the voice disorder and focuses on modifying or eliminating these causes. Symptomatic voice therapy modifies the deviant vocal symptoms identified by the voice pathologist, such as breathiness, low pitch, glottal attacks, and so on. The focus of psychogenic voice therapy is on the emotional and psychosocial status of the patient, which led to and maintained the voice disorder. The physiologic orientation of voice therapy relies on direct modification of respiration, phonation, and resonance to improve the balance of laryngeal muscle effort to the supportive airflow, as well as the correct focus of the laryngeal tone. Finally, the eclectic approach to voice therapy is the combination of any and all of the previous voice therapy orientations. Indeed, none of these philosophical orientations is pure. Much overlap is present, often leading, of course, to the use of eclectic voice therapy.

Clinical Voice Pathology

The role of the speech-language pathologist has expanded significantly in the evaluation and management of voice disorders. Indeed the "voice pathologist" has become an integral part of the team responsible for treating individuals with such disorders. This team is composed primarily of the laryngologist and voice pathologist, with other team members including relevant medical specialists, vocal coaches, and singing instructors. Never before in the history of the treatment of voice disorders have patients had the opportunity for such integrated multidisciplinary care. The physician's medical expertise combined with the voice pathologist's knowledge of speech and voice processes have significantly improved the accuracy of diagnosis and the management care of patients.

This text is designed to introduce and integrate the artistic nature of voice care with the scientific areas of knowledge that are necessary for the development of a "voice pathologist." Voice analysis and treatment is, indeed, a unique blend of art and science. The artistic nature of voice care involves sensitive human interactions. The vocal mechanism is quite strong and resilient physiologically but sensitive psychologically. The voice pathologist must develop a caring compassion, empathy, and understanding for the patient and the problems the voice disorder creates.

These interaction skills require that a person have the ability to listen not only to the characteristics of the voice quality, but also to what the patient says. In turn, gathering appropriate information related to the voice disorder is dependent on the interview skills of the voice pathologist. Despite many integral parts of a diagnostic voice evaluation, the patient interview remains the most valuable tool in the assessment and remediation of a voice disorder.

Considering the strong relationship between voice production and the emotional state of the patient, the voice pathologist must also develop effective counseling skills. It is common for patients with voice disorders to share personal information regarding their thoughts, feelings, and relationships. Often, this information must be discussed in depth as it relates to the voice problem. The role of the voice pathologist demands that professionals can discuss and consider sensitive issues related to voice. The voice pathologist must also be aware of the potential need to refer emotional concerns to other mental health care professionals, however.

Finally, developing and maintaining patient motivation is the "art" of clinical intervention. Motivational skill is the ability to instill action for change. Although many patients come to the voice pathologist highly motivated to improve voice production, some do not. The voice pathologist must have not only the ability to motivate the somewhat noncompliant patient, but also the creativity and perseverance to maintain motivation in those who proceed through the sometimes arduous tasks of therapy. In our experience, the ability to monitor progress through objective measures and laryngeal imaging procedures has significantly improved patient compliance and motivation.

The scientific nature of voice care involves a broad knowledge base including:

- normal anatomy and physiology
- laryngeal pathologies
- etiologic correlates
- diagnostic methods including:
  - perceptual assessment
  - vocal acoustics
  - vocal aerodynamics
  - laryngeal imaging techniques
- therapy methods

The voice pathologist must be completely familiar with the anatomy and physiology of the normal laryngeal mechanism, respiratory system, and supraglottic structures. Based on the specific physiologic needs of the patient, voice management approaches may be planned and implemented.

Knowledge of the laryngeal microstructure is also necessary to understand the many different laryngeal pathologies. The voice pathologist must learn to recognize various laryngeal pathologies, including their causes, signs, symptoms, and typical management approaches. Laryngeal pathologies encompass a broad range, from tissue lining changes of the vocal fold cover to neurologically induced, psychologically induced, or functionally induced changes in voice production.

The many causes of laryngeal pathologies also must be well understood by the voice pathologist. These causes include behavioral origins, medical etiologies, or psychologically based onset. The voice pathologist who recognizes the critical etiologic correlates will likely be very successful in discovering specific causes of voice disorders, which is the first step in successful remediation.

Recently, the ability to objectively measure many aspects of voice production has added important clinical tools in voice evaluation and management. Along with these tools comes the need to develop additional knowledge bases, including knowledge related to the science of voice acoustics, aerodynamics, and laryngeal imaging. Many commercial instruments are now available that provide multitudes of measures related to voice production. It is the responsibility of the voice pathologist to understand the science of the specific measures and to utilize the measures as only one part of the diagnostic voice evaluation. The clinical ear remains the most valuable perceptual assessment tool.

The practice of clinical voice pathology has a deep, rich, and interesting history that continues to rapidly evolve at this writing. Indeed, because of the greatly expanding bases of knowledge that are required to successfully manage voice disorders, the profession is steadily progressing toward specialty recognition. By combining the speech-language pathologist's natural artistic abilities related to human interaction skills with a strong scientific base, the voice pathologist is emerging as a specialist in the treatment of voice disorders. Improved patient care will be the ultimate result.

Our study of voice production begins in Chapter 2 with the anatomy and physiology of the mechanisms of voice. A complete understanding of this area of knowledge is an essential foundation in the preparation of the clinical voice pathologist.

References

1. Aronson A. *Clinical Voice Disorders: An Interdisciplinary Approach.* New York, NY: Brian C. Decker; 1980.
2. Boone D. *The Voice and Voice Therapy.* 2nd ed. Englewood Cliffs, NJ: Prentice-Hall; 1977.
3. Greene M. *The Voice and Its Disorders.* 3rd ed. Philadelphia, Pa: JB Lippincott; 1972.
4. Moore P. *Organic Voice Disorders.* Englewood Cliffs, NJ: Prentice-Hall; 1971.
5. Koufman J, Isaccson G. The spectrum of vocal dysfunction. In: Koufman J, Isaccson G, eds. *The Otolaryngologic Clinics of North America: Voice Disorders.* Philadelphia, PA: WB Saunders; 1991:985-988.
6. Moore P. Have the major issues in voice disorders been answered by research in speech science? A 50-year retrospective. *J Speech Hear Disord.* 1977;42:152-160.
7. Stemple J. *Voice Therapy: Clinical Studies.* St. Louis, Mo: Mosby Year Book; 1993.
8. Titze I. *Principles of Voice Production.* Englewood Cliffs, NJ: Prentice-Hall; 1994.
9. Hirano M. *Clinical Examination of Voice.* New York, NY: Springer-Verlag; 1981.
10. Kent R, Reed C. *The Acoustic Analysis of Speech.* San Diego, Calif: Singular Publishing Group; 1992.
11. Hixon T. *Respiratory Function in Speech and Song.* Boston, Mass: College-Hill Press; 1987.
12. Sapienza C, Stathopoulos E. Respiratory and laryngeal measures of children and women with bilateral vocal fold nodules. *J Speech Hear Res.* 1994;37:1229-1243.
13. Hirano M, Bless D. *Videostroboscopic Examination of the Larynx.* San Diego, Calif: Singular Publishing Group; 1993.
14. Stevenson S, Guthrie G. *A History of Otolaryngology.* Edinburgh, Scotland: E & S Livingstone; 1949.
15. Fink R. *The Human Larynx: A Functional Study.* New York, NY: Raven Press; 1975.
16. Wright J. *A History of Laryngology and Rhinology.* 2nd ed. Philadelphia, Pa: Lea and Febiger; 1941.
17. Chadwick G, Mann W. *The Medical Works of Hippocrates.* Oxford, England: Blackwell Scientific Publications; 1950.
18. Aristotle. *Historia Animalium.* Peck A, trans. Cambridge, England: Howard University Press; 1965.
19. Vesalius A. *De Humani Corporis Fabrica.* Basle; 1542.
20. Fabricius. *De Visiona Voce Auditu.* Venice; 1600.
21. Ryland F. *Treatise on the Diseases and Injuries of the Larynx.* London, England: Longmans; 1837.
22. Garcia M. Transaction Section of Laryngology. Paper presented at the VII International Congress of Medicine; 1881; London, England.

23. Czermak J. *Du laryngoscope et Son Emploi en Physiologie et Nen Medicine.* Paris, France; 1860.
24. Strohm M, Hicks D. The rationale for total human larynx transplantation. Paper presented at the Eleventh Annual Pacific Voice Conference; November 5-7, 1998; San Francisco, Calif.
25. Murphy A. *Functional Voice Disorders.* Englewood Cliffs, NJ: Prentice-Hall; 1964.
26. West R, Kennedy L, Carr A. *The Rehabilitation of Speech.* New York, NY: Harper & Brothers; 1937.
27. Van Riper, C. *Speech Correction Principles and Methods.* Englewood Cliffs, NJ: Prentice-Hall; 1939.

2

Anatomy and Physiology

Knowledge of the anatomy and physiology of the laryngeal mechanism is paramount to understanding voice disorders. This knowledge serves as a foundation for examining the larynx and evaluating phonatory function and is essential for recognizing the impact of specific pathologies on voice production. A solid understanding of the normal structure and function of the larynx is the basis for interpreting evaluative findings and developing appropriate voice treatment plans.

The larynx is essentially a cartilaginous tube that connects inferiorly to the respiratory system (trachea and lungs) and superiorly to the vocal tract and oral cavity (Figure 2-1). This orientation in the body is important, because it highlights the interactive relationship between these three subsystems of speech: the pulmonary power supply, the laryngeal valve, and the supraglottic vocal tract resonator. Because of the complexity and intricacy of the larynx and vocal folds, it is easy to focus on those structures as the "vocal mechanism," but it is essential to include breath support and vocal tract resonance in any clin-

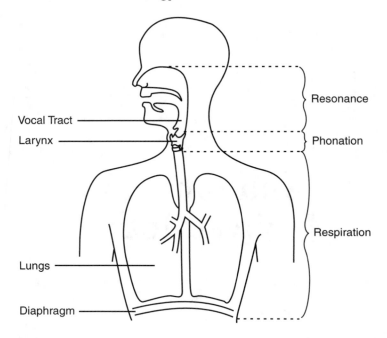

Figure 2-1. Orientation of the larynx in the body. Representation of three subsystems of voice: respiration, phonation, and resonance.

ical understanding of the anatomic and physiologic contributions to voice quality.

Indeed, the communicative function of the larynx relies heavily on the integration of this three-part system: respiration, phonation, and supraglottic resonance. Specifically, the lungs function as the power supply by providing aerodynamic (subglottal) tracheal pressure that blows the vocal folds apart and sets them into vibration. The vocal folds within the larynx provide the sound source for phonation, and they oscillate in a series of compressions and rarefactions, modulating the subglottal pressure and transglottal flow as short pulses of sound energy. The vocal tract serves as the resonating cavity, which shapes and filters the acoustic energy to produce the sound we recognize as human voice.[1-5]

Differential diagnosis of voice disorders requires careful assessment of these three components. Obviously, laryngeal health and overall function will influence the quality of voice production, but respiratory support and supraglottic resonance will also affect the speech product. For example, a patient with weak or inconsistent respiratory support will be unable to generate adequate vocal fold vibration to support normal vocal loudness or quality. Conversely, altering the shape and size of the vocal tract can result in improved vocal resonance by enhancing the phonatory sound source generated by the vocal folds.[6,7] The loss of any one of these elements would violate the potential for normal voice quality. The resulting voice product radiated from the lips is a truly interactive result of these subsystems, respiration, phonation, and resonance.

The Laryngeal Valve

The larynx consists of a complex arrangement of muscles, mucous membranes, and other connective tissue (Figures 2-2, 2-3, and 2-4 display the lateral, posterior, and coronal views of the larynx). Because the soft tissues of the larynx are responsible for airway preservation, the cartilage housing serves as a columnar protective shield for the laryngeal valve. Together, the muscles and cartilages create three levels of "folds," which serve as sphincters that provide both communicative and vegetative functions in the body.[1,2,8] The angles of closure are multidimensional and include the potential for valving in both a horizontal plane (eg, lateral to medial movements) and a vertical plane (eg, vertical compression).

The upper rim of the larynx is formed by the aryepiglottic folds, a strong fibrous membrane that connects the lateral walls of the epiglottis to the arytenoid cartilage complex. When the epiglottis cartilage folds posteriorly and inferiorly over the laryngeal vestibule, it separates the pharynx from the larynx and offers the first line of defense for preserving the airway. The second sphincter is formed by the ventricular folds, which are not normally active during phonation but may become hyperfunctional during effortful speech production or extreme vegetative closure. The ventricular folds are directly superior to the ventricle and the true vocal folds, forming a "double layer" of medial closure, if needed. The principle function of the ventricular sphincter is to increase intrathoracic pressure by blocking the outflow of air from

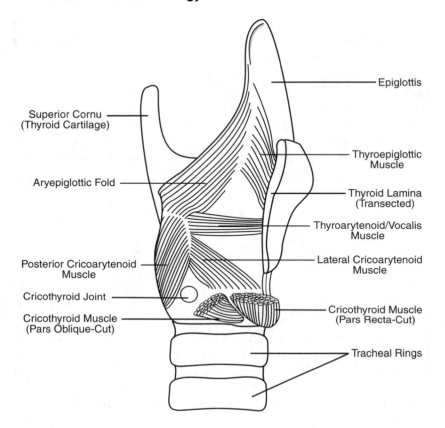

Epiglottis

Superior Cornu
(Thyroid Cartilage)

Thyroepiglottic
Muscle

Aryepiglottic Fold

Thyroid Lamina
(Transected)

Thyroarytenoid/Vocalis
Muscle

Posterior Cricoarytenoid
Muscle

Lateral Cricoarytenoid
Muscle

Cricothyroid Joint

Cricothyroid Muscle
(Pars Oblique-Cut)

Cricothyroid Muscle
(Pars Recta-Cut)

Tracheal Rings

Figure 2-2. Lateral view of the larynx.

the lungs. The ventricular folds compress tightly during rapid contraction of the thoracic muscles (eg, coughing or sneezing) or for longer durations when building up subglottic pressure to stabilize the thorax during certain physical tasks (e.g., lifting, emesis, childbirth, or defecation). The ventricular folds also add airway protection during swallowing.[1,2,8,9]

The third and final layer of this "folding mechanism" is the true vocal folds (Figure 2-4). For speech communication, the vocal folds provide a vibrating source for phonation. They also close tightly for nonspeech and vegetative tasks, such as coughing, throat clearing, and grunting. Thus, in a mechanical sense, the larynx and vocal folds function as a variable valve, modulating airflow as it passes through the vibrating vocal folds during

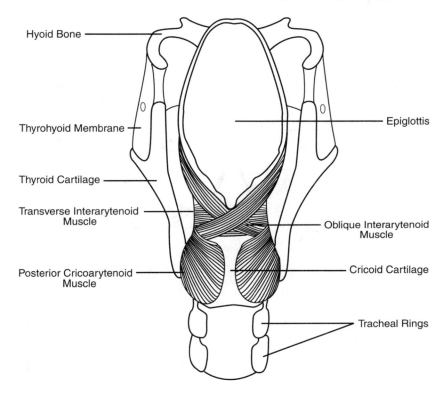

Hyoid Bone

Thyrohyoid Membrane

Thyroid Cartilage

Transverse Interarytenoid Muscle

Posterior Cricoarytenoid Muscle

Epiglottis

Oblique Interarytenoid Muscle

Cricoid Cartilage

Tracheal Rings

Figure 2-3. Posterior view of the larynx.

phonation, closing off the trachea and lungs from foods and liquids during swallowing actions, and providing resistance to increased abdominal pressure during effortful activities.[1,2,8,9]

Respiration for Phonation

Vocal fold vibration is the sound source that produces phonation and provides the speech signal. Phonation is dependent on the respiratory power that the lungs and the abdominal and thoracic musculature provide. The lungs are housed within the ribcage in the thorax and separated from the viscera (digestive organs in the abdomen) by a large, dome-shaped muscle called the diaphragm. The bottom of the lungs are attached to the top of

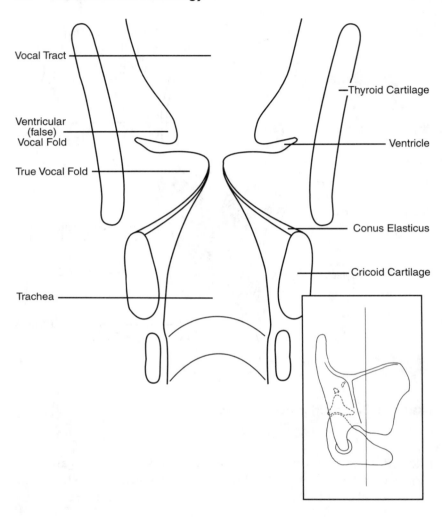

Figure 2-4. Coronal view of the ventricular and true vocal folds (Figure 2-4 insert: Coronal plane of Figure 2-4).

the diaphragm by a double-walled pleural lining. During inhalation, the diaphragm contracts (flattening downward in the body), compressing the viscera, and simultaneously pulling the lungs downward, thereby expanding the lung volume. As this lung volume expands, air is drawn passively into the lungs. During exhalation, the diaphragm relaxes and rises back up to its resting position, as passive elastic recoil pushes air out of the lungs and upward through the vocal folds and vocal tract. The vocal folds are abducted (opened) in the paramedian position (approximately 60%) during quiet exhalation, so no sound is generated. To exhale for speech, however, the vocal folds adduct (close) at midline, constricting the airflow stream as it exits the lungs. This aerodynamic energy sets the vocal folds into oscillation, creating the vibratory sound source that is phonation.[10,11] Without this airflow, no sustained phonatory sound source can be achieved. The interactive relationship between the subglottal air pressure buildup and transglottal airflow rate passing through the vibrating vocal fold valve influences the overall pitch, loudness, and quality of phonation.[4,5,11-13]

Vocal Tract Resonance

As sound waves generated by the vocal folds travel through the supraglottic air column into the pharynx, oral and nasal cavities, and across articulator structures such as the velum, hard palate, tongue, and teeth, the excitation of air molecules within this space creates a phenomenon called resonance. Resonance occurs when sound is reinforced or prolonged as acoustic waveforms reflect off another structure. The model of acoustic energy (phonation) traveling through a filter (vocal tract) modified in variable shape, size, and constriction characteristics (articulatory gestures) is the basis for Fant's Acoustic Theory of Speech Production.[14,15] This theory underlies our understanding of the three components of the acoustic speech product: glottal sound source, vocal tract filtering, and resonating characteristics.[14,15]

The shape and size of the vocal tract and its constrictions have a direct influence on the quality and strength of the acoustic product radiated from the lips and perceived by listeners. The sound of vocal fold vibration without the supraglottic resonating cavity (for example in intraoperative conditions or in excised larynx studies) reveals a flat, atonal buzz, devoid of any "ring" and completely unrecognizable as human voice. The contribution of this resonating filter is essential to creating the perceptual attributes of phonation, including pitch, loudness, nasality, and quality. Manipulating resonance characteristics by changing the vocal tract shape and oral posturing has been the study of vocal pedagogues, actors, and singers for several centuries.[6,7,11] Modifying resonance has also been applied directly to voice treatment methods in disordered speakers and professional voice users.[16,17]

Structural Support for the Larynx

The larynx is suspended in the neck from a single bone, the **hyoid.** Six laryngeal cartilages, three unpaired (**epiglottis, thyroid**, and **cricoid**) and three paired (**arytenoid, corniculate**, and **cuneiform**) provide structural support for the larynx and vocal folds (Figures 2-5 and 2-6). The **hyoid** bone marks the superior border of the laryngeal complex of muscles and cartilage. It articulates with the superior cornu of the thyroid cartilage and attaches to the thyroid through the thyrohyoid membrane. Although the hyoid serves as the muscular attachment for many extrinsic muscles of the larynx, it is notable as the sole bone in the body that does not articulate with any other bone. The **epiglottis** cartilage is shaped like a long leaf, with its base attached to the inner portion of the anterior rim of the thyroid cartilage. This attachment allows the blade of the epiglottis cartilage to fold along its midline and move forward and back, closing down inferiorly and posteriorly over the laryngeal vestibule. It forms the first level of the three tiers of a sphincteric folding mechanism to protect the airway from particles of food or liquid during swallowing. The epiglottis is composed of elastic cartilage and therefore does not ossify, or harden, with age. This composition is important because this structure must remain flexible throughout life to allow a pliable free edge to assist in closing the airway and diverting foods and liquids toward the esophagus.[1,2,9]

The **thyroid** cartilage forms a three-sided saddle-shaped curve. The thyroid cartilage is the anterior attachment of the true vocal folds at the internal rim of the anterior curve. Posteriorly are two superior cornu, or "horns" that extend upward to articulate with the hyoid bone, and two inferior cornu that articulate with the cricoid cartilage below it. The thyroid is composed of hyaline cartilage that ossifies and limits flexibility with age.[18,19] The lateral walls form quadrilateral plates, called **laminae** that attach at the anterior midline in a thyroid **notch** or prominence. In newborns, these laminae form a curve of about 130°, and the angle

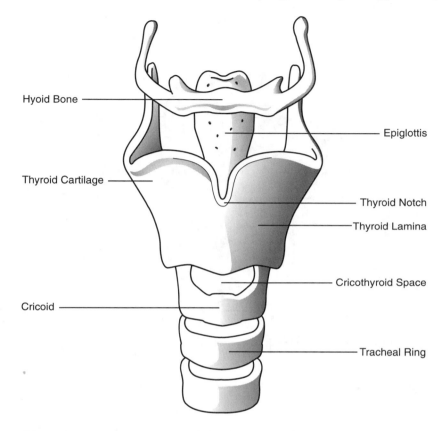

Figure 2-5. Anterior view of the laryngeal cartilages.

becomes more acute with age. A fully matured thyroid angle will be more acute for adult males (90°) than for adult females (110°).[20] In males, the thyroid notch will become more prominent anteriorly, resulting in the characteristic "Adam's apple." This thyroid notch can be seen or palpated at the front of the neck. Clinically, the position and movement of the thyroid notch can signal maladaptive extrinsic laryngeal muscle hyperfunction, including excessive muscle tension or misuse in voice pathologies.[17,21]

Below the thyroid cartilage is the **cricoid** ring, another hyaline cartilage. Its shape is described as a "signet ring," with a narrow anterior curve and broad posterior back. The cricoid has two sets of paired facets, or flat surfaces, that articulate with the adjacent thyroid and arytenoid cartilages. The cricothyroid joint con-

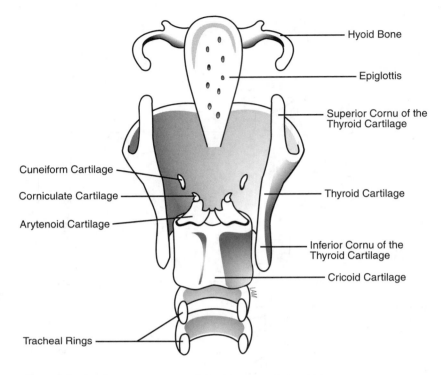

Figure 2-6. Posterior view of the laryngeal cartilages.

nects the lateral edges of the cricoid to the inferior cornu of the thyroid cartilage. The cricoarytenoid joints are positioned on the top of the posterior cricoid rim. Both the cricothyroid and cricoarytenoid joints are lined with a synovial membrane, which provides a connective tissue cushion for the joint, supplied with secretions for lubrication, blood supply, adipose cells, and lymph tissue. Both articular joint surfaces and the synovial joint membranes do display normal age-related deterioration, although no gender differences have been noted.[22] Figure 2-7 displays the articular facets of the cricoid cartilage. Inferior to the cricoid cartilage are the tracheal rings, which form the airway to the lungs.

The three paired cartilages are the **arytenoid**, **corniculate**, and **cuneiform** cartilages. The arytenoid cartilages are pyramid-shaped, with four surfaces: anterior, lateral, medial, and a base. The anterior angle projects forward at the base, forming the

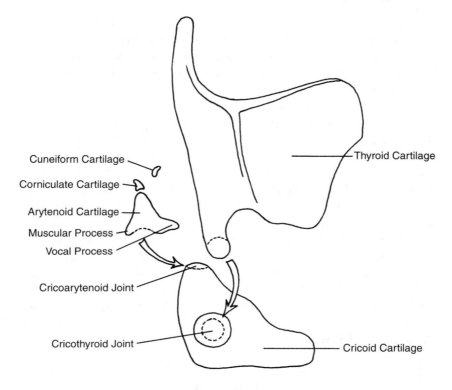

Cuneiform Cartilage

Corniculate Cartilage

Arytenoid Cartilage

Muscular Process

Vocal Process

Cricoarytenoid Joint

Cricothyroid Joint

Thyroid Cartilage

Cricoid Cartilage

Figure 2-7. Lateral view of the laryngeal joint attachments.

vocal process. The arytenoid is composed of hyaline cartilage, except for this vocal process, which has elastin cartilage at its tip.[18,19,21] This vocal process is the posterior point of attachment of the membranous portion of the true vocal folds and the beginning of the so-called cartilaginous portion of the vocal fold. The lateral arytenoid angle is the muscular process, which attaches to the intrinsic laryngeal muscles responsible for abducting and adducting the vocal folds. The medial arytenoid angle faces its arytenoid pair, forming an even surface for midline glottic closure. The base of the arytenoid cartilage is not flat, but rather a concave cylinder, to allow it to articulate smoothly with the humped (convex) superior surface of the posterior cricoid cartilage. The arytenoid base fits neatly over the posterior cricoid similar to a half-cylinder over a bar. The cricoarytenoid joint has two basic motions. First, it can rock anteriorly and posteriorly over the cricoid surface. Second, because the cricoid rim slopes downward laterally, the joint can also slide laterally. These rocking and sliding motions are a crucial mechanical feature of the larynx because these movements alter the orientation of the vocal process tips sufficiently to abduct, adduct, and stabilize the vocal folds. In response to intrinsic muscular contractions, the vocal process tips are pulled medially or laterally, which determines the position of the membranous fold and, consequently, the shape and size of the glottis. When the tips of the vocal process are directed medially (facing each other), normal vocal folds meet at midline and are closed (adducted). When vocal process tips are pointed laterally, the vocal folds are drawn open, and vocal fold abduction occurs.[1,2,8,22-24]

The corniculate cartilages (also called the cartilages of Santorini) are attached by a synovial joint to the superior tips of the arytenoids. The cuneiform cartilages (also known as the cartilages of Wrisberg) are embedded in the muscular complex superior to the corniculates. Both of these tiny cartilages consist of hyaline cartilage. They provide no clear function but may add structure and stability to preserve the airway.

Muscles

There are two logical groupings of the laryngeal muscles: extrinsic and intrinsic. Extrinsic laryngeal muscles are so named because they attach to a site on the larynx and to an external point, such as the hyoid bone, sternum, mandible, or skull base. The intrinsic muscles have both ends attached within the laryngeal cartilages. When contracted, all muscles increase tension and shorten, providing a "pull" between the attachments. The primary function of the extrinsic muscles is to influence laryngeal height or tension as a gross unit. For example, the larynx moves vertically as a whole in the neck for lifting, swallowing, phonating, and many vegetative acts. Extrinsic muscle manipulations also alter the shape and filtering characteristic of the supraglottic vocal tract, which modifies vocal pitch, loudness and quality.[1,2,17] The primary function of the intrinsic laryngeal muscles is to alter the shape and configuration of the glottis, by modifying the position and tension, and edge of the vocal folds.

These intrinsic laryngeal manipulations consist of adduction (closing), abduction (opening), and modifications in vocal fold length, tension, and thickness.[1,2,25] Both intrinsic and extrinsic muscle groups are necessary to accomplish the many vital and complex movements required for ventilation, airway protection, and communication, and are integral to maintaining a functioning laryngeal valve.

Extrinsic Laryngeal Muscles

The many extrinsic muscles of the larynx can be divided into two regional groupings: the suprahyoid above the hyoid bone and infrahyoid below the hyoid bone (Table 2-1; Figure 2-8). The location of many of the muscles can be identified based on their names, which describe the anatomical attachment. By knowing the attachments, one can predict the effect of individual muscle contraction (shortening) between those sites. The suprahyoid extrinsic laryngeal muscles include the stylohyoid, the mylohyoid, the digastric (anterior and posterior bellies), and the geniohyoid (not seen). The infrahyoid muscles include the thyrohyoid, the sternothyroid, the sternohyoid, and the omohyoid. The sternocleidomastoid muscle forms a broad sheath in the neck that extends from the sternum to the mastoid. In general, the infrahyoid muscles pull the hyoid bone and larynx to a lower position in the neck. The suprahyoid muscles raise the larynx by pulling the hyoid bone forward or backward and upward. This action is particularly important during a swallow, when laryngeal elevation can help protect the airway from aspiration.[2,8,9] Clinically, laryngeal elevation during phonation may be a sign of excessive extrinsic laryngeal muscle tension and is often an accurate indicator of hyperfunctional voice use.

Intrinsic Laryngeal Muscles

There are five intrinsic laryngeal muscles (Table 2-2), each of which attaches to cartilages in the larynx to modify the cricothyroid and cricoarytenoid joint relationships, and thereby affect the position, length, and tension of the vocal folds.[1,23] Specifically, these intrinsic muscles create two critical effects:

Table 2-1. Extrinsic Laryngeal Muscles

Muscle	Attachments	Function
Suprahyoid Muscles		
Stylohyoid	Temporal bone (styloid process) to hyoid	Raises hyoid bone posteriorly
Mylohyoid	Mandible to hyoid	Raises hyoid bone anteriorly
Digastric	Two bellies, anterior and posterior:	
Anterior:	Mandible to hyoid	Raises hyoid bone anteriorly
Posterior:	Temporal bone (mastoid process) to hyoid	Raises hyoid bone posteriorly
Geniohyoid	Mandible to hyoid	Raises hyoid bone anteriorly
Infrahyoid Muscles		
Thyrohyoid	Thyroid to hyoid	Brings thyroid cartilage and hyoid bone closer
Sternothyroid	Sternum to thyroid	Lowers thyroid cartilage
Sternohyoid	Sternum to hyoid	Lowers hyoid bone
Omohyoid	Scapula to hyoid	Lowers hyoid bone

- changing the position of the cartilage framework that houses the vocal folds
- altering the shape and configuration of the glottis, the opening between the vocal folds

As with the extrinsic muscles, the intrinsic muscles of the larynx are also identifiable by their names, which describe the cartilaginous attachments.

The **cricothyroid** is a broad, fan-shaped muscle that attaches inferiorly to the cricoid cartilage and superiorly to the thyroid cartilage. When the cricothyroid muscle contracts, it decreases the distance between these two cartilages, simultaneously lengthening

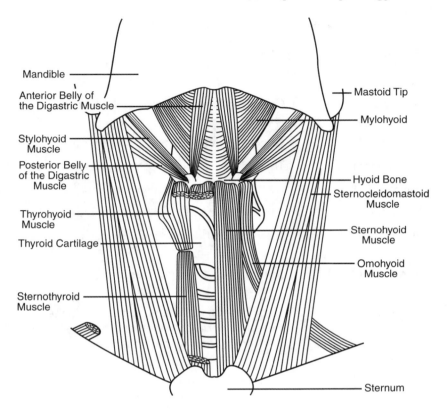

Mandible

Anterior Belly of
the Digastric Muscle

Stylohyoid
Muscle

Posterior Belly
of the Digastric
Muscle

Thyrohyoid
Muscle

Thyroid Cartilage

Sternothyroid
Muscle

Mastoid Tip

Mylohyoid

Hyoid Bone

Sternocleidomastoid
Muscle

Sternohyoid
Muscle

Omohyoid
Muscle

Sternum

Figure 2-8. Anterior view of the extrinsic laryngeal muscles.

and tensing the membranous vocal fold. (Figure 2-9). This vocal
fold lengthening is achieved as the thyroid cartilage is pulled inferiorly, as the cricoid is pulled superiorly, or by a combination of
these movements. The cricothyroid has two distinct muscle bellies,
pars recta (vertical) and **pars oblique** (angled). The exact function
of these two muscle bellies is not clear, but recent study[26] suggests
that pars recta and pars oblique function in variable patterns for
different speakers and at different portions of the fundamental frequency range. Regardless, cricothyroid contraction always reduces
the vibrating mass of the vocal fold by increasing its longitudinal
tension and limiting the vibratory wave to the thinnest portion of
the vocal fold, located at the medial edge. Therefore, the cricothyroid serves as the largest contributor to fundamental frequency
control, especially in higher tones.[1,2,9,11]

Table 2-2. Intrinsic Laryngeal Muscles

Muscle	Attachments
Cricothyroid (CT)	Cricoid to thyroid
Pars recta	Cricoid to inferior border of the thyroid lamina
Pars oblique	Cricoid to inferior cornu of the thyroid
Thyroarytenoid (TA)	Thyroid to arytenoid vocal process
(Thyro)vocalis	Medial portion of the thyroarytenoid
Thyromuscularis	Lateral portion of the thyroarytenoid
Lateral cricoarytenoid (LCA)	Lateral cricoid to arytenoid muscular process
Interarytenoid (IA)	Joins the left and right muscular processes of the arytenoids; two bellies:
Transverse	Unpaired muscle sheath, attaching to the lateral laminae of the left and right arytenoids, and running horizontally
Oblique	Paired muscles, coursing from the base of one arytenoid upward and across to the apex of the other, forming an X-configuration
Posterior cricoarytenoid (PCA)	Posterior aspect of the cricoid to arytenoid

The **thyroarytenoid** is attached anteriorly to the internal angle of the thyroid cartilage and posteriorly to the vocal process of the arytenoid. This muscle contains two compartments arranged in parallel. The lateral component is the **thyromuscularis**, whereas the medial component is the **thyrovocalis**, or simply, the **vocalis**. Often, the terms thyroarytenoid and vocalis are used interchangeably. Historically, the thyrovocalis (medial portion) was thought to exert greater control over phonation, whereas the thyromuscularis (lateral portion) contributed more to adduction. Recent study[27] has identified different types of muscle fibers in the two regions of this muscle. The lateral portion has more fast-acting muscle fibers; the medi-

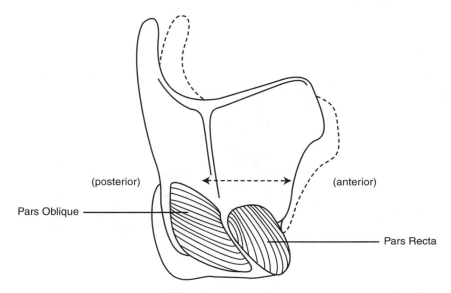

(posterior) (anterior)

Pars Oblique

Pars Recta

Figure 2-9. Action of the cricothyroid muscle.

al portion appears to have more slow-acting muscle fibers. The thyroarytenoid muscle is the actual "body" of the vocal fold. When contracted, it shortens the fold length by drawing the arytenoid cartilages anteriorly and thickens the vocal fold by increasing the mass of the vibrating medial edge. Thus, the thyroarytenoid contributes directly to lowering fundamental frequency, increasing loudness, and tighter glottic closure. Overall, this muscle contributes to control over the vocal fold shape and edge, as well as glottic closure patterns.[1,2,9,11,25]

The **lateral cricoarytenoid** is another broad, fan-shaped muscle that attaches the lateral side of the cricoid to the arytenoid muscular process. When the lateral cricoarytenoid contracts, it rocks the arytenoids anteriorly and slides them laterally. This movement redirects the vocal processes medially, bringing the membranous vocal folds to midline adduction (Figure 2-10). The lateral cricoarytenoid serves as one of the strongest vocal fold adductors (closers). The **interarytenoid** muscles are composed of two separate bellies, the **transverse** and the **oblique** portions. When these muscles contract, they shorten the distance between the arytenoid cartilages, thus

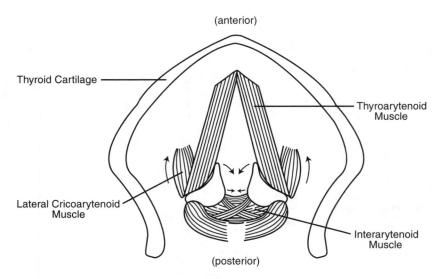

Figure 2-10. Action of the lateral cricoarytenoid and interarytenoid muscles (adduction).

serving as adductors and contributing to forceful closure of the posterior glottis (see Figure 2-8). The **transverse** (horizontal) belly is the only unpaired intrinsic laryngeal muscle; it attaches to the posterior plane of each arytenoid and brings the medial faces of the arytenoids together. The **oblique** (crossed) bellies attach at a 45° angle from the inferior border of one arytenoid to the superior border of its contralateral pair. When the bellies contract, the space between the corniculate and cuneiform cartilages decreases.[1,2,9,11]

The **posterior cricoarytenoid** is the sole abductor of the vocal folds. Its attachments are the posterior lamina of the cricoid and the muscular (lateral) arytenoid cartilage. When the posterior cricoarytenoid contracts, it abducts (opens) the vocal folds. Abductory movement when the arytenoids rock posteriorly to redirect the vocal processes laterally and separate the membranous portions of the vocal folds. The posterior cricoarytenoid abducts for respiration and during quick glottal opening gestures during unvoiced sound productions (Figure 2-11).[1,2,9,11]

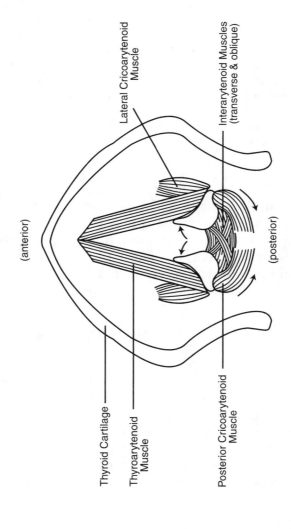

Figure 2-11. Action of the posterior cricoarytenoid muscle (abduction).

There are three "all except" rules that apply to the intrinsic ,cles of the larynx to help remember similarities and differ-u. .es among their functions:

- First, all muscles are paired, having a matched left and right muscle, except the transverse interarytenoid, which functions as a single unit, bringing the arytenoid carti- lages closer together.
- Second, all of the intrinsic muscles serve as adductors (bringing the vocal folds closer) except the posterior crico- arytenoid, the sole abductor (vocal fold opener).
- Third, all of the muscles are innervated by the recurrent laryngeal nerve except the cricothyroid muscle, which is innervated by the external branch of the superior laryn- geal nerve.

Recall that the importance of the intrinsic laryngeal muscles is their remarkable variability to modify the tone, posture, length, and shape of the vocal folds in a wide range of functions from forceful closure to complex phonation to quiet respiration. Table 2-3 summarizes the importance of each specific muscle function and indicates the effect of muscle contractions on abduction and adduction, vocal fold length and tension, and shaping of the medial edge.

Vocal Fold Microstructure

The membranous portion of the vocal folds is an intricate layered structure of five histologically discrete layers that vary in compo- sition and mechanical properties (Figure 2-12). This membranous structure oscillates (vibrates) to create sound in the larynx. The integrity of the vibrating pattern for phonation relies on a pliable, elastic structure. The different layers of vocal fold microstruc- ture[1,3,28-30] provide variable amounts of flexibility and stability.

Five Histologic Layers

The five histologic layers arranged from most superficial to deep- est are the epithelium, the superficial, intermediate, and deep lay- ers of the lamina propria and the vocalis muscle. The **epithelium**

Table 2-3. Intrinsic Laryngeal Muscle Functions

Parameters

Function	Adduction or abduction of the vocal folds
Length	Shortening or lengthening the true vocal folds
Thickness	Thickening or thinning the body of the vocal fold
Edge	Sharpening or rounding the free edge of the vocal fold
Tension	Increasing or decreasing stiffness of the vocal fold

Muscle Actions

	CT	TA	LCA	IA	PCA
Function	Tensor	Adductor	Adductor	Adductor	Abductor
Length	Longer	Shorter	Shorter	—	NA
Thickness	Thinner	Thicker	Thicker	—	NA
Edge	Sharper	Rounder	Rounder	—	—
Tension	Stiffer	Stiffer	—	—	—

CT = cricothyroid; TA = thyroarytenoid; LCA = lateral cricoarytenoid;
IA = interarytenoid; PCA = posterior cricoarytenoid; NA = not applicable.

is a mucosal covering of stratified squamous cells that wraps over the internal contents of the vocal folds. The epithelium is the thinnest of the five layers, consists of only six to eight cell layers, and has been described as a pliable capsule. The deep epithelial cell layer forms a border membrane to divide it from the lamina propria below it. The epithelium offers no mass and is totally compliant, but needs a thin layer of slippery mucous lubrication to oscillate best. The next three layers of the vocal fold form the **lamina propria**. This structure is composed of loose extracellular tissue (also called an extracellular matrix) composed of specialized proteins, carbohydrates, and lipids, and its composition will be discussed in a separate section.[31-33] The second histological layer is slightly more dense than the epithelium, although still loose and flexible. This is the **superficial layer of the lamina propria**, known commonly as Reinke's space. This superficial layer consists of a soft, slippery gelatinlike substance, which allows it to

MUCOSA

Epithelium ——————

Lamina Propria

    Superficial ——————
    (Reinke's space)

    Intermediate ——————

    Deep ——————

VOCALIS MUSCLE ——————

Conus Elasticus ——————

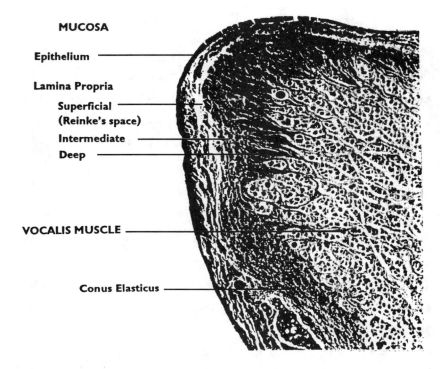

Figure 2-12. Layered microstructure of the vocal fold.

vibrate significantly during phonation. When the pliability or health of this layer is violated by vocal fold pathology, the vibratory waveform will be significantly impaired. There is a clear border between the superficial layer and the **intermediate layer of the lamina propria**, which lies below.[31-33] This intermediate layer is composed principally of elastic fibers, which can stretch to approximately twice the original length. Although this layer offers slightly more mass, it also vibrates during phonation. The fourth histologic layer is called the **deep layer of the lamina propria**. This layer is denser still and composed of collagen fibers. The tissues of the intermediate and deep layers of the lamina propria (third and fourth layers) together are known as the **vocal ligament**. These layers are not present in newborn vocal folds, and appear first between the ages of 1 and 4 years. The vocal ligament continues to develop throughout childhood until the larynx reaches full maturity at puberty.[34] Unlike the superficial layers, the transition between the deep layer fibers and the underlying vocalis muscle is irregular. The deep layer fibers are interspersed with muscle fibers to join these layers firmly together. This architectural fiber organization lends stability to the transition from lamina propria to muscle.[3,28] The fifth and final histologic layer is the **vocalis muscle**, which has been described previously. The vocalis forms the main body of the vocal fold and provides tonicity, stability, and mass. Furthermore, because of its nervous innervation, this muscle is the only true "active" tissue. The lamina propria and epithelium layers vibrate passively in response to aerodynamic breath support, but the vocalis muscle is the only portion of the true vocal fold that can contract and relax in response to neurologic control. Therefore, vibration of the vocalis is both active and passive.

The Extracellular Matrix

All three layers of the lamina propria contain an intricate extracellular matrix, composed of **fibrous proteins**, **interstitial proteins**, **carbohydrates**, and **lipids**. The fibrous proteins consist of **elastin** and **collagen** fibers that lie parallel to the vocal fold. These two fibrous proteins are found in different concentrations at different levels of the lamina propria, and each provides a separate contribution to the vibratory properties of the vocal fold cover. Elastin fibers predominate in the superficial and intermediate layers of the lamina propria, while collagen fibers are concentrated in the deeper layer. Elastin has a large dynamic range, allowing tissue to deform (stretch), yet return to its original shape. In contrast, collagen does not stretch easily but can tolerate stress and offers strength to the extracellular matrix. Accordingly, these denser fibers are found in deeper tissues.[32]

The interstitial proteins of the lamina propria consist of **proteoglycans** and **glycoproteins**. Less is known about the role of interstitial proteins of the lamina propria than fibrous proteins, but their role in vocal fold vibration seems to be related to control of tissue viscosity, layer thickness, and internal fluid content. One proteoglycan, called **hyaluronic acid**, appears throughout the lamina propria but has a larger concentration in the intermediate layer. Hyaluronic acid attracts water to form large, space-filling molecules that create a gel. The presence of hyaluronic acid affects overall tissue viscosity and seems to act as a cushion in the extracellular matrix, resisting compressive and shearing mechanical forces during vocal fold vibration. Hyaluronic acid, as with other proteoglycans in the lamina propria, has other known benefits, such as protecting cells from deterioration, assisting in tissue repair, and clotting. Interestingly, the concentration of hyaluronic acid in male vocal folds appears to exceed that of females by a 3:1 ratio. This gender difference corresponds to a thicker intermediate layer of the vocal fold lamina propria in males than in females. Clinically, this finding of a male predisposition for greater hyaluronic acid concentration in the lamina propria may begin to explain the difference in vocal fold injury types and prevalence in adult men and women.[33,35,36]

Glycoproteins, lipids, and carbohydrates have not been studied sufficiently in the lamina propria, and little is known about their functional role in the extracellular matrix. Only one glycoprotein, called **fibronectin**, has been seen extensively in the extracellular matrix. Fibronectin appears in both normal and injured vocal folds, and seems to play a role in wound healing.[33]

The Body-cover Theory of Vocal Fold Vibration

In summary, as the histological layers change from superior to inferior, from epithelium to three-layered lamina propria to muscle tissue, each level contributes a graduated change in mass and compliance for vibration. The epithelial layer is the most elastic component; subsequent layers form a complex transition to stiffer muscle tissue. Although the histologic layers present five distinct compositions, the functional differences for vibratory properties are not as discrete. As a general description, the layers are regrouped into three vibratory divisions: **cover** (epithelium and superficial layer of the lamina propria), **transition** (intermediate and deep layers of the lamina propria), and **body** (vocalis muscle). The theory of vocal fold vibration is based on these functional divisions, as described by Hirano.[1,28,30] The vibrating cover forms the compliant, fluid oscillation seen in vocal fold vibratory patterns, while the body provides the stiffer, underlying stability of vocal fold mass and tonus. The transition serves as the coupling between the superficial mucosa and the deep muscle tissue of the vocal fold during vibration. Thus, the body-cover theory of vibration accounts for the mass and stability provided by the vocalis muscle and deep layer of the lamina propria over which the compliant and flexible layers of the lamina propria and epithelium oscillate.[1,28,30]

This "undulation" or oscillation of the superficial vocal fold layers creates an infinitely variable ripple of tissue deformation and recoil. Vocal fold vibration is a complex waveform that challenges advanced vibration theory and modeling techniques. Some investigators have explored applications of chaos theory (fractal analysis) to vocal fold vibration, in an attempt to account for both the complexity and redundancy of vibratory patterns.[37] Clinically, it is useful to consider at least three vibratory phases of wave motion that can be seen from a superior view during endoscopy:

- horizontal (medial to lateral movements), as seen during the open and closing patterns of vibration
- longitudinal (anterior to posterior "zipperlike" wave), as seen in a front-to-back travelling wave
- vertical phase (inferior to superior opening and closing of the vocal folds), seen as an upper versus lower lip difference in some views of vocal fold vibration.[3,28,38]

Reports of mucosal wave amplitudes estimate the horizontal excursion (medial to lateral motion) during normal vocal fold vibration ranges from 1 to 2 mm. The vertical-phase change appears to be much larger, however, in the realm of 3 to 5 mm.[39] Clinically, only horizontal and longitudinal changes can be seen readily during most imaging techniques (ie, supraglottic view), although some close images of vocal folds will display vertical phase differences. This is an unfortunate limit, because experimental evidence suggests that this (mostly) unseen vertical-phase change in mucosal wave probably affects the overall vibratory waveform significantly.

Connective Tissues

Two special connective tissue structures support the vocal folds at points of greatest mechanical stress. First are the anterior and posterior **macula flava**, which are small oval bundles of elastic fibers and other connective tissues that provide stability to the end points of the membranous vocal folds. The anterior macula flava is found at the anterior attachments of the vocal fold to the collagenous fibers of the thyroid cartilage, whereas the posterior macula flava are positioned at the posterior attachments of the membranous vocal fold to the vocal process of the arytenoid cartilage. The second connective tissue is the **conus elasticus,** a strong membrane that serves as a supportive "shelf," arising from the subglottic tracheal wall, coursing superiorly and medially, and inserting into the vocalis muscle to support the inferior border of the vocal fold.[1,29]

Basement Membrane Zone

Recent investigations into the histochemical composition of the vocal folds have identified a transition area between the epithelium and superficial layer of the lamina propria. This region, known as the **basement membrane zone (BMZ),** was observed using electron microscopy and special histochemical staining techniques. The zone is composed of a complex organization of fibers and proteins in horizontal layers that attach the epithelial layer to the superficial layer of the lamina propria. This region between the epithelium and the superficial layer is a site of great mechanic shearing force and potential injury during vocal fold vibration. Accordingly, the BMZ consists of a series of anchoring fibers and provides a framework for supporting collagen fiber connections in the vocal fold mucosa and allowing the tissue to shift and glide. These anchoring fibers are composed of proteins and appear to be sensitive to the mechanical stress posed by vocal fold vibration. In fact, the BMZ displays evidence of mechanical trauma and shearing effects in injured vocal folds.[31,40]

Developmental Changes

In newborns, the larynx is situated high in the neck, with the cricoid positioned at the approximate level of C3 to C4 in the cervical column. Newborns breathe only through nasal passages in the first few months of life, thus allowing them to breathe and swallow simultaneously. As they grow in the first year, the larynx begins its descent in the neck, as the pharynx lengthens and widens. By puberty, the larynx descends to the level of C6 or C7. This descent of the laryngeal structures in the body, accompanied by skeletal facial growth and development, creates an expanded vocal tract, which contributes to the precipitous drop in fundamental frequency and resonance characteristics from childhood to physical maturation.[20]

The intrinsic larynx also undergoes dramatic changes from birth through puberty. Hirano, Kurita, and Nakashima[34] have examined the size and structure of the vocal folds across age ranges (Table 2-4). The vocal fold length of boys and girls appears to be similar until about age 10 years. After that point, there is a gradual but consistent gender development that changes both the overall length of the vocal folds and the covarying ratio between the membranous to cartilaginous portions of vocal folds. These changes do correlate with other standard indicators of physical maturation, including height, weight, and onset of puberty. In males, the rise in testosterone at puberty stimulates the anterior growth of the thyroid notch and wide growth of the pharynx.[20]

In newborn infants, the total vocal fold length ranges from 1.25 to 3 mm, and the ratio from membranous-to-cartilage portions is approximately 1.5:1. Because the newborn membranous vocal fold has no vocal ligament (intermediate and deep layers of the lamina propria) and, therefore, little stability, the greater

Table 2-4. Developmental Changes in the Larynx

	Newborns	*Adult Females*	*Adult Males*
Total	2.5-3 mm	11-15 mm	17-21 mm
Membranous	1.3-2 mm	8.5-12 mm	14.5-18 mm
Cartilage	1-3 mm	2-3 mm	2-3 mm
Membranous to cartilaginous ratio	1.5:1	4.0:1	5.3:1
Thyroid cartilage angle	130°	110°	90°
Cricoid level in the neck	C2-C3	C6	C7

Source: Hirano M, Kurita S, and Nakashima T[34]

ratio of cartilage-to-membrane length provides better mechanical protection of the airway. Recall that the vocal ligament emerges between the ages of 1 to 4 years and is fully developed by maturity. By adulthood, the female overall vocal fold length is 11 to 15 mm, whereas the male length is 17 to 21 mm. The ratio of membranous to cartilage portions is 4:1 in adult females and 5.5:1 in adult males.[20,34]

Geriatric Vocal Folds

Changes in vocal fold anatomy with aging have received increasing attention over the last decade. Voice pathologists have long been aware of the deterioration in voice quality, pitch, and loudness range and in endurance among geriatric speakers. Increased use of laryngeal imaging techniques has provided information about the common appearance of thinned (bowed) vocal folds in elderly patients, especially those who have no other explanation of pathology except advanced chronological age.[41,42] A large normative study also provided evidence of age-based changes in laryngeal and vocal fold appearance.[43] The clinical observation of these geriatric changes in voice quality and laryngeal appearance has been termed "presbylaryngeus," or aging larynx.

Histologic evidence of age-based changes in laryngeal anatomy is also available, but some researchers reported conflicting findings. Hirano, Kurita, and Nakashima[34] performed some of the early work and reported morphologic disorganization and breakdown of the collagen and elastin fibers in aging vocal folds. The intermediate layer of the geriatric vocal folds was observed to be looser and thinner, which could contribute to a loss of tissue bulk, resulting in the characteristic bowed appearance of geriatric glottic closure patterns. In a more recent study, Hammond et al[32,35,36] noted an increase in elastin fibers with age, from infant to geriatric years, with elastin fiber size and density increased in the superficial layer of the lamina propria, resulting in a thicker and less pliable layer structure. Some of this discrepancy between findings may be accounted for by different methodologies. Nonetheless, all studies confirm that the lamina propria decreases in flexibility and elasticity with age, due to increased cross-linking of fibers.

Neurologic Supply

Peripheral Innervation

The cranial nerve X, the **vagus**, innervates the larynx peripherally. Vagus means "wandering," and the name appropriately describes its circuitous and far-reaching route through the body to innervate sites from the skull to the abdomen. The vagus innervates the larynx via two important branches, the **recurrent** and **superior laryngeal nerves**, which contain all the sensory and motor fibers that supply the larynx (Figure 2-13). The first portion is the superior laryngeal nerve (SLN), which branches off the vagus near the nodose ganglia in the neck. After coursing alongside the carotid artery, the SLN forms internal and external branches. The internal branch inserts through the thyrohyoid membrane, superior to the vocal folds, and provides all the sensory information to the larynx. The external branch is a motor nerve to the cricothyroid muscle only.

The second branch off the vagus is the recurrent laryngeal nerve (RLN), which extends to the thorax, where it forms long loops through the heart before coursing superiorly back up under the thyroid gland and on to the larynx. The pattern of "recurrence" is different on the right and left sides of the body. The right RLN courses under the subclavian artery; the left RLN courses under the aortic arch before it reaches the larynx.[1,2,9,44] Consequently, these nerves (especially on the left) are susceptible to injury, and a patient with an unexplained idiopathic vocal fold paralysis should always be evaluated for possible cardiac, lung, or thyroid compromise to rule this out.

The RLN supplies all sensory information below the vocal folds and all motor innervation to the posterior cricoarytenoid, thyroarytenoid, lateral cricoarytenoid, and interarytenoid muscles. Two characteristics of the SLN and RLN ensure the ability of the intrinsic laryngeal muscles to move quickly and with great fine motor control. First, the laryngeal nerves have a high conduction velocity (second only to the eye), which allows rapid contractions. Second, the innervation ratio is low, meaning that many cells (estimated at 100 to 200) are innervating a single motor unit, allowing very fine motor control.[2,11,44]

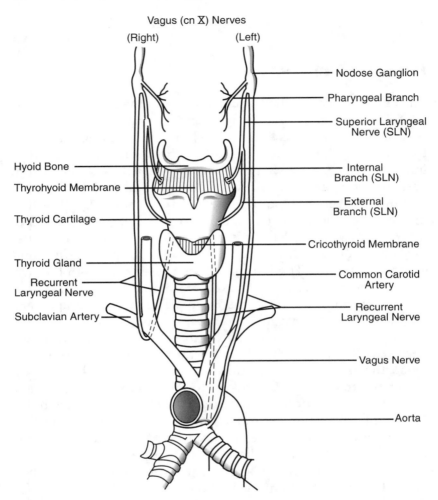

Figure 2-13. Vagus (cranial nerve X) innervation of the larynx.

Laryngeal Reflexes

A complex and detailed system of laryngeal reflexes exists for the principle function of airway preservation. Sensory receptors in the larynx are located in mucosal tissue, articular joints, and muscle. The sensory receptors in mucosal tissue respond to touch, vibration, changes in air pressure, and liquid stimuli. These receptors have the ability to elicit tight sphincteric closure to close off the trachea and lungs from foreign material in the upper airway. Muscle receptors are located most predominantly in the vocalis muscle and are also present in other intrinsic laryngeal muscles. Muscle spindles and other proprioceptive receptors have been identified in human vocal folds, but there appears to be some variability in the number and location of these muscular receptors in the larynx.[2,44,45] In the vocalis muscle, muscle spindles appear predominantly in the superior compartment of the muscle.[27] Overall, their presence suggests that the vocal fold muscles do have potential to exert differential control on muscle contraction and supply graduated changes in muscle length under variable stimuli.[44]

Another sensory response present in the larynx is a laryngeal reflex, which contracts rapidly to protect the airway from foreign materials or aspiration. Accordingly, these reflexes are triggered by receptors described above in the mucosal tissue, articular joints, and muscles. An extreme glottic closure reflex, called laryngospasm, can be triggered by stimuli reaching sites closer to the glottic level, and prolongation of this vocal fold adduction can pose a threat to ventilation.[2,13,44-46] A respiratory reflex that opens the vocal folds in rhythmic coordination with the diaphragm contraction has also been identified. In long-term tracheotomized patients, this rhythmic respiratory reflex appears to be suppressed.[46]

Central Nervous System Control

Central nervous system (CNS) mechanisms relay afferent (sensory) information from the larynx to the brain and send efferent (motor) commands from the brain to the body. In the larynx, these central nervous system relays and commands are not entirely understood. Because phonation is only one of the functional laryngeal tasks, there are enormously complex sensory and motor control relationships among the complex vegetative and communicative activities of the larynx in respiration, phonation, and deglutition. Furthermore, it is difficult to study the relevant anatomical structures in the larynx and function in vivo. Evidence suggests that afferent information sent from sensory receptors in the larynx to the CNS are transmitted by the internal branch of the superior laryngeal nerve, through the vagus to terminate in a region of the medulla called the nucleus tractus solitarius (NTS). This region contains areas that are involved in the control of respiration, laryngeal maneuvers, and swallowing. In anesthetized animal studies, NTS fiber activity has been shown to occur in phase with the timing of evoked swallowing or respiratory events. Other sensory fibers do not terminate in NTS, but continue to another section of the midbrain called the periaqueductal gray area (PAG).[44, 47] There is also some limited evidence of sensory projection from the larynx to even higher order centers (above the midbrain) in the cortex, including projections to the thalamus (a major sensory relay center), superiorly through the corona radiata, and finally to the postcentral gyrus of the cortex.

Conclusions from experimental work suggest that at least the midbrain level is required for vocalization, and that the PAG is a crucial center for voluntary control over vocalizations.[47] The PAG appears to project efferents (motor commands) through the nucleus retroambiguus (NRA) located in the medulla, which in turn projects to the motor nucleus ambiguus, located in the reticular formation. It has been suggested that this PAG-NRA projection may serve as a final common pathway for vocalization.[47] The nucleus ambiguus contains the central origins of the laryngeal motoneurons for all of the intrinsic laryngeal muscles. The localized site of cricothyroid motoneurons is more distinct than the motoneuron groupings of the other intrinsic muscles, which appear to converge in a general area. Motoneurons for esophageal and respiratory control are also located in the nucleus ambiguus. Studies that examine laryngeal motoneuron activity have found that units may be task-specific, for vocalization, inspiration, or a combination of expiration and vocalization.[2,44] Thus, the interaction between phonation, deglutition, and respiration is inherent to understanding the central pathways of laryngeal control, reflexive activity, and voluntary laryngeal maneuvers for nonspeech gestures and speech production.[2,44,47,48]

Blood Supply and Secretions

The internal fluid balance of the larynx is controlled by the blood supply, whereas external secretions control the external "hydration" of the vocal folds. The blood supply arises from the superior thyroid, superior laryngeal, and inferior laryngeal arteries. These arteries branch from the external carotid artery in the neck. Venous return is transmitted through the jugular vein.[1,2,9] Although vocal fold hemorrhages and varices may arise in some pathologic cases, there is limited blood supply to the superficial layers and epithelium of the vocal fold. The predominant blood supply is found in the intermediate and deep layers of the lamina propria and the vocalis muscle. Blood vessels run parallel to the vocal fold and are arranged similarly to the histologic layer organization in that larger arterial supply is found in the deeper layers, and smaller capillaries are seen in the lamina propria. When hemorrhage does occur, it creates an extra mass that inhibits vibration.[1,3]

Serous and mucous glands are located in the tissues lateral, superior (ventricle), and inferior to the vocal folds, again avoiding the medial edge.[49,50] Mucus propagation along the margin of the fold is assisted by the texture of the epithelial layer, which has microscopic irregularities that provide increased surface tension, thus holding the liquid to the membranous surface. As vocal folds vibrate, the thin liquid is dispersed along the vocal fold. This thin, watery, and healthy mucus contributes the characteristic "shine" seen on normal vocal folds. However, in dehydrated or pathologic conditions, the vocal folds may appear dry and dull, and thick clumps of white tacky mucus can appear, especially over lesion sites.[1,3,50]

Physiology of Phonation

Theory of Vibration

Vocal fold vibration is achieved based on the physical process of flow-induced oscillation,[1,4,5,11,51] where a consistent stream of air flows past the tissues, creating a repeated pattern of opening and closing (Figure 2-14). Van den Berg's classical description of the **aerodynamic-myoelastic** theory[52,53] allows that both airflow (aerodynamic) and muscular (myoelastic) properties account for the passive convergent and divergent motions of the vocal folds during phonation. This older theory recognizes the reciprocal role of the aerodynamic properties, subglottal pressure,

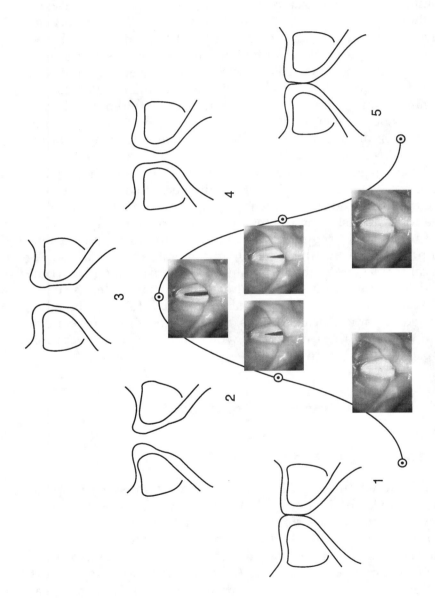

Figure 2-14. Vocal fold vibratory cycle.

and transglottal flow as they interact with the myoelastic resistance and elasticity provided by the vocal fold tissues. The theory holds that at the onset of phonation, subglottal pressure rises as expiratory forces are met by resistance from the adducted vocal folds. When pressure rises to overcome this resistance, the folds are blown apart and subglottal pressure diminishes, creating an increase in flow through the glottis. Because pressure and flow are inversely proportional, when flow increases, a momentary pressure drop occurs between the vocal folds, which also draws the vocal folds together, according to the Bernoulli principle. The elastic tissue recoil pulls the vocal folds back toward midline, completing a full cycle of vibration. With the vocal folds reapproximated, subglottal pressure builds again to repeat the process. The oscillation is achieved then by both aerodynamic contributions of the covarying pressure and flow and the mechanical properties of tissue deformation and collision posed by the elastic vocal fold tissues.[1,4,5,28]

Van den Berg's aerodynamic-myoelastic theory[53] provides some of the key elements of our understanding of vocal fold vibration. Nonetheless, current understanding of the complexities in both histologic tissue composition and vibratory mucosal waveforms has generated more advanced theories about vocal fold vibration. For example, Hirano's **body-cover** theory, mentioned previously, is the first recognition of the important role of the passive (nonmuscular) superficial layers (epithelium and lamina propria) to vocal fold vibration.[1,28]

Most recently, Titze[11] has expanded on these theories to describe the vocal folds as a flow-induced **self-oscillating** system, sustained across time by the aerodynamic forces of pressure and flow. Scherer,[4,5] Titze,[11,51] and others[52] have described a sequence of vocal fold oscillation that explains the interchange between these aerodynamic events and associated mechanical tissue response. Recall that pressure and flow are reciprocal in this context; when flow is high, pressure is low, and vice versa. In this model, respiration is the driving force that sets the vocal folds in motion (oscillation) and the interchange between pressure and flow at three critical sites keeps the vocal folds vibrating, as described below.

■ **Subglottal region**: At the area directly *beneath* the vocal folds, the "leading edges" of the folds are blown apart and set into motion by subglottal air pressure. As the vocal folds are blown open, **translaryngeal (glottal) flow** is positive. When the folds recoil to midline, flow is negative.

■ **Intraglottal space**: In the small space directly *between* the paired vocal folds, intraglottal pressure keeps the vocal folds oscillating as the convergent and divergent shaping of vocal folds in a back-and-forth motion is created by the alternating exchange of airflow and pressure peaks. When the vocal folds open, intraglottal pressure is positive, but dropping as flow increases. When the vocal folds close, intraglottal pressure is negative, but rising as flow is cut off by the closing glottis.

■ **Supraglottal air column**: At the outlet of the glottis, immediately above the vocal folds, the air molecules in the vocal tract are alternately compressed or rarified in a delayed response to the alternate pressure and flow puffs modulated by the vibrating vocal folds. In other words, these molecules in the vocal tract air column are pushed and released in response to the sound energy pulses released from the oscillating vocal folds. This asymmetrical "top-down" driving force transfers energy from the fluid (air pressure) down to the tissue (upper lip of the vocal folds) and assists in sustaining the oscillation.[4,5,11]

Fundamental Frequency Control

Several factors influence the rate of vocal fold vibration or fundamental frequency. The primary determinants of pitch control are vocal fold length and tension, including passive tension on the vocal fold cover and active stiffness of the vocal fold body. To achieve higher pitch, contraction of the cricothyroid muscle causes the vocal folds to lengthen and the medial edge to thin. To lower pitch, contraction of the vocalis shortens vocal fold length, decreasing tension on the cover and rounding the medial edge for greater amplitude of vibration. Two other factors appear to covary with fundamental frequency in predictable ways. First, subglottal pressure increases proportionally with increased fundamental frequency. Second, vocal fold vibratory amplitude motion is inversely proportional to the rate of vocal fold vibration: The higher the pitch, the smaller the amplitude.[1,4,5,11]

Intensity Control

The intensity of the glottal sound source increases proportionally with increased subglottal pressure and is achieved mechanically because of longer vibratory phase closure pattern and a wider amplitude of vibration. Intensity also tends to covary proportionally with fundamental frequency, although this is not a consistent relationship. Voice range profiles display the characteristic increase in intensity with increased fundamental frequency, for example. Finally, the vocal tract tuning or filtering characteristic can influence the loudness of the glottal source, as increased supraglottic resonance can increase the acoustic radiation of sound energy.[1,4,5,11]

Laryngeal Quality

Audio-perceptual judgments of voice quality are highly subjective, but generally, phonatory quality is affected by the integrity of the glottal valving waveform, as defined by regularity, symmetry, phase shape of tissue deformation across vibratory cycles, and the slope of the glottal flow waveform.[4,5] Deviations in the cycle-to-cycle slope and shape of the waveform characteristics will impair the resulting acoustic signal. The filtering characteristic of the supraglottic vocal tract will also enhance or detract from the perceived voice quality of the signal. In sum, the quality of voice relies on multiple factors, including compliant and symmetric biomechanic properties of the vocal folds, an adequate and consistent subglottic pressure and flow source, and appropriate vocal tract tuning characteristics.[1,4,5,11]

Summary

The many functions that the larynx serves, for both vegetative and communicative purposes, demonstrate the complexity of this remarkable organ. Research continues into the further definition of its anatomic and morphologic structure, its central and peripheral control mechanisms, and its physiologic function. The underpinnings of laryngeal anatomy and physiology are critical to understanding the relationship between voice pathologies, their consequential effects on voice production, and the recognition of reasonable rehabilitative planning. Additional chapters in this text will describe measurement tools that seek to define our understanding of vocal function and its relationship to voice production.

References

1. Hirano M. *Clinical Examination of Voice.* New York, NY: Springer-Verlag; 1981.
2. Kirchner JA. *Physiology of the Larynx.* Washington, DC: The American Academy of Otolaryngology-Head and Neck Surgery Foundation Inc; 1984.
3. Hirano M. Phonosurgical anatomy of the larynx. In: Ford CN, Bless DM, eds. *Phonosurgery.* New York, NY: Raven Press; 1991:25-42.
4. Scherer RC. Physiology of phonation: a review of basic mechanics. In: Ford CN, Bless DM, eds. *Phonosurgery.* New York, NY: Raven Press; 1991:77-94.
5. Scherer R. Laryngeal function during phonation. *NCVS Status Report.* 1991;7:171-186.
6. Acker BF. Vocal tract adjustments for the projected voice. *J Voice.* 1987; 1:77-82.
7. Lessac A. *The Use and Training of the Human Voice.* New York, NY: Drama Book Publishers; 1967.
8. Fink BR, Demarest RJ. *Laryngeal Biomechanics.* Cambridge, Mass: Harvard University Press; 1978.
9. Tucker HM. *The Larynx.* New York, NY: Thieme Medical Publishers Inc; 1987.
10. Hixon T. *Respiratory Function in Speech and Song.* Boston, Mass: College-Hill Press; 1987.
11. Titze IR. *Principles of Voice Production.* Englewood Cliffs, NJ: Prentice-Hall; 1994.
12. Gauffin J, Sundberg J. Spectral correlates of glottal voice source waveform characteristics. *J Speech Hearing Res.* 1989;32:556-565.
13. Davis PJ, Bartlett D Jr, Luschei ES. Coordination of the respiratory and laryngeal systems in breathing and vocalization. In: Titze IR, ed. *Vocal Fold Physiology.* San Diego, Calif: Singular Publishing Group; 1993: 89-226.
14. Fant G. The voice source: theory and acoustic modeling. In: Titze IR, Scherer RC, eds. *Vocal Fold Physiology.* Denver, Col: Denver Center for the Performing Arts; 1983:453-464.
15. Kent RD, Read C. *The Acoustic Analysis of Speech.* San Diego, Calif: Singular Publishing Group; 1992.
16. Verdolini-Marston K, Burke K, Lessac A, Glaze L, Caldwell E. A preliminary study on two methods of treatment for laryngeal nodules. In: Titze IR, ed. *Progress Report 4.* Iowa City, Ia: National Center for Voice and Speech; 1993:209-228.

17. Erickson D, Baer T, Harris KS. The role of strap muscles in pitch lowering. In: Bless DM, Abbs J, eds. *Vocal Fold Physiology.* San Diego, Calif: College-Hill Press; 1983:279-285.

18. Kahane JC. A survey of age-related changes in the connective tissues of the human adult larynx. In Bless DM, Abbs J, eds. *Vocal Fold Physiology.* San Diego, Calif: College-Hill Press; 1983:44-49.

19. Kahane JC. Connective tissue changes in the larynx and their effects on voice. *J Voice.* 1987;1:27-30.

20. Gray S, Smith M. Voice disorders in children. *NCVS Prog Rep.* 1996;10:133-149.

21. Rammage LA, Morrison M. Muscle tension dysphonia. Miniseminar presented at Annual Convention of the American Speech-Hearing Association; November 1998; Boston, Mass.

22. Kahane JC. Age-related changes in the human cricoarytenoid joint. In: Fujimura O, ed. *Vocal Fold Physiology.* Vol. 2. New York, NY: Raven Press; 1988:145-158.

23. Hirano M, Yoshida T, Kurita S, Kiyokawa K, Sato K, Tateishi O. Anatomy and behavior of the vocal process. In: Baer C, Sasaki S, Harris K, eds. *Laryngeal Function in Phonation and Respiration.* Boston, Mass: Little, Brown and Company; 1987:3-13.

24. Von Leden H, Moore P. The mechanics of the cricoarytenoid joint. *Arch Otolaryngol.* 1961;73:541-555.

25. Hirano M, Kiyokawa K, Kurita S. Laryngeal muscles and glottic shaping. In: Fujimura O, ed. *Vocal Fold Physiology.* Vol. 2. New York, NY: Raven Press; 1988:49-66.

26. McHenry M, Kuna S, Minton J, Vanoye C, Calhoun, K. Differential activity of the pars recta and pars oblique in fundamental frequency control. *J Voice.* 1997;11:48-58.

27. Saunders I, Han Y, Wang J, Biller H. Muscle spindles are concentrated in the superior vocalis subcompartment of the human thyroarytenoid muscle. *J Voice.* 1999;12:7-16.

28. Hirano M. Structure and behavior of the vibratory vocal folds. In: Sawashima T, Cooper D, eds. *Dynamic Aspects of Speech Production.* Tokyo, Japan: University of Tokyo Press; 1966:13-27.

29. Hirano M. Structure of the vocal fold in normal and disease states: anatomical and physical studies. In: Ludlow C, Hart M, eds. *ASHA Reports No. 11, Proceedings of the Conference on the Assessment of Vocal Pathology.* Rockville, Md: ASHA; 1981:11-30.

30. Hirano M, Matsuo K, Kakita Y, Kawasaki H, Kurita S. Vibratory behavior versus the structure of the vocal fold. In: Titze IR, Scherer, RM, eds. *Vocal Fold Physiology.* Denver, Colo: Denver Center for the Performing Arts; 1983:26-40.

31. Gray SD, Hirano M, Sato K. Molecular and cellular structure of vocal fold tissue. In: Titze IR, ed. *Vocal fold physiology.* San Diego, Calif: Singular Publishing Group; 1993:1-35.

32. Gray S, Titze I, Alipour F, Hammond T. Vocal fold extracellular matrix and its biomechanical influence. Part I: the fibrous proteins. *NCVS Status Prog Rep.* 1999;13:1-10.

33. Gray S, Titze I, Alipour F, Hammond T. Vocal fold extracellular matrix and its biomechanical influence. Part II: the interstitial proteins. *NCVS Status Prog Rep.* 1999;13:11-20.
34. Hirano M, Kurita S, Nakashima T. Growth, development, and aging of human vocal folds. In: Bless DM, Abbs J, eds. *Vocal Fold Physiology.* San Diego, Calif: College-Hill Press; 1983:22-43.
35. Hammond T, Gray S, Butler J, Zhou R, Hammond E. Age- and gender-related elastin distribution changes in human vocal folds. *Otolaryngol Head Neck Surg.* 1997;119:314-321.
36. Hammond T, Zhou R, Hammond E, Pawlak A, Gray S. The intermediate layer: a morphologic study of the elastin and hyaluronic acid contents of normal human vocal folds. *J Voice.* 1997;11:59-66.
37. Baken R. Irregularity of vocal period and amplitude: a first approach to the fractal analysis of voice. *J Voice.* 1990;4:185-197.
38. Hirano M, Yoshida T, Tanaka S. Vibratory behavior of human vocal folds viewed from below. In: Gauffin J, Hammarberg, B, eds. *Vocal Fold Physiology.* San Diego, Calif: Singular Publishing Group; 1994:1-6.
39. Titze IR, Jiang J, Hsaio S. Measurements of mucosal wave propagation and vertical phase difference in vocal fold vibration. *NCVS Status Prog Rep.* 1992;2:83-92.
40. Gray S. Basement membrane zone injury in vocal nodules. In: Gauffin J, Hammarberg B, eds. *Vocal Fold Physiology.* San Diego, Calif: Singular Publishing Group; 1991:21-28.
41. Biever DM, Bless DM. Vibratory characteristics of the vocal folds in young adult and geriatric women. *J Voice.* 1987;3:120-131.
42. Linville SE. Glottal gap configurations in two age groups of women. *J Speech Hear Res.* 1992;35:1209-1215.
43. Bless D, Glaze L, Campos G, Lowery D, Peppard R. Acoustic, aerodynamic, and stroboscopic measures of voice in normal speakers. *NCVS Status Prog Rep.* 1993;4:121-134.
44. Garrett JD, Larson CR. Neurology of the laryngeal system. In: Ford CN, Bless DM, eds. *Phonosurgery.* New York, NY: Raven Press; 1991:43-76.
45. Udaka J, Kanetake H, Kihara H, Koike Y. Human laryngeal responses induced by sensory nerve stimuli. In: Fujimura O, ed. *Vocal Fold Physiology.* Vol 2. New York, NY: Raven Press; 1988:67-74.
46. Suzuki M. Laryngeal reflexes. In: Hirano M, Kirchner JA, Bless DM, eds. *Neurolaryngology: Recent Advances.* Boston, Mass: Little, Brown, and Company; 1987:142-155.
47. Davis P, Zhang SP, Bandler R. Midbrain and medullary regulation of vocalization. In: Davis P, Fletcher N, eds. *Vocal Fold Physiology.* San Diego, Calif: Singular Publishing Group; 1996:121-136.
48. Larson CR, Wilson KE, Luschei ES. Preliminary observations on cortical and brainstem mechanisms of laryngeal control. In: Bless DM, Abbs J, eds. *Vocal Fold Physiology.* San Diego, Calif: College-Hill Press; 1983:82-95.
49. Gracco C, Kahane JC. Age-related changes in the vestibular folds of the human larynx: a histomorphometric study. *J Voice.* 1989;3:204-212.

50. Fukuda H, Kawaida M, Tatehara T, et al. A new concept of lubricating mechanisms of the larynx. In: Fujimura O, ed. *Vocal Fold Physiology.* Vol. 2. New York, NY: Raven Press; 1988:83-92.

51. Titze IR. Mechanisms of sustained oscillations of the vocal folds. In: Titze IR, Scherer RC, eds. *Vocal Fold Physiology.* Denver, Colo: Denver Center for the Performing Arts; 1983:349-357.

52. Berke G, Great B. Laryngeal biomechanics: an overview of mucosal wave mechanics. *J Voice.* 1993;7:123-128.

53. Van den Berg J. Myoelastic-aerodynamic theory of voice production. *J Speech Hear Res.* 1958;1:227-244.

3

Some Etiologic Correlates

Since West, Kennedy, and Carr[1] commented that there is always a reason for a voice disorder, voice pathologists have sought to identify those reasons with each new patient. Sometimes the causes are easily identified, such as in cases of vocal nodules in shouting children. At other times, finding the contributing causes of the disorder requires the skill of a highly experienced diagnostician. To enhance the successful outcome of the search, it is advantageous for those seeking the answers to be familiar with as many points of reference as possible. This chapter seeks to provide these reference points by discussing some of the more common etiologic factors associated with the development of voice disorders. These factors include the major categories of:

- vocal misuse
- medically related etiologies
- primary disorder etiologies
- personality-related etiologies

ETIOLOGIES OF VOCAL MISUSE

Vocal misuse (Table 3-1) refers to functional voicing behaviors that contribute to the development of laryngeal pathologies. These include behaviors of vocal abuse and the use of inappropriate vocal components, such as pitch, loudness, breathing strategies, phonation habits, and speech rate.

Vocal Abuse

Vocal abuse occurs whenever the vocal folds are forced to adduct too vigorously causing hyperfunction of the laryngeal mechanism. This hyperfunction, when repeated or habitual, may contribute to laryngeal tissue change, strain, and maladaptive behavior of the laryngeal musculature.[2,3] Brodnitz[4] suggested that sheer force, in the form of sudden and violent adduction of the vocal folds or a more persistent use of a vocally abusive behavior, is one of the main elements in the development of many voice disorders. Forceful behaviors associated with hyperfunction include excessive **shouting** and **loud talking,** such as children shouting on a playground or a factory worker talking loudly over machine noise. Vocal abuse also occurs during **screaming** and in the production of **vocal noises**. Vocal noises refer to those nonspeech laryngeal sounds that children make while playing. The standard sounds may include the roar of a car, truck, motorcycle, and

Table 3-1. Etiologies of Vocal Misuse

Vocally Abusive Behaviors	*Inappropriate Vocal Components*
Shouting	Respiration
Loud talking	Phonation
Screaming	Resonance
Vocal noises	Pitch
Coughing	Loudness
Throat clearing	Rate

spaceship engines; the piercing scream of sirens; and various growls, barks, and howls of animals.

One of the most prevalent forms of vocal abuse is incessant, habitual, nonproductive **throat clearing.**[5,6] In one study of 206 patients who were referred for voice therapy due to hyperfunctional voice disorders 141 (or 68%) presented with this abusive throat clearing behavior.[7] Vigorous, aperiodic adduction of the vocal folds, which occurs during even mild throat clearing, was observed through the classic, high-speed motion films of vocal fold vibration that Timcke, Von Leden, and Moore[8] produced.

Throat clearing may be either a primary or a secondary etiologic factor. As a primary factor, it may appear following a cold or respiratory infection, as described below:

> Mrs. M's voice evaluation revealed that she had never experienced vocal difficulties prior to contracting a cold 6 weeks earlier. Accompanying the cold had been excessive coughing and throat clearing. The cold symptoms and the cough subsided after 10 to 12 days, but Mrs. M unknowingly continued to harshly clear her throat. This caused a mild, persistent dysphonia. Indirect laryngoscopy performed during the 6th week revealed mild bilateral vocal fold edema. The subsequent voice evaluation identified continual throat clearing as the only etiologic factor associated with the persistent hoarseness. Habitual throat clearing was extinguished using a "hard swallow" modification approach (see Chapter 7), and the vocal folds returned to their normal structure and function allowing normal voice.

Throat clearing is often identified as a secondary abusive factor for patients who present with various laryngeal pathologies. Individuals frequently develop this behavior as a response to perceived laryngeal sensations. These laryngeal sensations may be caused by the presence of the pathology. Common sensations reported by patients include dryness, tickling, burning, aching, lump in the throat, or a "thickness" sensation. Patients often become hypersensitive to the laryngeal area as the result of the pathology. When this is the case, even normal sensations, such as those associated with drainage, become magnified, and a common response is habitual throat clearing. In these cases, throat clearing serves both as a symptom of the pathology and as a maintaining contributor to the disorder.

Coughing is also a vocally abusive behavior. Coughing may be the symptom of many different types of respiratory diseases, such as asthma, chronic obstructive pulmonary disease, or malignant lung lesions.[9,6] Coughing may also be a symptom of gastroesophageal reflux. When associated with a disease process, a physician treats coughing. Chronic cough, as with throat clearing, may be developed as a response to laryngeal pathology and is not always associated with disease processes. When this is the case, the voice pathologist often is called upon to extinguish this behavior as a part of the vocal management protocol.[10,11]

Inappropriate Vocal Components

Voice production is dependent on the interrelationship of many different physiologic components. These voicing components include respiration, phonation, and resonance, as well as the psychophysical components of pitch, loudness, and rate. It is expected that the presence of laryngeal pathology would modify any one or all of these components. Conversely, the functional misuse of any component or combination of components may cause a laryngeal pathology.

Respiration

In Chapter 2, we learned that vibration of the vocal folds is activated by the respiratory airstream overcoming the resistance of the approximated vocal folds, thus blowing the folds apart. The exchanges of pressure and flow interact with tissue compliance to draw the vocal folds back together, completing one vibratory cycle. Shipp and McGlone[12] demonstrated that the subglottic air pressure necessary to initiate phonation for normal conversational voice was between 3 and 7 cm of H_2O. Hirano[13] demonstrated that the normal airflow rate for voice production ranges from 50-200 ml/H_2O. When mass lesion, poor muscular control or incoordination, or neural problems compromise approximation of the vocal folds, airflow rates may increase, and subglottic air pressure is decreased. Hyperadduction of the vocal folds will produce the opposite effects.

Normal control of inspiration and expiration is necessary to support normal phonation. Aronson[14] suggested that the vast majority of voice patients use anatomically and physiologically normal respiration to support voice production. Nonetheless, certain functional respiratory habits and behaviors may lead directly to the development of a voice disorder. For example, a patient may habitually use a shallow, thoracic (chest) breathing pattern that does not support normal phonation. Low intensity and breathiness may characterize the resultant voice quality. Another functional breathing behavior that may contribute to the development of a voice disorder is the habit of speaking at the end of normal expiration. This behavior occurs when a person continues to speak when the normal tidal expiration has been completed. Speaking at the end of expiratory volume increases laryngeal muscle tension and contributes to vocal hyperfunction.

Phonation

The abusive hyperadduction of the vocal folds has previously been discussed. Patients who utilize hard glottal attacks and persistent glottal fry phonation may also demonstrate inappropriate phonation as a functional etiology.

Hard glottal attack, or glottal coup, describes one of three means by which phonation may be initiated. The hard attack is accomplished by complete and rapid adduction of the vocal folds, buildup of subglottic air pressure, and then explosion of the folds while initiating phonation.[15] Habitual use of a hard glottal attack usually causes an increase in laryngeal area muscle tension, as well as an increased and unnecessary impact on the vocal fold mucosa. The increased muscle tension requires a greater buildup of subglottic air pressure, all of which contributes to vocal hyperfunction.

The opposite of the hard glottal attack is the breathy or aspirate attack. When this mode of attack is used to initiate phonation, the vocal folds are abducted as exhalation for phonation begins and then only adduct after exhalation has been initiated, creating a moment of breathiness that is heard at the initiation of the vowel. Because of the poor glottic closure, the aspirate attack is also a voice misuse that may contribute to a voice disorder.

The third mode of vocal attack is the even or static attack. This is the most efficient means of initiating voice onset. With the static attack the vocal folds are nearly approximated as exhalation begins, permitting the onset of phonation to be smooth and effortless.

Glottal fry or pulse register is one of three vocal registers described by Hollien,[16] with the other two being *modal* and *loft* registers. Glottal fry is the lowest range of phonation along the frequency continuum and the least flexible. Production of glottal fry is characterized by tightly approximated vocal folds whose free edges appear flaccid.[17] The closed phase of the vibration cycle is long when compared with the total vibration cycle. The tighter closure requires a greater increase in subglottic air pressure, contributing to laryngeal hyperfunction. Persistent use of glottal fry, which has been described as sounding like a poorly tuned motorboat engine, will often cause vocal fatigue, laryngeal tension, and a "lump in the throat" feeling.

Opposite the pulse register is the **loft** register, which includes the higher range of the vocal frequencies including the falsetto. Persistent use of the loft register or falsetto voice is a maladaption of the normal voice physiology and can lead to voice pathologies, such as juvenile voice and functional falsetto. The range of frequencies normally used in speaking and singing comprise the **modal** register.

Resonance

Once sound is generated at the level of the vocal folds (the sound source), it then passes through a series of filters (the vocal tract) that dampen and enhance the sound and make each voice unique and distinctive to the owner of the voice. There is a wide range of acceptable voice resonance patterns, although the level of acceptability often is determined by geographic location, such as the Southern "twang." Certain resonance problems may have an organic basis, such as those resulting from velopharyngeal incompetence or a submucous cleft, whereas others are caused by functional disturbances. Functional resonance disturbances may be caused by the improper coupling of the pharyngeal, oral, and nasal cavities or the improper placement of the tongue and larynx.

Hypernasality or rhinolalia aperta occurs when vowels and voiced consonants are excessively resonated in the nasal cavity. This behavior occurs when the velopharyngeal port remains open during production of the phonemes other than the nasal consonants /m/, /n/, and /ŋ/. The increase in nasal resonance may or may not be accompanied by excessive nasal air emission, which is heard as a friction noise that accompanies the phonemes produced.

Denasality or rhinolalia clausa occurs when normal nasal resonance is not present on the phonemes /m/, /n/, and /ŋ/. The physical basis is an overclosure of the velopharyngeal port or an obstruction of the nasal cavity. The acoustic result sounds as if the speaker has a head cold.

Assimilative nasality occurs when the phonemes adjacent to the three nasal consonants are nasalized along with these sounds. The cause is presumed to be the premature opening of the port prior to the nasal consonant and a lingering opening of the port following the nasal consonant. This form of nasal resonance is often heard for a brief period following removal of large tonsils and adenoids.

Cul-de-sac nasality is a closed nasality in which all the vowels, semivowels, and nasals are produced with a hollow-sounding or dead-end resonance. This form of nasality is thought to be caused by obstruction in the anterior nasal cavity.

Retracted tongue and **elevated larynx** are anatomical postures that often accompany each other and contribute to altered resonance and laryngeal tension. When the larynx is elevated, the vocal tract will be shortened, thus raising all the formant frequencies. The increased extrinsic and intrinsic lingual muscle tension also tends to raise the fundamental frequency. The combination of these effects yields a higher pitched voice with a pinched resonance quality. Patients who exhibit these behaviors often complain of laryngeal aching and fatigue caused by the increased muscular activity.

Pitch

Pitch is the perceptual correlate of the fundamental frequency of voice. Misuse refers to pitch levels that are either too high, too low, or those that are lacking in variability. Habitual use of an inappropriate pitch may create laryngeal tension and strain. Patients we have treated who required direct pitch modification have included young men with pseudoauthoritative voices, speakers who frequently talk and lecture either in noisy locations or to large groups in less-than-adequate acoustical conditions, patients with other illnesses and emotional conditions, patients who have undergone vocal fold surgery who have not automatically made the appropriate pitch adjustments, male patients with functional falsetto, female patients with juvenile voice, and, transsexual patients.

Change in pitch is a common symptom of voice disorders, especially those associated with mass lesion or other vocal fold cover changes. Therefore, it seldom is appropriate from a therapeutic point of view to be concerned with direct pitch modification. Indeed, as the vocal fold mucosa improves, so too would the inappropriate pitch. To try to ascertain an "optimum" pitch from the pathologic voice would be frustrating. The various methods suggested to accomplish this task are flawed due to the presence of the pathology. Therefore, direct pitch modification is reserved for selected cases in which the use of an inappropriate pitch has been isolated as the *primary* etiologic factor associated with the development of the voice disorder.

Loudness

Loudness is the perceptual term that relates to vocal intensity. The inappropriate use of loudness is demonstrated in voices that are habitually too soft, too loud, or lack loudness variability. The vocally abusive behaviors of shouting and loud talking have been previously discussed. It is important to note that habitual use of an inadequate loudness level may also be a vocal misuse. Vocal intensity is determined by the lateral excursion of the vocal folds and the speed with which they return to approximate as dictated by the subglottic air pressure and the resultant airflow. When a person speaks very softly, the balance between the airflow and the muscular activity is disturbed. The decreased airflow causes more demands to be placed on the intrinsic muscle system, thus leading to possible vocal muscle strain and fatigue. Talking softly may be abusive if not well supported by the airstream.

Rate

As an etiologic factor, rate may contribute to laryngeal pathologies when speech is produced too rapidly. Faulty use of the laryngeal mechanism related to vocal hyperfunction is evident when speakers produce speech in too rapid a manner.[6] The patient who talks too fast typically does not use proper breath support, often talking on insufficient breath support. Increased rate may lead to vocal hyperfunction.

Rarely will a voice pathologist be presented with a voice disorder in which a single vocal component is isolated as the primary etiology. If inappropriate components are found to be the cause, a combination of components usually will be identified, with misuse of one being the predominant factor contributing to the voice disorder. Inappropriate components may also be the result of laryngeal pathologies that were caused by other etiologic factors. When this is the case, the components are recognized as the symptoms of the disorder (such as low pitch, glottal fry, breathiness, and so on).

Vocal misuse represents the most common etiologic factor identified in patients with voice disorders. Cooper[18] found that of 1406 patients, 36.6% had disorders associated with vocal misuse. Brodnitz[4] reported a figure of 25.8%. Voice therapy is particularly effective in the remediation of voice disorders caused by vocal misuse.

Medically Related Etiologies

This category of etiologic correlates refers to medical or surgical interventions that directly cause voice disorders and medical or health conditions and treatments that may indirectly contribute to the development of voice disorders (see Table 3-2). Voice pathologists' base of knowledge regarding these etiologic factors will aid them during the diagnostic process, especially when discussing the patient's medical history.

Direct Surgery

Direct surgical procedures are those that cause an insult to the anatomical structures responsible for phonation and resonance. These surgeries would include **total laryngectomy, hemi-laryngectomy, supraglottic laryngectomy, glossectomy,**

Table 3-2. Medically Related Etiologies

Trauma	Chronic Illnesses and Disorders
Direct surgery	Sinusitis
Laryngectomy (total, hemi, supraglottic)	Respiratory illnesses
Glossectomy	Allergies
Mandibulectomy	Medications
Palatal	Stomach disorder
Other head and neck	Nervous disorder
Indirect surgery	Endocrine disorder
Thyroid	Cardiac disease
Heart	Arthritis
Carotid	Alcohol and drug abuse
Lung	Smoking
Hysterectomy	
Intubation	
Mechanical trauma	
Burns	

mandibulectomy, palatal surgery, and other head and neck excisions such as radical neck dissection and pharyngeal surgeries. Most of these surgeries are conservation procedures designed to eradicate disease regardless of the effects on phonation. Vocal rehabilitation is essential following these surgeries and is described in Chapter 9.

Indirect Surgery

Surgery for other medical problems may indirectly contribute to the development of voice disorders. Because of the anatomical relationships of the **thyroid, heart, lungs, cervical spine,** and **carotid arteries** to the recurrent laryngeal nerves, the superior laryngeal nerves, and the branches of the vagus nerve, surgical procedures involving these structures may involve some trauma to the nervous supply of the larynx. Possible consequences may be a vocal fold paresis or paralysis and a loss of sensory innervation to the mucosal lining of the larynx.[19]

Women who have undergone a complete hysterectomy, including the uterus and both ovaries, may also experience vocal difficulties. A temporary or permanent lowering of the vocal pitch may be caused by hormonal changes. Some patients, in an attempt to maintain the "normal" higher pitch, place increased muscle strain on the laryngeal mechanism, thus setting the stage for the development of a voice disorder.

Finally, any surgery that requires general anesthesia and the placement of an endotracheal tube has the potential for causing mechanical trauma to the vocal folds.[20-22] Friedmann[23] suggested two different types of laryngeal injuries caused by intubation: (a) trauma to the mucosa over the vocal processes of the arytenoid cartilages in the posterior larynx and (b) trauma caused by constant pressure of the tube on the vocal process resulting in tissue necrosis. The result in either case is injury to the mucosa that covers the cartilage, with concomitant injury to the perichondrium. In an attempt to repair the damaged area, granulomatous tissue develops.[24] Treatment for this disorder will often involve a combination of medical, surgical, and voice therapy treatments.

Chronic Illnesses and Disorders

Many chronic illnesses and disorders and their treatments may contribute to the development of laryngeal pathologies. Because of the importance of these etiologic factors, Chapters 4 and 7 of this text deal with issues related to changes in vocal function associated with each of these disorders and illnesses in much greater detail. As outlined in Table 3-2, voice disorders may develop secondary to other systemic, cardiac, respiratory, immunologic, gastrointestinal, endocrine, inflammatory, and pharmacological influences.

For example, chronic **sinusitis** and other **upper respiratory infections**, although often limited to the supraglottic structures, may contribute to the development of hoarseness. Because the sinus drainage does not touch the vocal folds, it cannot be blamed for the hoarseness, although the patient may perceive it as the cause. Nonetheless, coughing and throat clearing, which often accompany these illnesses, are implicated in voice abuse and may be the direct cause of the voice problem. Medications used to treat these illnesses and their symptoms may also be implicated as a cause. **Antihistamines** are commonly used to dry the secretions but will also cause a reduction in the secretions of the salivary and mucous glands, thus contributing to potential dehydration of the vocal folds. **Anticough medications**, such as codeine and dextromethorphan, are also mucosal drying agents.[25]

Other, more chronic respiratory illnesses, such as **asthma**, **chronic obstructive pulmonary disease**, and **lung cancer** may directly or indirectly contribute to voice disorders. The increased responsiveness and hyperactivity of the trachea and bronchi in individuals with asthma may lead to transitory or prolonged episodes of wheezing, coughing, and dyspnea. Hoarseness may, therefore, result from vocal fold tissue lining abuse, poor respiratory support, and from the medications used to treat the condition. **Bronchodilators**, such as albuterol (Proventil and Ventolin), may have the side effects of tremor and nervousness. **Corticosteroid** inhalants may contribute to vocal fold bowing and an elevation of fundamental frequency.[26,27]

Chronic obstructive pulmonary disease (COPD) is a clinical term used to describe a group of diseases characterized by persistent slowing of airflow during exhalation. The most common of these diseases are emphysema and chronic bronchitis, both of which may cause the vocally abusive wheezing, coughing, dyspnea, and sputum expectoration. Again, medications used to treat these diseases may have a negative effect on the mucous membrane and the fluid secretion to the vocal folds.

Lung cancer may have a more direct effect on the functioning of the vocal folds. Indeed, a symptom of lung cancer is left vocal fold paralysis caused by damage to the vagus nerve. Radiation treatments, chemotherapy, and direct lung surgery may also violate the nervous supply to the vocal fold, as well as mucous secretion and internal hydration.

About one in every five persons in the United States has an **allergy** caused by something inhaled, ingested, touched, or injected. Severity may range from very mild to very severe to fatal. When an airborne allergen (a substance that elicits the allergic response) enters the body, it reacts with an antibody that is fixed to the surface of mast cells found in the nose, lungs, and skin. The allergen-antibody binding triggers the release of histamines, which are responsible for the allergic symptoms. The histamine causes contraction of smooth muscles, dilation of blood vessels, and stimulation of mucous glands to produce increased quantities of mucus.[28] Allergies may cause congestion and edema of the vocal folds, thus negatively affecting voice production. Treatments for allergies may include medicines such as antihistamines and topical steroids, with the side effects as previously described. Decongestants may also be utilized to decrease the edema of the mucous membrane. Long-term use of a vasoconstrictor, however, may show a diminished drug effect with the return of edema and congestion being greater than was previously present.[29] Persistent allergies may be treated through injections of the allergen designed to desensitize the patient to that allergen.

Gastrointestinal disorders may also negatively affect voice production. One of the most common disorders in this category is gastroesophageal reflux disease (GERD).[30] Reflux of the acidic stomach contents to the posterior larynx has been implicated in the symptoms of chronic hoarseness, voice fatigue, cough, chronic throat clearing, globus sensation (lump in the throat), and a sensation of choking. The burning of the posterior larynx may cause edema, ulceration, and granulation of the laryngeal mucosa and, when left untreated, may cause hyperkeratosis and even carcinoma of the larynx. In our practice and in practices across the United States, large numbers of patients have been diagnosed with GERD symptoms. A complete treatment regimen is described in Chapter 7.

The presence of lower intestinal disorders, such as spastic colon, irritable bowel syndrome, and diarrhea, may also be implicated in the development of voice disorders. Antispasmodic medications used for these disorders, such as atropine, scopolamine, and diphenoxylate hydrochloride, reduce glandular secretions and are drying agents.[25]

Patients who suffer with **emotional disorders**, such as emotional tension, depression, and anxiety, may also experience voice disorders for a number of reasons, including simple laryngeal area tension, poor respiratory support, and whole body fatigue from poor sleep habits, to name a few. Psychotropic medications prescribed for nervous tension, depression, psychotic disorders, and sleep disorders may have a negative effect on voice production because of drying and sedation. Some of these common drugs include Elavil, Pamelor, Prozac, and Paxil (antidepressants); Thorazine and Haldol (antipsychotics); and antihistamines that are often used for sleep disorders.

Endocrine dysfunction, such as hypothyroidism, hyperthyroidism, hyperpituitarism, amyloidosis, virilization, and minor hormonal changes associated with menstruation has also been implicated as a cause of voice disorders. Hoarseness, vocal fatigue, pitch changes, loss of range, breathiness, reduced loudness, and pitch breaks have all been observed in individuals with endocrine disorders.[31-35]

Cardiac and **circulatory problems** may also contribute to the development of voice disorders. We previously discussed the potential negative surgical effects on the recurrent laryngeal nerve. Medications used to control high blood pressure, such as methyldopa, reserpine, and captopril, are drying agents and their diuretic effect could potentially result in dryness and irritation of the mucous membrane of the vocal folds.[25]

Arthritis, an inflammatory disease of the body's synovial joints, has also been implicated in the development of voice disorders. The symptoms of cricoarytenoid joint arthritis are hoarseness, a laryngeal fullness feeling, and pain associated with the inflammation of the joint. In more severe cases, the joint may be fixed (cricoarytenoid ankylosis) and imitate the appearance of a vocal fold paralysis. The severity of the symptoms is dependent on the severity of the arthritis.

Finally, the negative effects of **smoking**, **alcohol abuse**, and **illicit drug use** on the vocal mechanism cannot be denied. Minimally, the heat and chemicals from tobacco smoke cause erythema, edema, and generalized inflammation of the vocal tract. Even more threatening is the contribution tobacco smoke makes to the development of laryngeal carcinoma. Other conditions that smoking can cause include polypoid mucosal changes and the precancerous conditions of leukoplakia and hyperkeratosis (Chapter 4).[36] Sataloff [34, 35] reported that marijuana smoke is particularly irritating, causing considerable vocal fold mucosal response. He also noted that cocaine could be extremely irritating to the nasal mucosa, causing increased vasoconstriction and altering mucosal sensation, resulting in decreased voice control and a tendency toward vocal abuse.

Alcohol is a vasodilator and thus may cause drying of the mucous membrane of the vocal folds. In addition, it is a central nervous system depressant that, when abused, results in symptoms of incoordination, dysarthria, and impaired judgment. Alcohol use may also aggravate GERD.

Caffeine is also a drug. It is a central nervous system stimulant, which has the potential to cause hyperactivity and tremor. In addition, it decreases laryngeal secretions causing laryngeal dehydration. As with alcohol, caffeine has a relaxation effect on the upper esophageal sphincter, and it can promote gastroesophageal reflux.

Smoking and drug and alcohol abuse may directly cause laryngeal pathologies. These chronic external and internal irritants are extremely abusive to the vocal mechanism and have been implicated as causes of many pathologies, from chronic laryngitis to laryngeal neoplasm. In addition to the direct abuse of inhaled chemicals, many smokers also have a "smoker's cough," which adds additional vocal abuse to compound the problem.

When dealing with medically related etiologies, the appropriate physician specialist must identify and treat the primary medical condition. The voice pathologist often proves helpful in identifying for the physician behaviors that may or may not be associated with the medical condition, thus adding to the diagnostic process. Improvement of the medical condition does not automatically improve the concomitant voice disorder. Voice evaluation and therapy proves to be a valuable asset to many patients exhibiting other surgical or medical conditions.

Primary Disorder Etiologies

This major etiologic category includes embryological, physiologic, neurologic, and anatomical disorders (see Table 3-3) that have vocal changes as secondary symptoms of the primary disorder. Included in this category are **cleft palate** and **organic velopharyngeal insufficiency**, with their characteristic hypernasal vocal components. An inappropriate high pitch and a pharyngeal resonatory focus frequently characterize the vocal components of

Table 3-3. Primary Disorder Etiologies

Cleft palate

Organic velopharyngeal insufficiency

Deafness

Cerebral palsy

Neurological disorders

Trauma

people with profound hearing loss. Boone[37] found that 17- and 18-year-old male subjects with deafness had a mean fundamental frequency 54 Hz higher than the same measure for males of the same age with normal hearing. Individuals with a severe-profound sensorineural hearing loss often speak with the tongue retracted toward the pharyngeal wall, creating a disturbance in normal voice resonance.

The voices of individuals with **cerebral palsy** will vary widely because the neurologic damage is not related to one form of neurologic lesion.[38] Individuals presenting with cerebral palsy often speak with a labored, monotonous, and strained phonation with a limited frequency range. Control of intensity, caused by body positioning and respiratory support limitations, may also be problematic. These symptoms are also similar to the unpredictable effects of traumatic brain injuries (TBI).

Many voice symptoms are present in a wide range of neurologic disorders. In his exceptional review of dysphonias associated with neurological disease, Aronson[14] reported that technically, neurologic voice disorders are dysarthrias and are most often embedded "in a complex of respiratory, resonatory, and articulatory dysarthric signs" (p. 77). The neurological disorders with associated voice symptoms are discussed in detail in Chapter 4.

Accidental **trauma** is the final cause of a voice disorder listed in the category of Primary Disorder etiologies. Blunt or penetrating injuries to the larynx often cause edema, fractured laryngeal cartilages, joint dislocations, and lacerations. These injuries may be caused by automobile accidents and sports-related injuries, stabbing and gunshot wounds, strangulation, and, on rare occasions, traumatic intubation injuries. Inhalation of flames, gasses, and fumes and swallowing of caustic substances also may cause serious traumatic injury to the laryngeal mucosa. The primary concern related to severe trauma of the larynx is the establishment and maintenance of an adequate airway. Voice therapy will follow recovery from the acute stage of the injury.

As primary disorders, these conditions require appropriate medical, surgical, educational, and rehabilitative interventions. The voice pathologist will most often serve as a part of a team attempting to modify the voice, swallowing, articulation, and language components of these various disorders.

Personality-related Etiologies

The final major etiologic category is that of personality-related causes of voice disorders (see Table 3-4). Voice is a sensitive indicator of emotions, attitudes, and role assumptions.[39] Indeed, the quality of voice often directly suggests the way a person feels physically and emotionally. The resulting vocal symptoms may simply reflect a whole-body tension that causes a more specific hypertonicity of the intrinsic and extrinsic laryngeal muscles and, ultimately, a tension dysphonia. In other cases, the symptoms may be a sign of a much more serious underlying psychological disorientation.[40] In either case, the tensions and stresses of everyday life may contribute directly to the abnormal functioning of the sensitive vocal instrument.

Environmental Stress

Environmental stress represents the many occurrences in human life that can cause emotional and physical stresses, provoking vocal disorders in some individuals. For example:

Table 3-4. Personality-related Etiologies

Environmental stress

Conversion behaviors

Identity conflict

Mrs. S, an attractive 60-year-old woman, was referred by the laryngologist with the diagnosis of mild bilateral vocal fold edema. She complained of a chronic "hoarseness" and "tiredness" in her voice after only minimal use. Her general voice quality was described as mildly dysphonic, characterized by habitual use of low pitch, breathiness, and intermittent glottal fry phonation. During the voice evaluation, no *vocally abusive behaviors, medically-related causes,* or *primary disorders* were identified. Without further interview, we may have surmised that the cause of this disorder was the use of the inappropriate vocal components of pitch and respiration.

The social history, however, revealed that Mrs. S's husband had died just 2 months prior to the evaluation. She was in the process of trying to close his affairs and sell the house they had shared for 36 years. As you would now expect, this patient was experiencing what may be called an *emotional dysphonia* due to the depression and stress she was experiencing. The laryngeal muscular tension caused by her generalized hypertonicity led to the use of inappropriate vocal components, which physically contributed to the development of vocal fold edema. Nonetheless, the major cause of this disorder was the environmental stress.

Conversion Behaviors

At times, environmental stress may become so severe that avoidance behaviors are developed to counteract stressful situations. These avoidance behaviors become an unconscious substitution of a somatic symptom, involving the sensory or motor nervous systems, for the unpleasant or intolerable emotional event or conflict.[39] In the psychiatric literature, these behaviors are referred to as psychological conversion disorders.[41] As a cause of voice disorders, the conversion behavior may manifest as whispering, muteness, or unusual dysphonias. For example:

Mrs. P was a 36-year-old homemaker and mother of two sons ages 14 and 16 years. She was referred by the laryngologist with the diagnosis of normal appearing vocal folds. Her voice quality, which she had experienced for 6 weeks, was aphonic with intermittent periods of phonation in the form of a high-pitched squeak.

The social history, gathered during the evaluation, revealed that Mrs. P's 16-year-old son recently had been arrested for theft. Until this unfortunate occurrence, he had been a model youth making good grades in school and had participated in sports, drama, and other positive social activities. Mrs. P's vocal difficulties began about the time of his arrest. This was apparently her psychological reaction to this intolerable, stressful situation. Voice therapy was successful in returning the patient's voice to normal within the first session (see Chapter 7).

Identity Conflict

The final personality-related etiology is that of identity conflict. Aronson[14] stated that psychosexual conflicts are neither signs of environmental stress nor conversion reactions to stressful life problems. Identity problems are embedded in the fabric of the personality. Persons who experience difficulties in establishing their own personalities may present with voice problems as a result. These may include maintaining a high-pitched falsetto in the postadolescent male; or a weak, thin, juvenile-sounding voice in an adult female; or the desire of the male-to-female transsexual to raise the pitch of her voice. We would strongly caution the reader that although some individuals with these vocal disorders may present with psychological conflicts, the majority do not. Indeed, the voice problem may simply be a learned response or the conscious desire to project a particular image. (The pathologies associated with the etiology of identity conflict are discussed in Chapter 4.)

Voice disorders that are the result of personality-related etiologies are particularly amenable to voice therapy. At times, psychological referral and family counseling may be necessary and appropriate. The voice pathologist must realize the limitations of direct voice therapy and make referrals to mental health professionals as necessary. It has been our experience that, in the majority of cases, patients with personality-related voice disorders are well managed by the voice pathologist.

Summary

This chapter has presented some of the etiologic correlates of voice disorders in a categorical manner. It should be understood, however, that most voice disorders have more than one contributing etiologic factor. One of the rewards of working with patients who have voice disorders is the challenge of discovering the pertinent parts of the etiologic puzzle. The perceptual symptoms of many voice pathologies are similar, but the causes for those symptoms are many. The voice pathologist achieves success by finding the causes and then modifying or eliminating them, thus resolving the pathology and improving the voice. Chapter 4 discusses the various laryngeal pathologies that develop as a result of these etiologic factors, and Chapters 5 and 6 present ways of discovering these etiologic correlates.

References

1. West R, Kennedy L, Carr A. *The Rehabilitation of Speech*. New York, NY: Harper and Brothers; 1937.
2. Koufman J, Isaccson G. The spectrum of vocal dysfunction. In: Koufman J, Isaccson G, eds. *The Otolaryngologic Clinics of North America: Voice Disorders*. Philadelphia, Pa: WB Saunders; 1991.
3. Stemple J, Stanley J, Lee L. Objective measures of voice production following prolonged voice use. *J Voice*. 1995;9:127-133.
4. Brodnitz F. *Vocal Rehabilitation*. 4th ed. Rochester, NY: American Academy of Ophthalmology and Otolaryngology; 1971.
5. Greene M. *The Voice and Its Disorders*. 3rd ed. Philadelphia, Pa: JB Lippincott; 1972.
6. Wilson D. *Voice Problems of Children*. Baltimore, Md: Williams and Wilkins; 1979.
7. Stemple J, Lehmann D. Throat clearing: The unconscious habit of vocal hyperfunction. Paper presented at: American Speech-Language-Hearing Association National Convention; November 1980; Detroit, Mich.
8. Timcke R, Von Leden H, Moore P. Laryngeal vibrations: measurements of the glottic wave, Part 2: Physiologic variations. *Arch Otolaryngol*. 1959;69:438-444.
9. Irwin R, Curley F. The diagnosis of chronic cough. *Hospital Practice*. 1988;23:82-96.
10. Blager F, Gay M, Wood R. Voice therapy techniques adapted to treatment of habit cough: a pilot study. *J Comm Disord*. 1988;21:393-400.
11. Stemple J. *Voice Therapy: Clinical Studies*. St. Louis, Mo: Mosby Year Book; 1993.
12. Shipp T, McGlone R. Laryngeal dynamics associated with voice frequency change. *J Speech Hear Res*. 1971;14:761-768.
13. Hirano M. *The Clinical Examination of Voice*. Vienna, Austria: Springer-Verlag; 1981.
14. Aronson A. *Clinical Voice Disorders: An Interdisciplinary Approach*. New York, NY: Brian C Decker; 1980.
15. Jackson C, Jackson C. *Diseases of the Nose, Throat and Ear*. Philadelphia, Pa: WB Saunders; 1959.
16. Hollien H. On vocal registers. *J Phonetics*. 1974;2:125-143.
17. Zemlin W. *Speech and Hearing Science: Anatomy and Physiology*. 3rd ed. Englewood Cliffs, NJ: Prentice-Hall; 1988.

18. Cooper M. *Modern Trends in Voice Rehabilitation.* Springfield, Ill: Charles C Thomas; 1973.

19. Ballenger J. *Diseases of the Nose, Throat, Ear, Head and Neck.* 13th ed. Philadelphia, Pa: Lea and Febiger; 1985.

20. Balestrieri F, Watson C. Intubation granuloma. *Otolaryngol Clin North Am.* 1982;15:567-579.

21. Peppard S, Dickens J. Laryngeal injury following short-term intubation. *Ann Otol Rhinol Laryngol.* 1983;92:327-330.

22. Whited R. Laryngeal dysfunction following prolonged intubation. *Ann Otol Rhinol Laryngol.* 1979;88:474-478.

23. Friedmann I. Granulomas of the larynx. In: Paparella M, Shumrick D, eds. *Otolaryngology. Head and Neck.* Vol. 3. 2nd ed. Philadelphia, Pa: WB Saunders; 1980:2449-2469.

24. Doyle P, Martin G. Paradoxical glottal closure mechanism associated with postintubation granuloma. *J Voice.* 1991;5:247-251.

25. Martin F. Tutorial: drugs and vocal function. *J Voice.* 1988;2:338-344.

26. Watkin K, Ewanowski S. Effects of triamcinolone acetonide on the voice. *J Speech Hear Res.* 1979;22:446-455.

27. Williams A, Baghat M, DeStableforth C, Shenoi P, Skinner C. Dysphonia caused by inhaled steroids. Recognition of a characteristic laryngeal abnormality. *Thorax.* 1983;38:813-821.

28. Spiegel J, Hawkshaw M, and Sataloff R. Allergy. In: Sataloff R, ed. *Professional Voice: The Science and Art of Clinical Care.* New York, NY: Raven Press; 1991:153-157.

29. Colton R, Casper L. *Understanding Voice Problems: A Physiological Perspective for Diagnosis and Treatment.* Baltimore, Md: Williams and Wilkins; 1990.

30. Olson N. Laryngopharyngeal manifestations of gastroesophageal reflux disease. In: Koufman J, Isaccson G, eds. *The Otolaryngologic Clinics of North America: Voice Disorders.* Philadelphia, Pa: WB Saunders; 1991.

31. Aronson A. *Clinical Voice Disorders: An Interdisciplinary Approach.* 3rd ed. New York, NY: Brian C Decker; 1990.

32. Damste P. Voice changes in adult women caused by virilizing agents. *J Speech Hear Disord.* 1967;32:126-132.

33. Gould W. Vocal cords can speak of hormonal dysfunction. *Consultant.* 1972;12:101-102.

34. Sataloff R. Endocrine dysfunction. In: Sataloff R, ed. *Professional Voice: The Science and Art of Clinical Care.* New York, NY: Raven Press; 1991:201-205.

35. Sataloff R. Patient history. In: Sataloff R, ed. *Professional Voice: The Science and Art of Clinical Care.* New York, NY: Raven Press; 1991:69-83.

36. Wynder E, Stellmann S. Comparative epidemiology of tobacco-related cancers. *Cancer Res.* 1977;37:4608-4622.

37. Boone D. Modification of the voices of deaf children. *Volta Rev.* 1966; 68:686-692.

38. Greene M, Mathieson L. *The Voice and Its Disorders.* 5th ed. London, England: Whurr Publishers; 1989.

39. Morrison M, Rammage L. *The Management of Voice Disorders.* San Diego, Calif: Singular Publishing Group; 1994.

40. Kinzl J, Bierl W, Rauchegger H. Functional aphonia. A conversion symp-

tom as a defensive mechanism against anxiety. *Psychother Psychosom.* 1988;49:31-36.

41. Aronson A, Peterson H, Litin E. Psychiatric symptomotology in functional dysphonia and aphonia. *J Speech Hear Disord.* 1966;31:115-127.

4

Pathologies of the Laryngeal Mechanism

Voice disorders arise when an individual's quality, pitch, or loudness differs from voice characteristics typical of speakers of similar age, gender, cultural background, and geographic location. The range of etiologies of voice disorders is large, and these differences may result from a variety of factors. Structural, medical, or neurologic alterations of the respiratory, laryngeal, and vocal tract mechanisms may create a voice disorder. Other pathologies develop following maladaptive or inappropriate voice use. Another type of voice disorders occurs in direct response to psychogenic factors.

The complementary relationship among these various physical, voice use, and psychogenic influences ensures that most voice disorders and laryngeal pathologies will have contributions from more than one etiologic factor and that there is considerable overlap among these three groupings.[1-3] For example, inappropriate vocal behaviors or excessive vocal demands may generate organic pathology (eg, polyps or nodules). Psychological trauma or excessive emotional stress may accompany the onset of spasmodic dysphonia. Voice disorders that emerge during an upper respiratory infection may persist long after the cold has resolved, presumably because of the effortful phonation and other maladaptive vocal behaviors adopted by the speaker during the cold. These typical case scenarios highlight the overlapping influences of an original etiologic factor, whereas other secondary components serve to maintain the voice disturbance. Consequently, treatment alternatives are also eclectic and can include medical or surgical intervention, voice rehabilitation therapy, psychological counseling, or a combination approach. This chapter presents general descriptions and differential diagnostic signs of the most common voice disorders and considers the underlying contributions from medical, surgical, behavioral, rehabilitative, and psychosocial components.

Incidence of Voice Disorders

The incidence of voice disorders is difficult to establish because figures vary dependent upon age, gender, and occupation. Verdolini[3] reported a prevalence of 3% to 10% in the general population. LaGuaite[4] studied 428 otolaryngology patients, aged 18 to 82 years, and found that 7.2% of the males and 5% of the females had some form of laryngeal pathology. Herrington-Hall et al[5] studied a group of 1262 patients who sought evaluation from several otolaryngologists and also reported gender differences in the prevalence of laryngeal pathologies. Ten years later, Coyle examined an additional 1158 new patient records to expand and replicate the study.[6] These studies concurred that the most frequent voice pathologies for patients seeking treatment from otolaryngologists are benign vocal fold lesions (such as nodules, polyps, and edema) and functional voice disorders (including diagnoses of symptoms of vocal fatigue and hoarseness). The most recent study also added a prominent diagnostic category: reflux laryngitis. Other diagnoses of vocal fold paralysis, carcinoma, and vocal fold bowing also were frequent but occurred more often in elderly speakers. In general, pathologies occurred more frequently in older populations, with the largest group of patients ranging in age from 45 to 64 years. Females sought treatment for voice disorders more frequently than did males, and overall, laryngeal pathologies were significantly more common in females than in males.

Occupations also affect incidence of voice disorders.[7] In a study of school teachers[8] 32% self-identified as having had a voice disorder, compared with only 1% of other occupations sampled. Overridingly, occupations that place persons at risk for voice disorders are those that require voice production to conduct the work, such as professional voice use (acting, singing, and other vocal performances), telemarketing, and reception service. Threats increase when persons must talk over loud ambient noise, as in the case of aerobic instructors, factory workers, stock traders, and restaurant servers.

Prevalence of specific laryngeal pathologies also varies with the speaker. In the Herrington-Hall study, the pathologies most common in younger adults (22-44 years) were vocal nodules and edema. Polyps and dysphonia without visible pathology were most common during middle age (45-64 years), whereas vocal fold paralysis was the most common pathology associated with more advanced age (>64 years). Interestingly, cancer of the larynx was evenly distributed between the middle and advanced age groups. The most common pathologies in females were nodules and psychogenic disorders. Males presented with cancer, leukoplakia, and hyperkeratosis in far greater numbers than did females. Specific prevalence of vocal pathology varied among age ranges of males. For example, males between infancy and 14 years presented with vocal nodules more often than they did with other disorders. The most common pathology for males between 25 and 44 years was edema. Between ages 45 and 64 years, males sought evaluation for polyps, and after 64 years, vocal fold paralysis was most prevalent. Females presented with edema, polyps, and nodules most frequently during young adulthood (22-44 years) and middle adulthood (45-64 years).[5]

Estimates of voice disorders for children are also variable but tend to exceed estimates for adult speakers.[9,10] Typical prevalence rates range from as low as 6% to as high as 23%. In a study describing laryngeal disorders in children evaluated by otolaryngologists, Dobres et al[11] found the most common pathologies to be subglottic stenosis, vocal nodules, laryngomalacia, dysphonia without visible organic pathology, and vocal fold paralysis. Much of these data were collected from physicians located within a major children's medical center, however, where more extreme medical conditions were treated.

Pathology Classifications

There is no optimal approach to organizing and classifying the broad and ever-increasing range of laryngeal pathologies and voice disorders. Recognizing that many potential facets influence voice disorders, a complete listing of the pathologies presented in this chapter is contained in Table 4-1, and five separate classifications are presented here:

1. Structural changes in the vocal fold
2. Neurogenic voice disorders
3. Systemic disease contributors to laryngeal pathology
4. Disorders of voice use
5. Idiopathic voice disorders

Structural Changes of the Vocal Fold

Pathologies of the vocal fold include those that cause any alteration in the histological structure of the vocal fold. Usually, preliminary diagnosis of laryngeal pathologies relies on the visual appearance of the vocal folds. For this reason, it is essential that voice professionals are familiar with the normal appearance of the vocal folds (Figures 4-1 and 4-2). Changes in the mucosal layers or in the vocal fold muscle body will affect the mass, size, stiffness, flexibility, and tension of the vibrating mechanism; they also will alter the glottal closure pattern during phonation. Any one of these vocal fold changes has the potential to alter vocal quality, pitch, and loudness.[12] Differential diagnosis of the voice disorder etiology usually is made through careful visual examination of the lesion, but the history of voice use, disorder onset, course, and remission will also contribute important information critical to understanding the source of the problem and the indications for treatment.

The audio-perceptual quality of voice in patients with any lesion varies tremendously as a function of the lesion severity,

Table 4-1. Pathology Classifications

Structural Changes of the Vocal Fold
Nodules
Polyps
Vascular lesions: vocal hemorrhage and varix
Reinke's edema/polypoid degeneration
Laryngitis: acute and chronic
Granuloma/contact ulcer
Congenital and acquired cysts
Papilloma
Congenital and acquired webs
Sulcus vocalis
Presbylaryngeus
Epithelial hyperplasia: leukoplakia and hyperkeratosis
Epithelial dysplasia: carcinoma
Neurogenic Voice Disorders
Recurrent laryngeal nerve paralysis
Bilateral abductor paralysis
Bilateral adductor paralysis
Unilateral abductor paralysis
Unilateral adductor paralysis

(continued)

Table 4-1. (continued)

Neurogenic Voice Disorders (continued)
Superior laryngeal nerve paralysis
Bilateral paralysis
Unilateral paralysis
Spasmodic dysphonia
Adductor type
Abductor type
Essential vocal tremor
Other neurologic disorders
Myasthenia gravis
Dystonia
Multiple sclerosis
Huntington's chorea
Parkinson disease
Amyotrophic lateral sclerosis
Systemic Disease Influences on the Larynx and Voice
Pharmaceutical effects
Endocrine influences
Growth hormone
Thyroid function
Sex hormonal imbalances

Table 4-1. (*continued*)

Systemic Disease Influences on the Larynx and Voice (*continued*)
Immunologic diseases
Rheumatoid arthritis
Allergies
Infectious disease
Candida
Respiratory diseases
Esophageal reflux
Disorders of Voice Use
Muscle tension dysphonia
Vocal fatigue
Vocal abuse and misuse
Ventricular phonation
Puberphonia/mutational falsetto
Transgender voice
Conversion aphonia
Idiopathic Voice Disorders
Paradoxical vocal fold motion
Congenital airway anomalies
Subglottic stenosis
Laryngomalacia

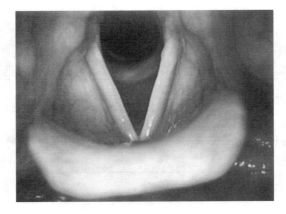

Figure 4-1. Normal vocal folds (abduction). From Abitbol[96(p83)] (See also Plate 1)

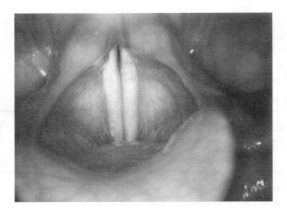

Figure 4-2. Normal vocal folds (adduction). From Abitbol[96(p83)]

the patient's habitual voice use pattern, and any compensatory strategies he or she may adopt. These compensatory strategies include both productive and maladaptive changes. Productive changes might include improved breath support, enhanced vocal tract tuning, or appropriate loudness and pitch changes. Maladaptive compensatory adjustments include effortful phonation, poor tone focus, or inappropriate pitch and loudness.

Often, certain perceptual attributes are salient for many types of vocal fold lesions. Rarely will a distinctive audio profile discriminate differentially the type of vocal fold impairment. Typical voice complaints include dysphonia (eg, increased breathiness, roughness, increased strain or effort with phonation, intermittent voice breaks or aphonia), loss of pitch and loudness range, and vocal fatigue.

Vocal Nodules

Vocal nodules (Figures 4-3 and 4-4) are one of the most common benign vocal fold lesions. Nodules represent an inflammatory degeneration of the superficial layer of the lamina propria with associated fibrosis and edema. These lesions are usually bilateral and vary in size from as small as a pinhead to as large as a pea. Nodules are usually located on the medial edge between the anterior one third and posterior two thirds of the true vocal fold, or at the point of greatest amplitude of vocal fold vibration. At least two types of nodules have been described, acute and chronic. Acute nodules arise from traumatic or hyperfunctional voice use and appear rather gelatinous and floppy, as the overlying squamous epithelium is normal. Chronic nodules appear harder

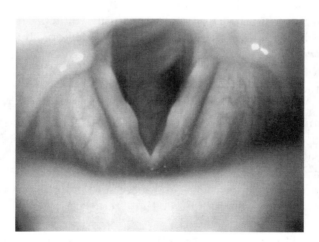

Figure 4-3. Vocal nodules (abduction). From Abitbol[96(p141)] (See also Plate 2)

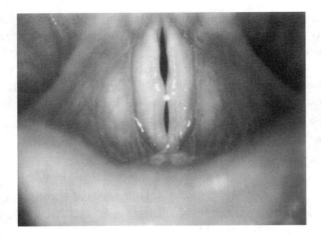

Figure 4-4. Vocal nodules (adduction). From Abitbol[96(p141)] (see also Plate 3)

and more fixed to the underlying mass of the mucosa because of increased fibrosis and a thickened epithelium. During vibration, the mass and stiffness of the vocal fold cover are increased, but the mechanical properties of the transition and body may not be affected.[12-15]

Nodules can occur at any age, but occur most frequently in both male and female children and in female adults. Nodules are rarely present in adult males. The resulting effects on voice can be variable, depending on the extent of the lesions, the length of time since onset, and any accompanying laryngeal inflammation. The symptoms of vocal nodules include mild to moderate dysphonia characterized by roughness, breathiness (caused by anterior and posterior glottal gaps that result from the approximating nodules) and increased laryngeal muscle tension. Nodules occur commonly in untrained singers, especially in those using inappropriate vocal technique. Aronson and others[1,16] have asserted that most individuals with nodules are talkative, socially aggressive, and tense, and may have acute or chronic interpersonal conflicts that generate tension, anxiety, anger, or depression.

The first line of management for vocal nodules is voice therapy. When nodules are removed surgically without the benefit of voice rehabilitation therapy, they may quickly recur. Even the chronic nodule may resolve when the patient follows the appropriate management program. When nodules do not respond to therapy in the patient who has been compliant with voice therapy, surgical management may be required, followed by postsurgical voice rehabilitation. If the patient has had repeated or longstanding vocal fold trauma, it is common to observe residual scarring on the vocal fold. In these conditions, vocal fold surgery may be necessary to restore the healthy mucosa, followed by voice conservation and voice rehabilitation therapy.

Bastian[13] has reported that nodules may also be accompanied by vascular vocal fold lesions, including hemorrhage, varix (mass of tortuous blood vessels), or hematoma resulting from injury of the small blood vessels in the traumatic lesion site. Under these acute conditions, lesions may respond to a rapid course of oral steroids. Typically, however, nodules do respond positively to voice therapy,[14,17] and medical therapies or phonosurgery are not usually needed.

Polyps

A vocal fold polyp (Figures 4-5 and 4-6) is a fluid-filled lesion that develops in the superficial layer of the lamina propria, usually (but not necessarily) in the middle one third of the membranous vocal fold. Most polyps have an active blood supply, which may account for their sudden onset and rapid increase in size. Although polyps most often occur unilaterally, they may also appear bilaterally and may present in sessile (blisterlike) or pedunculated (attached to a stalk) forms.[12,13,15] As with nodules, the cause of vocal fold polyps is thought to be acute vocal trauma or some form of voice abuse. However, most polyps occur in adults and these lesions are seen rarely in children. Vocal symptoms will vary significantly from mild to severe dysphonias depending on the type and location of the polyp and its interference with glottic closure. A pedunculated polyp may not affect phonatory quality if the lesion falls below the vibrating edge of the vocal folds, for example. Whenever a polyp interferes with vocal fold closure and vibration, dysphonia will result. Large vocal fold polyps can also obstruct the glottis and create audible inspiration. A polyp will cause the mass of the vocal fold cover

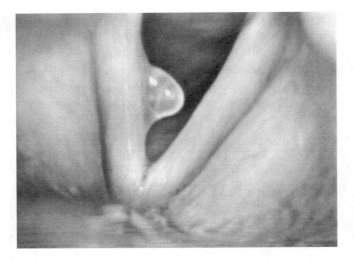

Figure 4-5. Translucent polyp. From Abitbol[96(p164)]

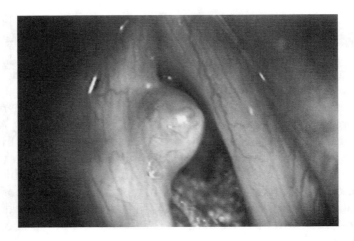

Figure 4-6. Sessile polyp. From Abitbol[96(p165)]
(See also Plate 4)

to increase, but the stiffness of the cover will vary with lesion size and duration. In general, stiffness is decreased when edema is the primary cause but increased when a hemorrhagic blood vessel is "feeding the lesion." Occasionally, a proliferation of collagen fibers or cyst development will accompany polyps. Unlike nodules, polyps often require surgery, especially if rapid improvement is not seen following stringent voice conservation. The combination approach using phonosurgery and voice rehabilitation therapy is optimal.[13]

Reinke's Edema and Polypoid Degeneration

Reinke's edema (Figures 4-7 and 4-8) occurs when the superficial layer of the lamina propria (also known as Reinke's space) becomes filled with viscous fluid because of long-standing trauma. In its most severe form, the entire membranous portion of the vocal folds become infiltrated with thick, gelatinous fluid, giving them the appearance of enlarged, fluid-filled bags or balloons. This extreme form is called polypoid degeneration. Both Reinke's edema and polypoid degeneration are caused by chronic misuse of the laryngeal mechanism, and consistent precursors include long-term vocal abuse and smoking.[19] Because this excessive swelling affects the entire length of the vocal folds, glottic closure is usually complete. The mass and stiffness of the vocal fold cover are increased markedly, but the vocal

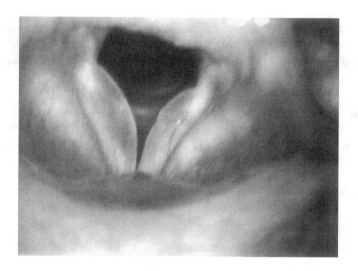

Figure 4-7. Reinke's edema (early). From Abitbol[96(p268)] (See also Plate 5)

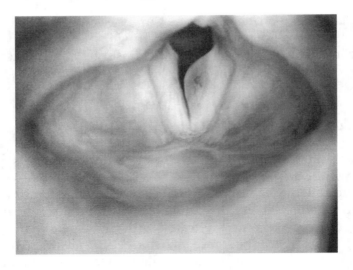

Figure 4-8. Reinke's edema (advanced). From Abitbol[96(p263)] (See also Plate 6)

fold body appears unaffected by these superficial tissue changes. Unlike other laryngeal pathologies, Reinke's edema and polypoid degeneration tend to result in consistent changes in voice quality, including mild to moderate dysphonia, characterized by low pitch and a husky hoarseness. This voice quality has traditionally been described as a "whiskey" or "smoker's" voice. Treatment for polypoid degeneration and Reinke's edema is usually surgical excision, using a lateral incision to extract the superfluous contents while protecting the medial edge of the vocal fold.[13,19] Voice therapy is valuable both preoperatively in identifying the causes for the pathology and postoperatively for reestablishing good vocal hygiene and improved voice production. Most patients have become accustomed to the low-pitched vocal roughness, and they should be made aware preoperatively of the dramatic change in voice quality that will occur following surgery. In postoperative therapy, clinicians can assist the patient in using their "new" voice correctly.

Vascular Lesions: Vocal Hemorrhage, Hematoma, and Varix

Vascular vocal fold lesions, including hemorrhage, hematoma, and varix (Figure 4-9) occur because of some traumatic (usually acute) injury to the small blood vessels of the vocal fold. Often, a hemorrhage occurs when a small capillary on the superior surface of the vocal fold ruptures, causing a bleed into the superficial layer of the lamina propria (Reinke's space). A hematoma is the accumulation of blood that has leaked from the vessel. A varix is a mass of blood capillaries that appears as a small, longstanding "blood blister" that has hardened over time, creating an adynamic segment in the vocal fold and contributing to loss of pitch and loudness range. It may also appear as a blunt end of a varicose vein, seen on the surface of the vocal fold after the hemorrhage has resolved.

All of these resulting injuries create mucosal stiffness and, in more severe cases, scarring of the vocal fold cover, causing significant acute dysphonia at the time of the bleed and continued dysphonia in the period after the injury. When other

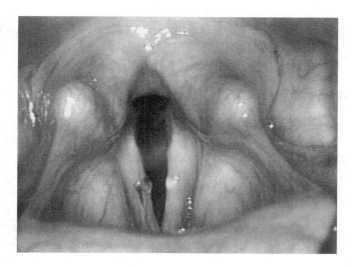

Figure 4-9. Vocal fold vascular lesions. From Abitbol[96(p228)] (See also Plate 7)

laryngeal inflammation or edema accompanies vocal fold hemorrhage and hematoma, the submucosal vocal fold space may also combine with the vascular trauma to create a mass lesion, resulting in marked dysphonia.[13] A varix may cause an asymmetry in the amplitude of vibration and the mucosal wave, as seen stroboscopically. The effects on voice vary, depending on the extent and length of time since onset. A varix in the nonprofessional voice is usually not cause for concern. Nonetheless, even this slight disruption in normal vocal fold function may be significant for those who depend on their voices professionally.

Although a vocal fold hemorrhage can occur in anyone, Sataloff[18] suggested that it appears to be common among premenstrual women using aspirin products. The treatment of choice is strict voice rest and conservation, which, in most cases, results in spontaneous resolution of the hematoma. Without care, the treatment may yield a worse result than the original problem. Other treatment for these vascular lesions may include a rapid course of steroids, or, in the case of an unresolved varix, microexcision of the lesion using careful laser vaporization. Voice therapy following resolution of these lesions is useful to restore voice quality, endurance, and range. Some patients also demonstrate an understandable fear in reentering their normal vocal activities. The voice pathologist's support and guidance can be instrumental in directing the patient to full voice use.

Laryngitis: Acute and Chronic

The term laryngitis is used to describe an inflammation of the vocal fold mucosa, causing mild to severe dysphonia with lowered pitch and intermittent phonation breaks. In severe cases, aphonia may result. The cause of acute laryngitis is unknown, but it is usually associated with upper respiratory viruses and bacterial infections.[4,19,21] The most effective treatments for acute laryngitis include external and internal hydration, antibiotics if prescribed, and rest. Occasionally, a cough suppressant may be prescribed to limit additional damage to the vocal folds. Because many patients will not feel pain with repeated coughing, they may unknowingly injure their voices further because they are not aware of the potential vocal fold damage from severe or prolonged coughing.

Children may experience an even more serious response to acute laryngitis involving a narrowing of the subglottic airway causing a sharp cough, hoarseness, and inspiratory stridor. Parents who have experienced these sudden and somewhat frightening symptoms know that this illness is croup (laryngotracheobronchitis).[20] Croup attacks last a variable period from 30 minutes to an hour or more; repeated attacks are common.

Chronic laryngitis (Figure 4-10) is a condition of long standing laryngeal mucosal inflammation, viscous mucus, and epithelial thickening that is unassociated with infection. Voice quality is mildly to severely dysphonic depending on the severity of the mucosal and epithelial change. Other symptoms include laryngeal fatigue and nonproductive coughing and throat clearing, but local pain is seldom present. The causes of chronic laryngitis include repeated episodes of acute laryngitis, vocal misuse and abuse, smoking, and poor laryngeal hydration. Air pollutants, airborne allergies, the use of dehydrating medications, gastroesophageal reflux disease, and repeated vomiting associated with bulimia have also been implicated as etiologic factors. The

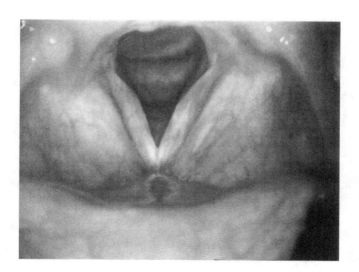

Figure 4-10. Chronic laryngitis. From Abitbol[96(p290)] (See also Plate 8)

typical treatment for chronic laryngitis is to identify and eliminate potential causative factors. Voice therapy is often useful in identifying specific etiologic correlates and devising compensatory strategies to modify these harmful elements.

Granuloma and Contact Ulcer

Granulomas (Figures 4-11 and 4-12) are highly vascular lesions that develop as the result of tissue irritation in the posterior larynx, usually on the vocal process of the arytenoid cartilage. These lesions often are associated with three predisposing conditions. First, granulomas may develop because of the presence of esophageal reflux,[22,23] which is thought to irritate the tissues of the posterior larynx and predispose this area to injury or ulceration (eg, contact ulcer). Second, many granulomas form following laryngeal intubation for surgery or for long-term airway ventilation. Finally, contact ulcers and granuloma have been associated with persistent voice misuse, especially the use of a pressed, low-pitched voice quality. Unless the lesion is large, the presence of a granuloma does not affect the membranous vibra-

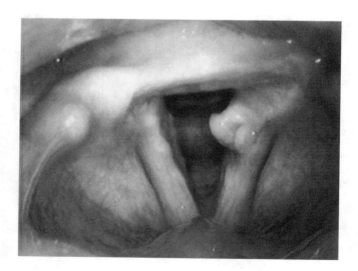

Figure 4-11. Unilateral contact granuloma. From Abitbol[96(p206)] (See also Plate 9)

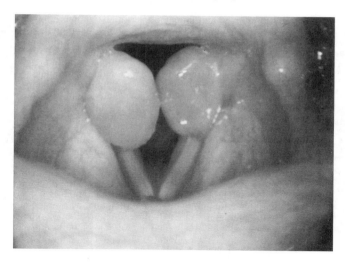

Figure 4-12. Bilateral contact granuloma. From Abitbol[96(p202)] (See also Plate 10)

tion of the vocal fold. Nonetheless, many patients complain of "throat" pain, restricted pitch ranges, and voice fatigue. Sataloff[21] suggested that reflux most likely contributes to the development of all forms of granulomas and that the first line of treatment should be an antireflux regimen. If medical treatment does not resolve the granuloma, then surgery may be considered. However, granulomas are known to be persistent lesions that often recur. Because the lesion is located in an area of constant movement and mechanical pressure during vocal fold adduction, the potential for chronic irritation and recurrence is high. Voice rehabilitative therapy must include a reduction of the medial compression of the vocal folds, and long-term compliance with antireflux behaviors.[21-23]

Congenital and Acquired Cysts

Cysts are fluid-filled, sessile growths (Figures 4-13 and 4-14) that can be present congenitally or acquired later in life, but there are no clear etiologic factors. These epithelial sacs may occur anywhere in the membranous portion of the true vocal fold, in the laryngeal ventricle, or in the ventricular folds. Vocal fold cysts

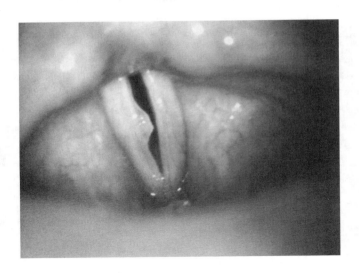

Figure 4-13. Vocal fold cyst (mucosal). From Abitbol[96(p180)] (See also Plate 11)

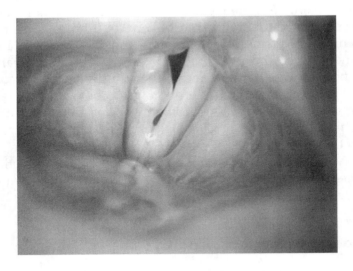

Figure 4-14. Vocal fold cyst (intracordal). From Abitbol[96(p176)] (See also Plate 12)

are embedded in the superficial layer of the lamina propria as the result of a blocked mucosal gland duct, with occasional extension into the intermediate and deep layers of the fold.[12] They appear as a whitish oval form, sometimes transparent below the epithelium. Although cysts usually occur unilaterally, bilateral cysts may be present. Because cysts often arise in the medial edge of a fold, contralateral tissue thickening may occur as a result of vibratory interference. Thus, a combination of tissue changes occurs because of the presence of a primary (cyst) and secondary (contralateral) irritation. These tissue changes may give the erroneous appearance of bilateral lesions, so that a unilateral vocal fold cyst may be easily misdiagnosed as bilateral vocal fold nodules. Cysts create a stiff adynamic segment over the lesion site that is visible during stroboscopic imaging. Stroboscopic observation of vocal fold vibration often is helpful to detect the increase in mass and stiffness of the vocal fold cover to differentiate cysts from nodules.[15]

As with other mass lesions, cyst size and severity will influence the extent of voice quality changes, from mild to moderate dysphonias to near aphonia in the case of large cysts. Because of the predominant stiffness characteristics posed by these lesions, even a small cyst may have a significant negative effect on the singing voice. Cysts do not respond to behavioral voice therapy, and the definitive treatment is surgical excision, usually from a superior and lateral approach to avoid scarring of the medial edge of the vocal fold.[24,25] Postoperative rehabilitative voice therapy may also aid in recovery.

Papilloma

Papillomas (Figure 4-15) are wartlike lesions that develop in the epithelium and invade deeper into the lamina propria and vocalis muscle. These lesions have a cellular composition of stratified squamous epithelium with connective tissue cores. Papillomas are persistent tumors thought to be caused by viruses, although no clear etiology has been established. They tend not to be transmitted between family members, nor has any genetic pattern been identified. Papillomas are usually found equally in both genders of children,[26-30] usually appearing

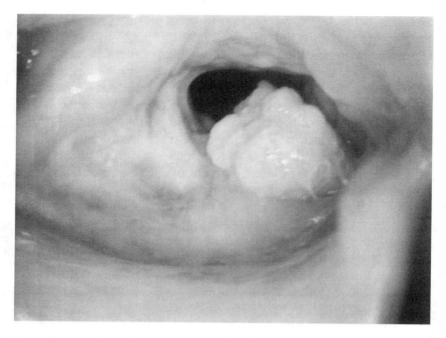

Figure 4-15. Papilloma. From Abitbol[96(p211)] (See also Plate 13)

between the ages of 2 and 4 years. Less frequently, the disorder can begin in adult years, and the incidence of adult onset is increasing. In children, the development of papilloma usually decreases with age, and often papillomas may disappear altogether during puberty.

The lesions affect the mass and stiffness of the cover, transition, and body of the vocal fold, resulting in severe dysphonia.[14] Because of the diffuse locations and rapid spread of the papilloma, medical treatments are aggressive, including interferon therapy and laser excision. Multiple laser surgeries are often required to control these tumors, and these repeat procedures can create vocal fold scarring, thus producing a secondary voice disorder. Most worrisome, however, is the fact that papillomas are known to spread within the upper airway, involving the larynx, trachea, and bronchus, potentially leading to compromised respiration and occasionally death. Because of the diffuse locations of these growths and the speed at which they tend to proliferate, tracheostomy is sometimes required to guarantee the patient a functional airway. Some risk of spread to the tracheostomy area has also been reported, however.[31]

The role of voice therapy in treatment of papilloma is twofold. There is some evidence that papilloma spread and severity may be reduced in patients who avoid hyperfunctional voice use and reduce excessive medial compression of the vocal folds.[31] Second, treatment may be required to assist patients in recovering appropriate or optimal voice quality postsurgery, especially when vocal folds are scarred by multiple procedures. The resulting voice quality may range from mild dysphonia to complete aphonia, depending on the extent of the disease and the aggressiveness of the required treatment(s).

Congenital and Acquired Webs

Webs of the vocal folds occur when there is a tissue bridge between the two vocal folds at the anterior commissure. Congenital webs (Figure 4-16) arise when the vocal folds fail to

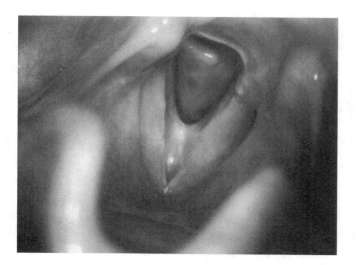

Figure 4-16. Anterior congenital web. From Abitbol[96(p376)] (See also Plate 14)

separate during the 10th week of embryonic development. Webbing may occur anywhere from the anterior to the posterior glottis. If the web is complete at birth, airway compromise is a threat. More commonly, webbing of the anterior glottis causes various degrees of dyspnea and stridor, depending on the extent of the web.[19,20,26,28,31] Phonosurgery is conducted to separate the web, using a keel to maintain separation of the raw edges of the folds and to avoid reformation of the web caused by postoperative scarring. The keel is removed after several weeks. During the healing period, the airway is maintained via a tracheostomy. Voice therapy to encourage proper development of voice pitch and quality may have a role in postoperative rehabilitation.

The voice qualities of children with congenital webs will range from normal voice to a severe dysphonia, again depending on the length and thickness of the web. In some cases, virtually no effects are noted in either breathing or voice quality. Occasionally, a congenital web may go undetected in males until puberty, when the vocal pitch fails to lower because of the reduced vibratory length of the folds.

Other small acquired webs (Figure 4-17) may develop in the anterior commissure in the postoperative period following vocal

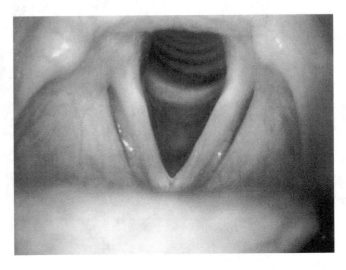

Figure 4-17. Anterior microweb. From Abitbol[96(p372)]

fold surgeries that involve the anterior membranous portion of the folds or following vocal trauma. These microwebs, also called synechias, occur when irritation of the anterior commissure reheals as a small fibrotic web. The effect of this microweb on voice quality can be variable, and surgical management is occasionally warranted, especially in elite performers.[32]

Sulcus Vocalis

A vocal fold sulcus (Figure 4-18) is a ridge or furrow that runs the entire length of the medial surface of the membranous portion of the vocal fold. The sulcus involves the superficial layer of the lamina propria, causing the vocal fold edge to appear bowed and resulting in a characteristic spindle-shaped gap. Sulci usually occur bilaterally, although a unilateral sulcus can occur. When a sulcus is present, the stiffness of the vibrating cover is significantly increased. The deeper structures of the vocal fold are not involved.[12,32,33]

There is no clear etiology for sulcus vocalis. One proposed theory is that vocal fold sulci develop following abnormal

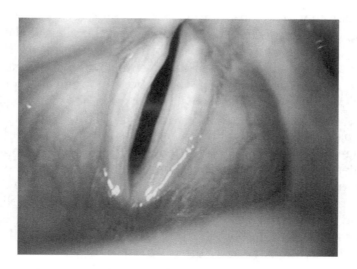

Figure 4-18. Sulcus vocalis. From Abitbol[96(p390)] (See also Plate 15)

embryologic maturation of the vocal fold cover, resulting in a furrowed appearance of the membranous vocal fold edge. Apparent acquired onset of sulcus vocalis is also possible, especially as a result of laser surgery, aging changes, and vocal fold paralysis.[12,32,33] Sulcus vocalis can be difficult to identify reliably because the furrow is often overlooked without stroboscopic imaging. Even with the advantage of stroboscopy, the sulcus may be missed because of a loosely tethered overlying flap of mucous membrane that obscures the view of a midline furrow.

Voice quality with the presence of a vocal fold sulcus may be mild to severely dysphonic depending on the stiffness of the fold and the size of the glottal gap resulting from the sulcus. Surgeons have attempted various techniques to remove the sulcus with mixed results.[34] Direct voice therapy focused on increased vocal efficiency without excessive strain has yielded voice improvement for some patients, but no characteristic treatment of choice has emerged for this pathology.

Presbylaryngeus

Presbylaryngeus means aging voice and is thought to be a voice disorder that develops during normal processes of laryngeal aging, including decreased respiratory efficiency, loss of elasticity of the vocal fold mucosa, and possibly deterioration of the tone of the vocal fold body. Also, ossification of the hyaline laryngeal cartilages may contribute to slight deviations in range and speed of intrinsic laryngeal adjustments. The perceptual effect of these aging changes is decreased loudness, pitch instability, and decreased voice quality. Presbylaryngeus appears to begin after the age of 65 and may be forestalled in individuals who are in excellent physical condition[35] or speakers who have professional voice training and have remained active vocal users. The classic appearance of the vocal folds in presbylaryngeus is a slightly bowed glottal gap during vibration, presumably because of loss of vocal fold bulk in both body and cover.[36] Voice rehabilitative therapy may improve voice quality dramatically in patients with presbylaryngeus unassociated with other medical problems.

Epithelial Hyperplasia: Leukoplakia and Hyperkeratosis

Epithelial hyperplasia is a general term that describes abnormal mucosal changes in the vocal folds. These changes usually occur in response to combinations of hyperfunctional voice use and chemical irritants, especially alcohol and tobacco use. Two vocal fold pathologies seen in adults, typically classified as precancerous lesions, are leukoplakia and hyperkeratosis. These lesions appear as hyperplastic and irregular thickening of the epithelium and may enter and involve the superficial layer of the lamina propria of the vocal fold. Lesions that invade the intermediate and deep layers of the lamina propria often signal early carcinoma.[14] The lesions are usually bilateral but can occur unilaterally. They increase the mass and stiffness of the cover of the fold while leaving the transition and the body unaffected.

Leukoplakia (Figure 4-19) is a prediagnostic term that means "white plaque" and describes the appearance of a thick white substance that covers the vocal folds in diffuse patches,

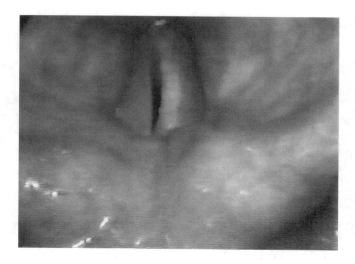

Figure 4-19. Leukoplakia (See also Plate 16).

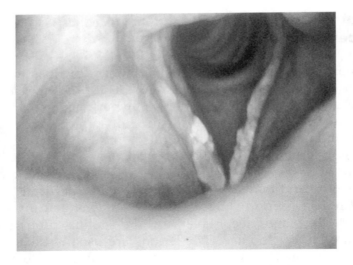

Figure 4-20. Hyperkeratosis. From Abitbol[96(p296)] (See also Plate 17)

usually on the superior surface of the vocal fold as opposed to midline margins. The pathology of leukoplakia is variable and may include both benign and malignant lesions. Hyperkeratosis (Figure 4-20) is a layered buildup of keratinized cell tissue and is distinctive for its leaflike appearance and consists of a horny overgrowth of irregular margins on the vocal folds.[12]

Both of these lesions are treated as cautionary signs for possible future malignancy. Patients are instructed to avoid future exposure to tobacco smoke, chemical inhalants, and other irritants.[37] Usually, phonosurgery will be conducted to confirm the diagnosis with a small biopsy and to remove the hyperplasia from the vocal fold mucosa. Voice therapy often is used to ensure that voice conservation strategies and vocal hygiene are in place and to assist in recovery of voice quality and modification of the behaviors that contributed to the causes.

Epithelial Dysplasia: Carcinoma

Cancer of the larynx (Figure 4-21) is potentially the most devastating of all laryngeal pathologies because of the life threatening implications of the disease and the potentially devastating effect

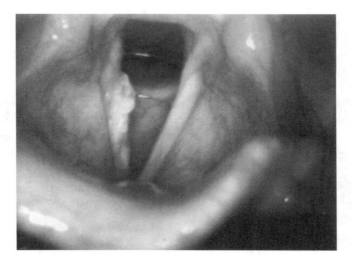

Figure 4-21. Carcinoma. From Abitbol[96(p310)]
(See also Plate 18)

on vocal communication if a total laryngectomy must be performed to remove the malignancy. The most common symptom of this pathology is persistent hoarseness. Rarely, sensations of laryngeal pain or referred pain to the ear may be present in later stages in the development of the disease. In advanced disease, the extent of the tumor may create airway compromise, swallowing problems, or both.

Most laryngeal carcinomas are of the squamous cell type and originate from the epithelium. If the lesion develops further, it will invade the deeper layers of the vocal fold including the vocalis muscle, which will affect the mass and stiffness of all affected mechanical layers.[12] Vocal symptoms will vary from a very mild to severe dysphonia depending on the location and the extent of the tumor.

Laryngeal carcinoma is thought to be caused by chronic irritation of the laryngeal epithelium and mucosa by such agents as tobacco smoke and alcohol, but it rarely may have other etiologies. Carcinoma can also occur in other sites of the larynx external to the true vocal folds. Whenever a suspicious lesion is identified in the laryngeal area, a surgical biopsy is conducted to excise a tissue sample for histopathological analysis and a definitive diagnosis. Once the presence of malignancy is confirmed, treatment options include radiation therapy or surgical excision, chemotherapy, or a combination approach.

Increasingly, head and neck surgeons are assessing tumor size and if possible, using laryngeal preservation surgeries for appropriate candidates,[38,39] so that the tumor can be excised without sacrificing one or both vocal folds. Laryngeal preservation allows a continued primary vibratory source of phonation from the remaining or reconstructed sites. Regardless of the management approach, the voice pathologist plays an important role in preparing the patient and the family for the consequences of the various forms of surgery and in the subsequent delivery of appropriate laryngeal or alaryngeal voice rehabilitation (see Chapter 9).

Neurogenic Voice Disorders

Neurogenic voice pathologies are those voice disorders directly caused by an interruption of the nervous innervation supplied to the larynx, including both central and peripheral insults. Some of these disorders are confined to voice and laryngeal manifestations (eg, vocal fold paralysis), whereas others may reflect a larger deterioration of many motor control systems, including broader impairment of respiration, resonance, swallowing, and other functions beyond the head and neck (eg, progressive neurogenic disease).

Recurrent Laryngeal Nerve Paralysis: Unilateral and Bilateral

Vocal fold paralysis is the most common neurogenic voice disorder. Vocal fold paralysis may be bilateral or unilateral and is typically caused by peripheral involvement of the recurrent laryngeal nerve and less commonly of the superior laryngeal nerve. More proximal involvement of the vagus (cranial nerve X) would affect the muscles supplied by both the recurrent and superior laryngeal nerves. The location of the lesion along the nerve pathway will determine the type of paralysis, and the resultant voice quality. There are many possible etiologies of vocal fold paralysis including surgical trauma, cardiovascular disease, neurological diseases, and accidental trauma. Historically, estimates of idiopathic vocal fold paralysis were approximately 30% to 35%.[40] More recently, Kelchner et al examined records for 117 patients with unilateral adductor paralysis and identified a 16.3% incidence of idiopathic onset, which is lower than historic estimates.[41] The authors speculated that improved diagnostic techniques (eg, imaging studies) may account for the smaller number of patients for whom onset appeared truly "idiopathic." In cases of idiopathic onset of paralysis, patients frequently report that hoarseness began following a viral infection.

Patients with unilateral vocal fold paralysis (Figures 4-22 and 4-23) present with varied vocal symptoms, ranging from mild to severe dysphonia. The characteristic perceptual symptoms of paralysis are breathiness, low intensity, low pitch, and intermittent diplophonia. These vocal impairments result from irregular and incomplete valving of the pulmonary airstream

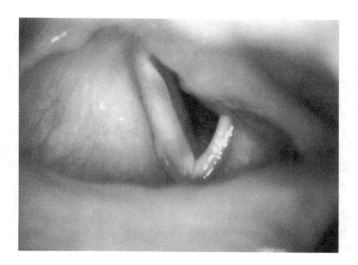

Figure 4-22. Unilateral left vocal fold paralysis (abduction). From Abitbol[96(p344)] (See also Plate 19)

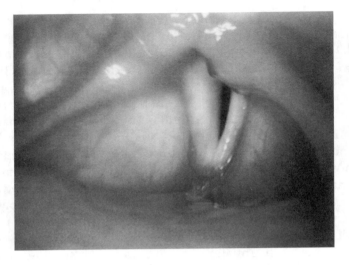

Figure 4-23. Unilateral left vocal fold paralysis (adduction). From Abitbol[96(p344)] (See also Plate 20)

through the glottis during the production of sound. Two physical dimensions account for this loss of vocal power and quality:

1. inadequate closure of the vocal folds at midline, as the paralyzed vocal fold remains lateral to the midline and cannot meet its contralateral fold, and
2. loss of vocal fold body and tonicity, resulting in bowing, flaccidity, and weakness of the paralyzed fold.

Both factors contribute to the asymmetric, aperiodic, and incomplete vibratory closure during phonation seen in patients with unilateral vocal fold paralysis. Because the recurrent laryngeal nerve serves both adductor and abductor functions of the vocal folds, in either unilateral or bilateral paralysis the location of the paralyzed fold has important implications for the nature and severity of the associated voice impairment.

The most serious form of vocal fold paralysis is a bilateral impairment. When vocal folds are paralyzed in the adducted position (at midline), they cannot open (abduct) to create sufficient airway for respiration. This critical condition is called **bilateral abductor paralysis** and requires that an adequate airway be established surgically, often through a tracheostomy. Surgical manipulation of one arytenoid cartilage will also create sufficient airway by either removing the arytenoid entirely or suturing it laterally.[40] With these arytenoid procedures, care must be taken to protect the airway to prevent possible aspiration. If an arytenoid lateralization is performed, voice quality will be weakened considerably.

When bilateral paralysis occurs with vocal folds positioned laterally in an abducted paramedian position, ventilation is no longer a concern, but airway protection becomes a much larger threat because of failure of the vocal folds to close to avoid aspiration. This condition is termed **bilateral adductor paralysis**, and in this configuration, neither voice production nor airway protection can be achieved satisfactorily. Patients with this form of paralysis often require gastrostomy tube feedings because of insufficient airway protection. They may also need augmentative communication aids to compensate for the complete aphonia. Both speech amplifiers and electrolarynx devices have been used to augment the "whispered" voice. Six to nine months following the onset, contracture and fibrosis of the folds may occur, causing the folds to be drawn closer to the midline and permitting a harsh breathy phonation. This development also improves airway protection during swallowing. A new problem of a limited airway may develop, however.

When unilateral paralysis occurs with the vocal fold in the midline position (but failing to abduct) mild airway and voice disturbances result, as compared to the other scenarios described here. In **unilateral abductor paralysis**, the paralyzed fold remains at the midline, but the contralateral fold abducts and adducts normally, allowing both airway protection and quasi-normal speech and voice production. This positioning of the paralyzed fold will reduce the size of the airway, and during strenuous activity, some inspiratory stridor may be evident. Overall, this paralysis does not severely compromise the patient's respiratory status. Voice quality for contextual speech will remain near normal; however, the patient may experience difficulty in building the necessary subglottic pressure for increased vocal loudness because of the laxness of the paralyzed fold.

Unilateral adductor paralysis is the most common type of vocal fold paralysis, with the paralyzed fold resting in an abducted or paramedian position whereas the contralateral fold adducts and abducts normally. As might be expected, the position and vertical level of the paralyzed fold and the size of the resulting glottal gap determine the effect of the paralysis on phonation. Voice quality is usually characterized by breathiness and diplophonia. The ability to build subglottic air pressure is also impaired resulting in decreased vocal intensity and the inability to be heard in even low levels of background noise.[42] Patients with this pathology often complain of physical fatigue resulting from the increased effort to produce voice and the breathlessness associated with phonation. Treatment approaches for unilateral adductor paralysis include a large range of behavioral, surgical, and combination approaches, all of which are described in Chapter 7.

Superior Laryngeal Nerve Paralysis: External Branches

Paralysis of the superior laryngeal nerves occurs much less frequently than does paralysis of the recurrent laryngeal nerves, possibly because of their much shorter course through the body. Thyroid disease and thyroid surgeries may create temporary or permanent paralysis of the superior laryngeal nerve. Unlike recurrent laryngeal nerve paralysis, the diagnosis of superior laryngeal nerve paralysis may not be readily observable and is often difficult to ascertain. Bilateral paralysis of the cricothyroid muscles is rare and often must be confirmed through the use of EMG studies. If paralysis should occur, the vocal folds will lack their normal tone and will not lengthen sufficiently during attempts at increased pitch production. Voice quality is limited in frequency and intensity range and stability.[43]

Unilateral superior laryngeal nerve paralysis may result in an oblique positioning or an overlap of the folds because of the unequal rocking of the cricothyroid joint. The overlap creates a gap between the folds that directly limits the midline closure pattern during vocal fold vibration and further decreases the ability to build subglottic air pressure, thus limiting vocal intensity. Often these voice disturbances are not noticeable during connected speech production, but the laxness of the affected fold creates an imbalance that reduces the speaker's ability to increase and control pitch. Most patients with unilateral paralysis of the superior laryngeal nerve complain of vocal fatigue and the inability to sing.[43] Although there is no medical treatment for superior laryngeal nerve paralysis, voice therapy may be utilized for educational and voice conservation purposes.

Spasmodic Dysphonia: Adductor and Abductor Types

Spasmodic dysphonia remains a curious and unresolved voice disorder because of its uncertain etiology and treatment potential. Spasmodic dysphonia is a descriptive term for a family of symptoms, all of which include some form of strained, strangled, and effortful voice production. The cause of this disorder has been debated for many years. Although early descriptions linked the disorder to a psychoneurosis,[44-46] more recent evidence has demonstrated a neurologic origin.[47-49] Dedo et al[50] reported information from 12 spasmodic dysphonia patients who underwent examination by a neurologist. Of these patients, 6 showed signs of neurologic disturbances including postural tremor, blepharospasm, idiopathic torsion dystonia, and buccolingual dyskenesia. Blitzer and Brin[49] offered strong evidence that spasmodic dysphonia should be considered a focal dystonia specific to the larynx and similar to other dystonias such as blepharospasm and torticollis. Theories abound, but neither definitive etiology nor structural defect has been identified.

The most recent evidence about spasmodic dysphonia (SD) suggests that it is a focal dystonia of the central motor system, extrapyramidal in origin, presumably caused by a supranuclear lesion locus in proximity of the basal ganglia. Comparative examination of signs and symptoms of SD with the dysarthrias and brain imaging studies[47] and brainstem conduction studies[48] support this theory. As with other focal dystonias, SD is characterized by abnormal involuntary movements that are action-induced and task specific. Thus, SD affects the movement patterns of the larynx during voicing, resulting in abnormal and involuntary co-contraction of the vocalis muscle complex, despite normal laryngeal and vocal fold structure.

There are two principle types of spasmodic dysphonia: adductor type and abductor type. Adductor spasmodic dysphonia is the more common and results in a severely hyperfunctional voice, including a "strained-strangled" quality, multiple pitch or voice breaks and occasional voicing "blocks" of tension or effort that interrupt the continuity of phonation. Struggle is often a salient feature of voice onset patterns. The laryngeal behavior is characterized by an intermittent, tight adduction of the vocal folds creating a strained, forced voicing behavior. When examined through indirect laryngoscopy, the vocal folds appear normal in structure and function. Intermittent periods of normal phonation may occur during speech production, during both laughter and angry outbursts of speech, and while singing. Some patients are able to reduce the frequency and severity of the spasms when talking at a pitch level that is slightly higher than normal. The majority of patients with adductor spasmodic dysphonia find it difficult, if not impossible, to shout. Many patients with adductor type spasmodic dysphonia complain of physical fatigue, tightness of the neck, back, and shoulder muscles and shortness of breath caused by their efforts to phonate through the closed glottis. The severity of the symptoms of adductor spasmodic dysphonia varies within and among individuals. Some patients experience only a mild interruption in normal phonation, whereas others may be rendered voiceless by the severity of the spasms. In the more severe cases, patients may compensate by whispering or phonating on inspired air. Secondary behaviors similar to those observed in stutterers, such as head jerking, eye blinking, and vocalized starters, may also develop.[51]

Abductor spasmodic dysphonia is a virtual "mirror image" of the adductor type. Phonation is interrupted by a sudden, involuntary period of aphonia, which is accompanied by a burst of air, as the vocal folds spasm in the abducted position. The voice is characterized by involuntary breaks and intermittent aphonia, with uncontrolled prolonged bursts of breathy phonation. Voice onset may appear normal, and then loss of voice ensues with continued speaking. The vocal fold spasms appear to occur primarily during the production of unvoiced consonants[1] and can occur during all positions within words, on whole words, and on several words in succession. Patients often report that their voices improve when they are angry, when they increase their intensity, or when they alter their pitch. Voice quality worsens when they are anxious or fatigued.

For both types of SD, these speech-related symptoms may coexist with apparently undisrupted nonspeech laryngeal maneuvers, including singing, laughing, coughing, throat clearing, and humming. Symptoms may be exacerbated with psychosocial stress or increased speech demands but persist regardless of the patient's emotional state.[1] The incidence of spasmodic dysphonia is unknown, but is thought to be relatively low. The disorder is said to occur equally in men and women with the most common onset in middle age. Rarely, symptoms of spasmodic dysphonia can occur in adolescence. Some patients experience a rapid onset associated with the occurrence of a traumatic event. Others report a more gradual onset following hoarseness associated with an upper respiratory infection. Still others appear to present with an idiopathic spasmodic dysphonia. The severity of the vocal symptoms appears to peak within the first year following the onset of the disorder.

Many patients with spasmodic dysphonia have experienced long and discouraging searches first for a diagnosis of the disorder and then for a treatment to cure or reduce the symptoms. To this end, patients may have seen several otolaryngologists, neurologists, psychologists, and speech pathologists. They may have received voice therapy, psychotherapy, psychological counseling, stress reduction interventions, drug therapies, EMG and thermal biofeedback, relaxation training, acupuncture, hypnosis, and faith healing. Unfortunately, none of these approaches has proved to be consistently effective in relieving the vocal symptoms. In the past two decades, a specialized form of chemodenervation has been used with good success to treat spasmodic dysphonia. Percutaneous injections of botulinum toxin (BOTOX) into the intrinsic laryngeal muscles have provided temporary reprieve from symptoms of spasmodic dysphonia. A full discussion of this treatment approach is presented in Chapter 7.

Because spasmodic dysphonia represents a complex of symptoms rather than a specific diagnosis, the disorder can be difficult to identify empirically.[52] Perceptual attributes of SD may be similar to those of other organic, functional, or psychogenic voice disorders. The history of onset does not provide differential clarification, as both SD and functional or conversion voice disorders may arise following excessive, prolonged, or extreme vocal demands or following a period of unusual stress, trauma, or emotional upset. Thus, decisions about the presence and management of SD patients require careful examination of the individual's speech and voice symptoms across time, attending to the consistency, severity, and resistance to change following traditional treatment methods.

Organic (Essential) Vocal Tremor

Essential tremor is a central nervous system disorder that is characterized by rhythmic tremors (4 to 7 cycles/second) of various body parts including the larynx. Tremor may involve the head, arms, neck, tongue, palate, face, and larynx either in isolation or in combinations. In some patients, the tremor may only be observed when the affected body part is being used (intentional tremor), whereas other patients will exhibit the tremor behavior even at rest. The onset of essential tremor is usually gradual and begins most commonly in the fifth or sixth decade of life. The disorder occurs most frequently in males, is often hereditary, and is often accompanied by other neurological signs.[53-55]

Laryngeal tremor is most noticeable during prolonged vowels because the rhythm of the tremor is easily discerned. Connected speech may be negatively affected as well. In some cases the tremor is so severe that it causes voice stoppages similar to those of spasmodic dysphonia. Indeed, these two disorders, which may coexist, are often mistaken for one another. The differential voice diagnosis can be made during sustained vowel trials. Under these conditions, spasmodic dysphonia will usually display normal sustained phonation (in severe cases, brief intermittent strain-strangled spasms may break through), whereas organic vocal tremor will display the characteristic rhythmic modulations during phonation.

The principle perceptual features of organic tremor are regular wavering of pitch and intensity, measurable during sustained pitch productions at a range from 4 to 7 Hertz. In severe forms, voice breaks may be noticeable. In addition to the persistent perceptual features, the laryngeal tremor is visible during sustained phonation during the laryngeal examination. This disorder is exclusive of tremor in other neurologic processes, such as Parkinson and cerebellar disease. There is no successful treatment for essential vocal tremor. Patients with coexisting SD and essential vocal tremor who receive BOTOX commonly report relief from the focal dystonia, without any change in tremor activity.

Other Neurologic Disorders

Neurologic disorders that affect the larynx do not occur in isolation and, as such, voice impairments will accompany other disordered motor speech functions, including respiration, articulation, resonance, and prosody. Indeed, many of the hallmark diagnostic signs and symptoms are based on clusters of perceptual attributes and deficits of the speech pattern. The range and type of neurologic voice problems are as varied as the underlying dysarthrias, and detailed summaries of the associated vocal characteristics have been compiled.[1,56-59] The classic audio-perceptual attributes of voice production in neurologic disease are often diagnostic in combination with findings from the neurologic examination.

Therapy for neurologic disorders that affect voice production is compensatory and will not reverse the underlying neuropathy but may help maximize the patient's communicative skills. The range of laryngeal deficits that may present in association with neurologic disorders is broad and certainly encompasses both voice quality and supralaryngeal (articulation, resonance, and prosody) factors. These problems include vocal fold hypoadduction, hyperadduction, phonatory instability, and incoordination of both prosody and voice-voiceless contrasts. Thus, treatment may address both focal voicing behaviors (eg, increasing loudness, reducing strained quality) or global speech targets (increasing respiratory support, increasing intelligibility). Table 4-2 displays the voice characteristics associated with different types of dysarthria. Following the table is a description of voice characteristics typical of the more common neurologic disorders that are referred to the voice pathologist.

Myasthenia Gravis

Myasthenia gravis is a lower motor neuron impairment that is characterized by rapidly deteriorating voice quality and flaccid dysarthria caused by muscle weakness. Persons with myasthenia gravis may have symptoms confined to the larynx (myasthenia laryngis), but more commonly they experience broad-based

Table 4-2. Voice Deviations Associated With Dysarthrias

Type	Audio-Perceptual Characteristics	Examples
Flaccid	Vocal fold hypoadduction resulting in weak, breathy phonation; reduced loudness; diplophonia; hypernasality; and nasal emission	Myasthenia gravis
Spastic	Vocal fold hyperadduction resulting in low pitch; strained-strangled, effortful, and harsh phonation; slow speech rate	Dystonia
Ataxic	Irregular, random variations in pitch, loudness, prosody, and speech rate, including excess and equal stress	Cerebellar disorders
Hyperkinetic	Vocal dystonia; respiratory irregularities resulting in random and sudden changes in pitch and loudness, tremor, myoclonus, intermittent aphonia	Multiple sclerosis Huntington's chorea
Hypokinetic	Monopitch and loudness, hypernasal, imprecise articulation, weak phonation and limited vocal endurance; rapid speech rate	Parkinson disease
Mixed	Symptoms of both spastic and flaccid dysarthria characteristics	Amyotrophic lateral sclerosis

speech decline during prolonged speech tasks or concentrated repetitions. Voice characteristics include vocal weakness, breathiness, and limited pitch and loudness range.[1,56,57] These symptoms improve following rest. Medical treatment may help manage and reduce the symptoms of myasthenia gravis. The focus of voice therapy is to maintain and conserve voice efficiency, often through augmentative amplification.

Dystonia

Vocal dystonia will result in spastic dysarthria including a characteristic harsh and strained voice quality, slow speech rate, and intermittent aphonia. Spastic dysarthria is also present in speech and voice of patients following various types of upper motor neuron diseases, cerebrovascular accidents (CVA), and traumatic brain injury.[57] Depending on the prognosis for recovery or improvement, spastic dysarthria may spontaneously resolve or ultimately lead to continued speech and voice decline. The focus of voice therapy is to relieve excessive tension in the laryngeal musculature and foster relaxed and fluid phonation during speech.

Multiple Sclerosis

Multiple sclerosis is an example of hyperkinetic dysarthria affecting both speech and voice. This disorder is a progressive demyelinating disease that results in both sensory and motor impairments of the limbs, which can spread to include the vocal tract and other head and neck musculature. Speech characteristics, if affected, are characterized by effortful bursts of phonation and intermittent aphonia. Abnormal speech rate, altered prosody, and decreased articulatory precision may affect speech intelligibility in severe stages of the disease; dysphagia may be present.[57,60] Behavioral voice treatment for this and other degenerative diseases is usually palliative, with focus on preserving functional communication. In terminal stages, cognitive decline may preclude effective behavioral compensation.

Huntington's Chorea

Huntington's chorea is a slow, progressive neurologic disease characterized by upper motor neuron signs of dysarthria, including hyperkinetic, strained-strangled voice. Severe symptoms often include erratic bursts of phonation. In terminal stages, most patients are anarthric, and respiratory and swallowing difficulties are common.[1,56,57] Compensatory and maintenance voice therapy is useful to forestall effects of inevitable decline and to monitor changes in speech, respiration, and swallowing. Augmentative communication may be useful in later stages of the disease.

Parkinson Disease

Parkinson disease is an extrapyramidal disorder that affects both speech and voice production and represents a common form of hypokinetic dysarthria. Phonation is characterized by monopitch and monoloudness, with weak, breathy voice and occasional vocal tremor. Speech intelligibility may be reduced, especially in advanced stages of the disease. Diagnosis is made upon neurological examination, following exclusion of other neurologic processes, including laryngeal dystonia.[1,56,57,61] Medical treatments with some degree of success are available to patients with Parkinson. Recently, the use of the Lee Silverman Voice Therapy behavioral program has provided strong evidence of outcome success in improving the loudness and intelligibility of speech in patients with idiopathic Parkinson disease. The central targets of this program are loud productions of steady state phonation conducted in a rigorous exercise routine, including multiple trials daily. Despite the focus on respiration and phonatory loudness, treatment effects have generalized to increased articulatory strength, precision, and intelligibility, as well as improved vocal loudness and quality.[61]

Amyotrophic Lateral Sclerosis

Amyotrophic lateral sclerosis (ALS) is a degenerative neurological disorder with primary pathology of both upper and lower motoneurons, including spread to the motoneurons of the spinal cord, brainstem, and cortex. Symptoms of ALS represent the speech and voice characteristics of mixed dysarthria. Muscle weakness, fasciculation and atrophy provide evidence of lower motor neuron involvement, whereas spasticity, strain, and effortful speech signal the effects of upper motor neuron impairment. Dysarthria and dysphagia occur in persons with ALS during terminal stages of the disease. The dysarthria is described as a mixed spastic-flaccid type.[1,56,57,62-65] Features of spastic dysarthria include slow speech rate, strained-strangled voice, and reduced stress and prosody. Features of flaccid dysarthria include hoarse, breathy voice, consonant distortions, and short phrases. Hypernasality may be a feature of both spastic and flaccid dysarthria. The voice of patients with ALS has sometimes been described as "wet" or "gurgly" or having a tremor or flutter on vowel prolongation.[1] Individual variability is great, however, and longitudinal assessment may be most useful for reliable description of perceptual features.[62,64] Although voice therapy may address compensatory strategies, there is no successful medical or rehabilitative treatment identified for ALS.

Systemic Disease Influences on the Larynx and Voice

Focal or regional influences of the head, neck, upper back, and throat can influence laryngeal health, specifically vocal fold vibration during phonation. Musculoskeletal tension in the throat, temporomandibular joint problems, swallowing difficulties, blunt trauma to the neck, chin, or jaw are all examples of the possible local insults that may influence the laryngeal mechanism and subsequent voice quality. Furthermore, there is increasing evidence from both clinical and research settings that systemic or "whole body" influences may also affect the larynx and voice production.[19,20,66] Imunologic and neurologic disorders, infectious diseases, and pharmacologic agents are all examples of systemic processes that may alter voice production.

To understand the relationship between body systems and the larynx, some researchers have examined normal and pathologic fluctuations of systems and measured vocal function as a dependent variable. For example, Orlikoff[67,68] examined acoustic perturbations as a function of cardiac status, including heart-beat, and suggested that stability of systemic blood flow may influence fine measures of laryngeal control. Other researchers have used acoustic analysis to mark the varying periods within the female hormonal cycle.[69-71] Further studies addressing the relationship between hormonal levels and vocal function have supported the interpretation of a time-varying effect on voice performance based on fluctuations in hormone activity. This research supports a longstanding clinical impression among professional voice performers, notably singers, that range, quality, stability, and endurance of phonation can be affected by the hormonal cycle. Finally, an increasing number of clinical studies have provided evidence of the time-locked association between certain disease processes and effects on voice quality.

There are three basic treatment alternatives available for patients with medical pathologies affecting voice: medical (pharmacologic) therapy, phonosurgery, and voice rehabilitation. In many cases, the primary therapy will be medical, although some counsel in the area of voice rehabilitation and conservation will be appropriate as a second-order treatment. The voice pathologist plays a supportive role in this context by assisting in the correct diagnosis and prognosis for change based on the assessment of laryngeal anatomy, vocal fold vibratory pattern, vocal function measurement, and rehabilitative options for voice treatment. Collaboration between otolaryngologists and voice pathologists continues to expand through joint assessment of the laryngeal image and vocal function, efficacious cotreatment alternatives that include both phonosurgery and voice rehabilitation, as well as clinical delivery models that encourage a team approach to patients with voice disorders. More than ever, it is critical that the voice pathologist be aware of the medical pathologies in an otolaryngology patient population that affect the larynx and especially voice production.

Pharmaceutical Effects on Voice

The effects of medications on voice performance and vocal function have not been explored exhaustively. Martin[72] reviewed some general characteristics of medications, their predicted influence on the body, and possible effects on to the larynx. Four drug actions common in medications that treat organic vocal pathologies are listed below. These include drugs that influence

1. **airflow**, including **bronchodilators**, which expand the diameter of bronchioles in the lungs to increase the oxygen and carbon dioxide exchange during respiration. These medications are common for treatment of allergies, asthma, and other forms of upper respiratory compromise.
2. **fluid level in tissues**, especially **diuretics, corticosteroids** and **decongestants**, which use separate chemical actions to reduce edema of tissues because of local inflammation.[73]
3. **upper respiratory secretions** using agents that reduce secretions, such as **antihistamines, antitussives** (cough suppressants), and **antireflux** medications.
4. **vocal fold structure**, through long-term use of **hormonal therapies**, especially testosterone, which results in permanent deepening of the pitch of the voice.

Endocrine Influences

Growth Hormone

Because the endocrine glands secrete hormones that are responsible for body growth and development, certain endocrine disorders can alter or limit voice quality because of changes in vocal fold development. These processes may first become apparent at puberty, when anticipated changes in body growth and associated changes in voice are most prominent. This growth and development will accompany predicted maturation of the larynx and vocal folds, and generally, changes that create fluctuating voice stability during puberty will resolve without long-term disturbance.[74] In females, ongoing cyclic changes that fluctuate with puberty onset, pregnancy, menstrual cycle, and menopause may alter voice production during certain times. During menstruation, for example, the resulting edema may result in dysphonia, reduced pitch and loudness range, and loss of stability of phonation. In the postmenopausal years, female fundamental frequency and other structural changes in the vocal fold appear more prominent, affecting voice quality and endurance. In some women, and often in elite female vocal performers, variations in vocal range and stability correspond to changes in hormonal cycles, such as occur during premenstrual periods, pregnancy, and menopause. In theory, all of these cyclic changes have the potential to influence voice production throughout the lifespan.[18]

Thyroid Function

Thyroid disorders affect the entire chemical and emotional balance of the body, so medical, intellectual, and affective influences are all possible. Hyperthyroidism results from excessive secretions of the thyroid gland and is managed either through surgical excision or radioactive iodine treatment. Hypothyroidism, or reduced thyroid hormone production, may be treated medically using thyroid replacement therapy. Thyroid function also affects voice production, but the predicted vocal outcomes are not clear. Various physical signs and perceptual attributes have been associated with hypothyroidism, including hoarseness, low pitch, coarse, and gravelly vocal symptoms caused by thickened or edematous vocal folds and altered fluid content in the lamina propria.[1,19,20,75] Other patients with this diagnosis have reported a persistent, unexplained dry cough. Perceptual features of hyperthyroidism include slight vocal instabilities including "shaky" voice, breathy quality and reduced loudness. Because the voice disorder arises from a primary medical etiology, treatment is referred back to the appropriate medical specialist.

Sex Hormonal Imbalances

As a general rule, hormonal imbalances produce the greatest effect on vocal pitch, as seen with diagnoses of arrested or aberrant development of gender maturation and reproductive functions. Virilization is the abnormal secretion of androgenic hormones, resulting in male gender characteristics in females. The vocal effects are low pitch, hoarseness, and occasionally voice breaks.[18,19] Other specific hormone therapies, including estrogen replacement, androgens, testosterone, and oral contraceptives may alter voice quality. This sensitivity to hormonal changes is more common in females than it is in males.

Color Plates

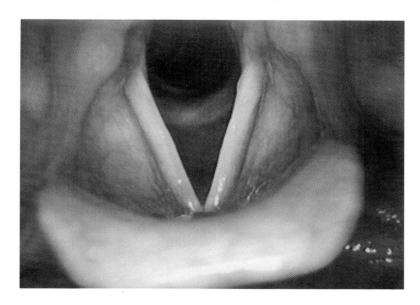

Plate 1. Normal vocal folds (abduction). From Abitbol (p. 83)

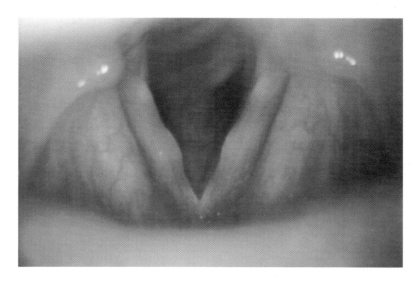

Plate 2. Vocal fold nodules (abduction). From Abitbol (p. 141)

Plates 1, 15, 17-21, and 24 are reprinted with permission from *Atlas of Laser Voice Surgery*, by J. Abitbol, 1995. San Diego, Calif: Singular Publishing Group. Page numbers in Plate legends refer to page numbers in source.

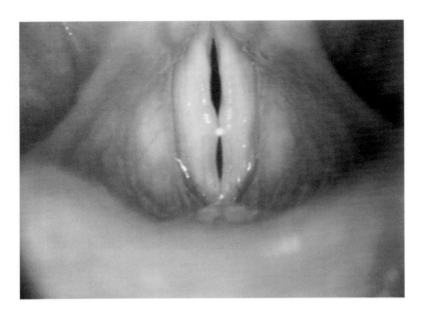

Plate 3. Vocal nodules (abduction). From Abitbol (p. 141)

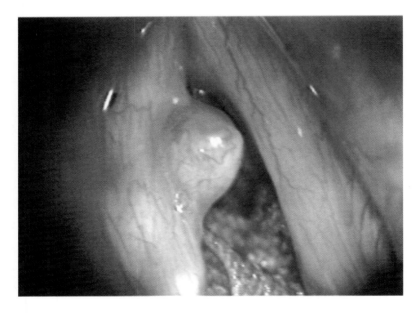

Plate 4. Sessile polyp. From Abitbol (p. 165)

Clinical Voice Pathology

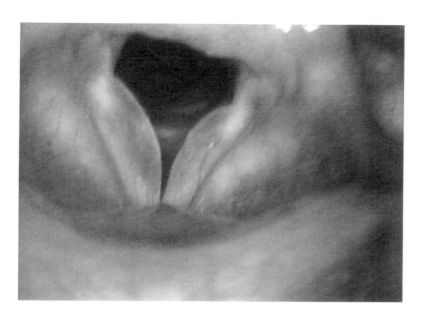

Plate 5. Reinke's edema (early). From Abitbol (p. 268)

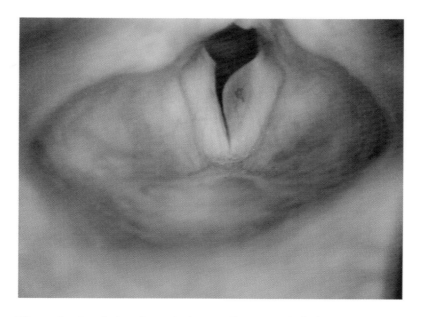

Plate 6. Reinke's edema (advanced). From Abitbol (p. 263)

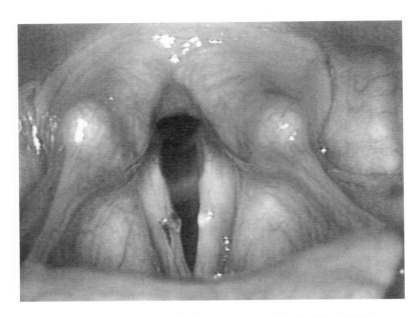

Plate 7. Vocal fold vascular lesions. From Abitbol (p. 228)

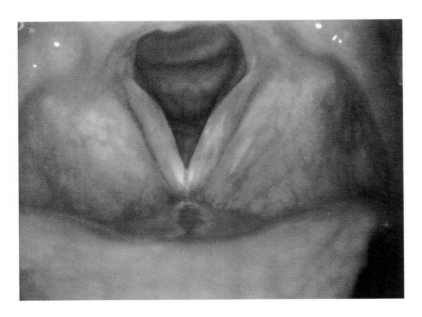

Plate 8. Chronic laryngitis. From Abitbol (p. 290)

Clinical Voice Pathology

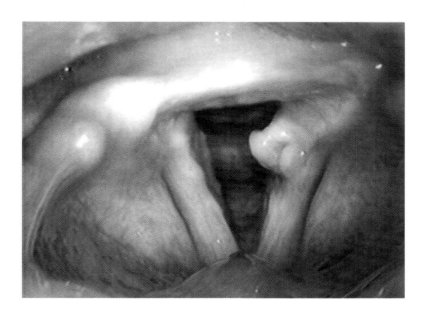

Plate 9. Unilateral contact granuloma. From Abitbol (p. 206)

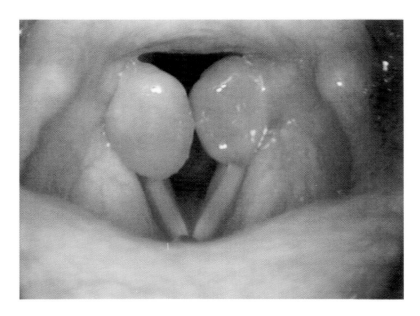

Plate 10. Bilateral contact granulomas. From Abitbol (p. 202)

Color Plates

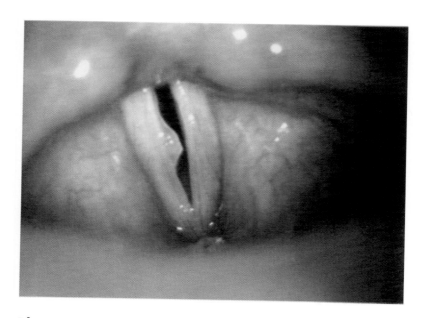

Plate 11. Vocal fold cyst (mucosal). From Abitbol (p. 180)

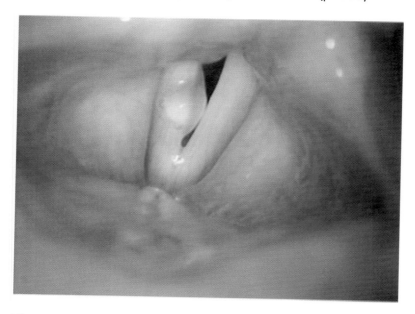

Plate 12. Vocal fold cyst (intracordal). From Abitbol (p. 176)

Clinical Voice Pathology

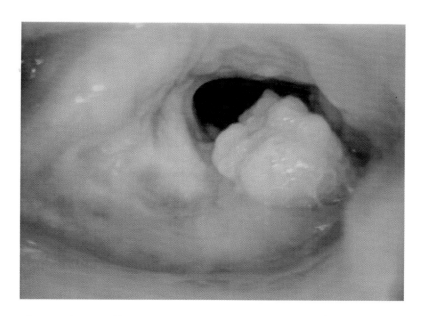

Plate 13. Papilloma. From Abitbol (p. 211)

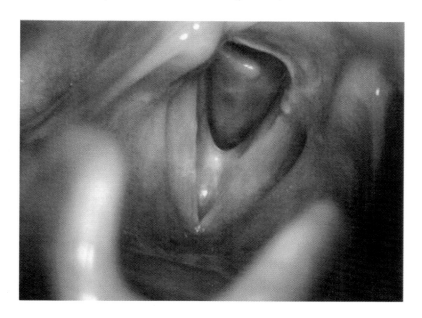

Plate 14. Anterior congenital web. From Abitbol (p. 376)

Color Plates

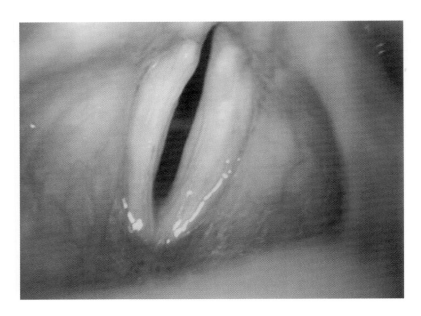

Plate 15. Sulcus vocalis. From Abitbol (p. 390)

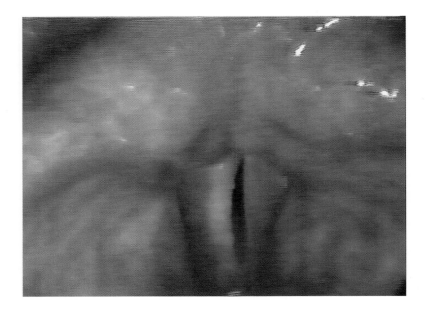

Plate 16. Leukoplakia.

Clinical Voice Pathology

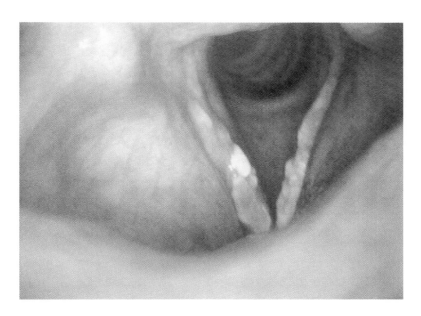

Plate 17. Hyperkeratosis. From Abitbol (p. 296)

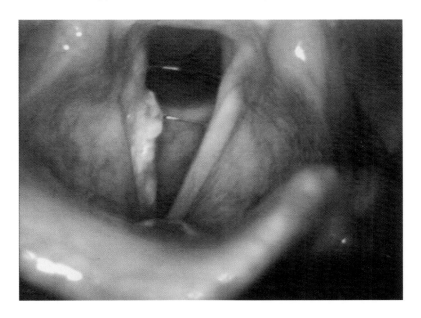

Plate 18. Carcinoma. From Abitbol (p. 310)

Color Plates

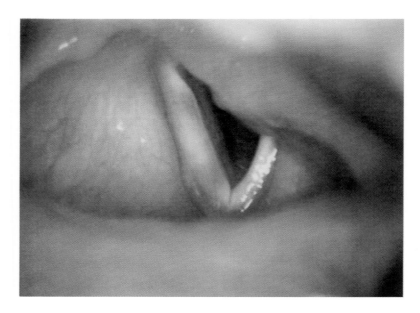

Plate 19. Unilateral left vocal fold paralysis (abduction). From Abitbol (p. 344)

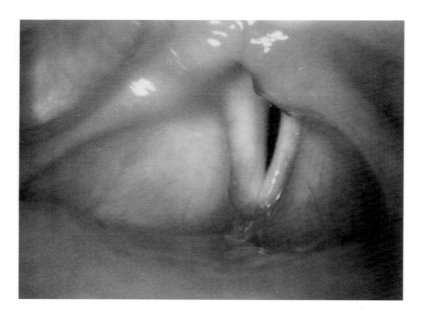

Plate 20. Unilateral left vocal fold paralysis (adduction). From Abitbol (p. 344)

Clinical Voice Pathology

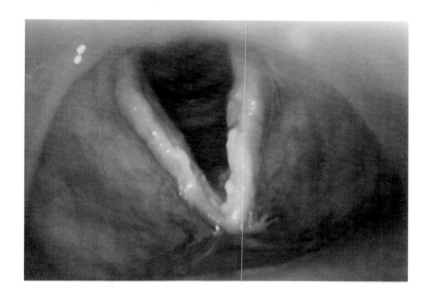

Plate 21. Fungal infection. From Abitbol (p. 292)

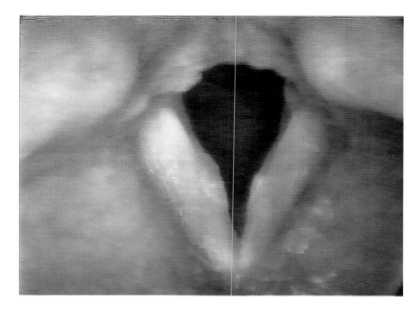

Plate 22. Reflux esophagitis.

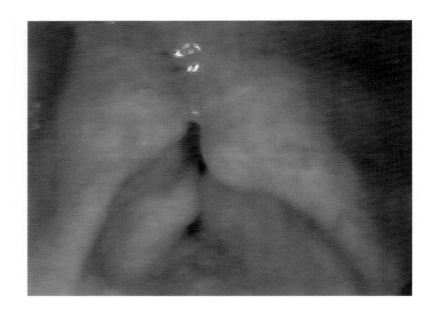

Plate 23. Ventricular phonation.

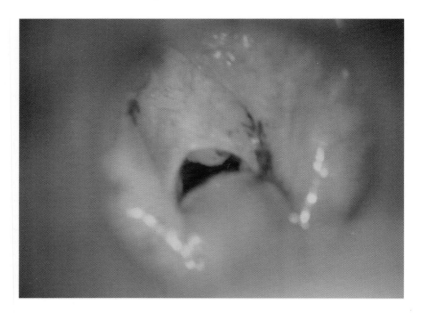

Plate 24. Laryngeal stenosis. From Abitbol (p. 367)

Clinical Voice Pathology

Behavioral voice therapy can be used to augment the "feminine" quality of voice and speech. Treatment with estrogen or other hormonal therapy may improve voice quality, but pitch changes are usually permanent.

Immunologic Disorders

Voice disorders seem to occur in persons with immunologic disease but without other obvious contributing etiologies (eg, vocal abuse, laryngeal pathology). Although there is little evidence about the potential effects of these immunologic disorders on laryngeal health and voice quality, clinicians who work in medical settings are familiar with the potential for voice change and deterioration in patients with lupus, Sjögren's disease, mixed connective tissue disease, and other autoimmune disorders. The changes in voice quality are not predictable, and certainly not every patient with these diagnoses will exhibit voice complaints. Most often, patients who are referred to clinic with these disorders describe throat pain during talking, symptoms of vocal fatigue, loss of voice quality, endurance, or range. Rheumatoid arthritis and allergies are presented here as representative examples of two common immunologic disorders that have been associated with voice problems.

Rheumatoid Arthritis

Rheumatoid arthritis is a chronic immunologic and inflammatory disorder that disrupts the normal structure and function of synovial joints, including the cricoarytenoid and cricothyroid joints of the larynx. When affected, laryngeal function for both respiration and voice production may be compromised by pain, swelling, and, in the most severe form, mechanical fixation of the joints. Inflammation of the vocal fold may be accompanied by a bright red appearance of the arytenoid cartilages during symptomatic periods. Medical treatments include antiinflammatory and corticosteroid drugs. Rarely, fixation of the arytenoid joint(s) creates an acute airway compromise and results in the need for tracheotomy or unilateral arytenoidectomy for airway preservation.[76-78]

Allergies

Allergies represent another group of immunologic disorders that can affect voice production because of the associated inflammation or irritation of the pharynx and nasal mucosa. Increased mucus production, nasal drainage or congestion, and edema of the respiratory mucosa will alter vocal tract resonance and may inhibit phonation if excessive secretions reach the level of the vocal folds.[79,80] It is common for patients who have allergies to experience symptoms of chronic cough, throat clearing, inflamed nasal and pharyngeal tissues, and other respiratory ailments that may contribute to voice disorders. Often, symptoms vary with the severity of the allergic response and may cycle with seasons, pollen counts, and specific exposures. Secondarily, the medications and treatments prescribed to treat allergies may also negatively influence voice production because of increased dehydration (antihistamines) and prolonged use of steroid inhalers, which has an uncertain effect on vocal folds.[80]

Infectious Diseases

Certain infectious diseases, whether viral, bacterial, or fungal in origin, can also create or aggravate voice problems because of chronic laryngitis and occasionally, granulomas. A large variety of infectious diseases provoke manifestations in the upper airway, including symptoms of chronic cough, irritation, edema, and eruptions of the mucous membranes of the larynx and pharynx. Some examples include pneumonia, sinusitis, and tuberculosis. The associated dysphonia generally resolves following antibacterial treatment of the microorganism.[81,82]

Candida

Some patients with infectious disease are prone to overgrowth of oral and pharyngeal candida, or yeast, and fungal laryngeal infections may arise (Figure 4-24). Because normal yeast is present in the larynx, pharynx, and trachea, this overgrowth can be particularly troublesome to treat, especially if the patient is immunocompromised due to other primary disease. Treatment is conducted using antifungal medications. In immunocompro-

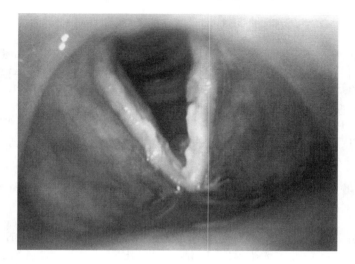

Figure 4-24. Fungal infection. From Abitbol[96(p292)] (See also Plate 21)

mised patients, a prolonged course (ie, several months) may be required for full therapeutic effect. Candida is also a common finding in patients with human immunodeficiency virus (HIV) who exhibit symptoms of hoarseness, dry mouth, and mild chronic laryngitis caused by a depressed immunologic system and repeated upper respiratory infections.[83]

Respiratory Diseases

Respiratory disease, including asthma, chronic obstructive pulmonary disease, and croup (acute laryngotracheobronchitis) all result in acute or chronic symptoms of dyspnea, with audible inhalatory stridor and expiratory wheeze. If associated laryngeal edema is excessive, the pediatric airway may be threatened because of its smaller dimension. Although voice quality is clearly a secondary concern relative to ventilatory needs and airway preservation, any compromise of the respiratory power behind vocal fold vibration will have deleterious effects on phonation.[19,20,74,81] Treatment for these disorders usually includes bronchodilators and inhaled steroids, to suppress the symptoms of dyspnea and laryngeal edema, if present. As with other systemic disease, improvement in voice production is generally commensurate with overall return of respiratory function.

Gastroesophageal Reflux Disease (GERD)

Reflux esophagitis (Figure 4-25) may result in both dysphonia and throat pain, especially if the irritation of the laryngeal mucosa is so great that granuloma tissue or contact ulcers have erupted.[24] Usually, the effects of reflux esophagitis are confined to the posterior larynx and may be indicated clinically by erythema or hyperplasia of the interarytenoid rim of the glottis. Formal assessment can be conducted using a transnasal pH monitor to assess the rise of gastric acids in the esophagus over a 24-hour period.[84-86] Pharmaceutic management with over-the-counter or prescription antacids, coupled with a behavioral antireflux protocol, can generally bring symptoms under control. Recently, otolaryngologists have augmented the effects of antacids with aggressive medical treatment of GERD using other medications, including proton pump inhibitors and H2 blockers. Other behavioral aspects of an antireflux protocol may include recommendations for changes in diet, losing excess weight, eliminating caffeine, alcohol, and other substances that can aggravate or inhibit digestion, wearing loose clothing that does not bind the midriff, elevating the head of the bed at night, and avoiding unnecessary bending in activities such as bowling or gardening.

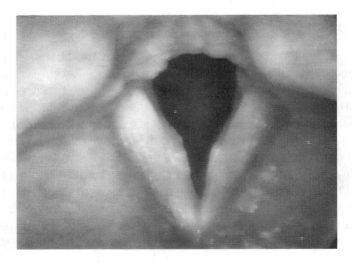

Figure 4-25. Reflux esophagitis (See also Plate 22).

Disorders of Voice Use

Pathologies associated with inappropriate voice maladaptations or patterns are another source of vocal pathology. Unlike organic laryngeal pathologies, disorders of voice use refer to dysphonia that occurs despite the presence of an essentially normal vocal fold cover and intact neurologic function. These pathologies include the various psychogenic voice disorders, as well as those associated with the functional misuse of the laryngeal musculature in voice production.

Muscle Tension Dysphonia

Morrison and Rammage[87,88] first described muscle tension dysphonia, and the diagnosis is characterized by variable symptoms of voice disruption accompanied by observable tension or stiffness of the neck, jaw, shoulders, and throat. Patients with muscle tension dysphonia often report periodic pain in the sites of the larynx, neck, and other areas. Also, the incidence of concomitant psychosocial stress or other interpersonal conflicts has been determined as a commonly associated feature of this disorder. Behavioral voice rehabilitative therapy is useful for relieving symptoms and restoring appropriate vocal technique in patients with this disorder.

Vocal Fatigue

Vocal fatigue is a frequent descriptor for a well-known set of symptoms, including deteriorated vocal quality, decreased endurance, loss of frequency and intensity control, and complaints of effortful, unstable, or ineffective voice production. Clinically, these symptoms are among the most common complaints from patients who are referred for unexplained voice disorders. Understanding vocal fatigue is complicated by its many signs and symptoms, as well as a lack of thorough understanding of the pathogenesis of the complaint. Theories about the existence of so-called muscular fatigue in the larynx have given rise to the term laryngeal myasthenia or myasthenia laryngis.[89,90] The terms are intended to reflect the sensation of tiredness that patients report following attempts to vocalize, although there is no experimental evidence to associate these valid clinical symptoms with either central or peripheral muscle fatigue. Other potential factors that may influence sensations of fatigue include strain of the nonmuscular laryngeal tissues (ligaments, joints, membranes), increased viscosity of the vocal fold cover caused by friction and shearing forces, loss of internal hydration and cooling in the laryngeal tissues, and loss of subglottal pressure because of respiratory fatigue.

Clinically, patients with complaints of vocal fatigue will exhibit vocal folds that appear normal under indirect laryngoscopy. Symptoms of the disorder include dryness in the mouth and throat; pain at the base of tongue, throat, and neck; sensations of "fullness" or a "lump" in the throat; shortness of breath; and effortful phonation. When observed stroboscopically, the folds often demonstrate an anterior glottal chink, a decrease in the amplitude of vibration, and a phase asymmetry.

We still do not fully understand the mechanism of laryngeal muscle fatigue, which underscores the need for better clinical definition of diagnostic indicators for this disorder. Regardless of the definition, the clinical signs and symptoms of vocal fatigue are well known to patients and clinicians alike. The treatment for symptoms of the disorder using physiologic voice therapy has proved promising and effective and is described in detail in Chapter 7.

Vocal Abuse and Misuse

These terms have long been subject to disagreement and dispute by voice professionals, and other labels have been proposed, including "phonotrauma" and "repetitive strain injury."[3] The essential components of vocal abuse and misuse are prolonged, effortful, and maladaptive vocal behaviors, usually based on excessively loud or aggressive voice production, sharp glottal attack (voice onset), inappropriate technique for voice or singing, and aggressive laryngeal vegetative maneuvers, including throat clearing, coughing, or grunting. Some forms of abuse and misuse rise from at-risk situations or environments, including the need to talk above loud ambient noise or to talk for long periods of time or unhealthy vocal demands placed on persons through external occupational demands. Vocal abuse and misuse often result from poor or ineffective training in vocal technique, including insufficient respiratory support, excessive laryngeal tension during phonation, and failure to achieve proper oral resonant focus. Across time, the aggregate effect of these poor vocal behaviors, whether produced knowingly or unknowingly, is traumatic injury to the vocal fold cover, sometimes to the extent that benign lesions will form.[1,89]

Ventricular Phonation (Plica Ventricularis)

During phonation, a great amount of supraglottic muscle tension occasionally is created in the laryngeal area, causing a pull of the ventricular ligaments and approximation of the ventricular folds (Figure 4-26), which are also known as the false vocal folds. In the extreme case, the ventricular folds may actually be the source of vibration for voice production. During normal vocal fold vibration, the ventricular folds are at rest, superior and lateral to the true vocal folds. False vocal fold phonation, as a functional behavior, may be caused by physical and emotional tension. In addition, it has been used as a compensatory voice

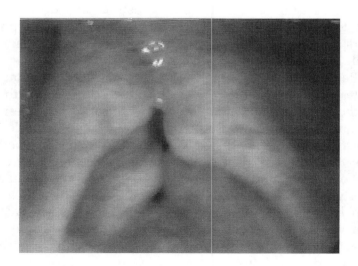

Figure 4-26. Ventricular phonation (See also Plate 23).

source when other serious pathologies make it difficult or impossible to phonate using the true vocal folds.[1]

The voice quality of ventricular phonation is typically a moderate to severe dysphonia characterized by low pitch, roughness, and strain. When true vocal fold vibration is physically possible, the ventricular phonation can benefit from treatment including counseling and vocal re-education through direct voice therapy. Many patients are referred to the voice pathologist with the diagnosis of plica ventricularis. One common pitfall should be noted: this diagnosis often is made erroneously when the false folds compress because of the laryngeal exam, thus obstructing the view of the true vocal folds. In this case, the vibratory source continues to be the true vocal folds, but because of the medial compression of the false folds, the diagnosis of ventricular phonation is made.

Puberphonia: Mutational Falsetto and Juvenile Voice

The laryngeal mechanism goes through a dramatic change in both males and females during puberty. The male voice lowers about one octave during mutation and the female voice lowers two to three semitones. When this acoustic change does not take place following the normal physical maturation, puberphonia occurs. The male is said to have a mutational falsetto and the female a juvenile or childlike voice.

Researchers have suggested many causes for mutational falsetto, including attempts to resist the natural growth into adulthood, a strong feminine self-identification, the desire to maintain a competent childhood soprano singing voice, and embarrassment when the voice lowers dramatically, perhaps earlier than those of their peers.[1] Falsetto voice also may be the result of muscular incoordination and dysfunction without other underlying etiology. Usually, these clinical signs include an elevated larynx and high-postured tongue that alters vocal tract resonance. The juvenile voice of the postadolescent female is recognized less commonly than mutational falsetto because the vocal symptoms of this disorder are less dramatic for the female. Women who demonstrate a juvenile voice may have resisted the transition into adulthood or may have habituated this altered laryngeal and vocal tract posture.

The voice qualities associated with these pathologies are typically mild dysphonias characterized by high pitch, low intensity, cul-de-sac nasality, and breathiness. Physiologically, this is caused by persistent hyperfunction of the cricothyroid muscles with a pronounced elevation of the entire larynx.[1,88] Because of the inability to compress the vocal folds well, patients with these disorders often are not able to build appropriate subglottic air pressure to increase intensity. Common complaints are associated with an inability to shout or to compete with background noise and with voice fatigue. Young males may also demonstrate raspy voice qualities as they attempt to lower the pitch level in the presence of the muscular positioning of the folds and larynx for the falsetto. Mutational falsetto and juvenile voice are most often identified during the first few postadolescent years, with the social consequences being more negative for the male. Occasionally these pathologies are not identified until the adult years, when it often is more difficult to attain and maintain normal voice pitch and resonance. Nonetheless, voice therapy is the treatment of choice with these disorders. Usually appropriate pitch and resonance can be triggered in the first therapy session, but subsequent therapy is needed to familiarize and stabilize the "new" voice as the patient's own.

Transgender Voice

Patients who elect to proceed with gender reassignment (male to female or female to male) do not present as voice disorders per se. Nonetheless, these patients need to alter voice production so that listeners will perceive the speaking voice as appropriate for the desired gender. These patients can benefit from behavioral therapy and occasionally from phonosurgery. Treatments are targeted specifically for the defined need posed by the patient's gender transition. Usually, the transgendered voice patients will seek goals to modify vocal pitch, quality, and prosody in voice, while making simultaneous adjustments in speech articulation and language patterns to create and maintain a communication style consistent with the desired gender.[91]

Psychogenic Conversion Aphonia and Dysphonia

The patient who whispers or presents with an unusual voice quality despite having a neurologically and anatomically normal laryngeal mechanism may have the pathology of conversion aphonia or dysphonia. Onset is normally sudden with many patients relating the disorder to symptoms of a cold or flu that often is accompanied by a "sore throat." The majority of conversion voice disorders occur in women,[1,5,6] but men, women, and children of all ages are subject to conversion disorders of the voice.

Stress and tension induce a psychological conversion reaction. This reaction response is a direct attempt to draw attention away from the real problem. It permits the individual to focus on the voice instead of the true source of the stress or emotional conflict. These voicing behaviors are unconscious methods of avoiding the strong interpersonal conflicts that cause the stress, depression, or anxiety.[1,92]

Once the maladaptive aphonia or dysphonia has habituated, patients believe that they have truly lost the ability to normally produce voice. On occasion, by the time patients seek help from the laryngologist or voice pathologist, the need for the conversion reaction has diminished significantly and they are ready for the voice problem to be resolved. Although some patients continue to receive secondary gain from the disorder and resist all therapy modifications, the majority will respond quickly to direct voice therapy.

Idiopathic Voice Disorders

Paradoxical Vocal Fold Motion

Although paradoxical vocal fold motion is not a primary vocal complaint, the disorder is marked by inappropriate adduction of the vocal folds during inspiration, resulting in inhalatory stridor, which can be confused with upper respiratory disorders including asthma. Patients will perceive episodic shortness of breath, often during periods of active exercise. Although the episodes are typically self-limiting, they have the potential to create airway distress and often frighten patients. In severe cases, the disorder may result in chronic dyspnea, requiring a tracheostomy.[93]

The etiology for paradoxical vocal fold motion is unknown, but a large percentage of patients with these symptoms have other respiratory diagnoses, including asthma, allergies, or frequent upper respiratory infections. Other etiologies associated with this disorder include esophageal reflux, panic or anxiety disorders, and neuromuscular dyskinesia. Recent evidence suggests that some latent differences in laryngeal movements are detectable in persons with paradoxical vocal fold motion even during asymptomatic periods.[94] Treatment for paradoxical vocal fold motion is frequently successful and includes behavioral techniques to interrupt the cycle of adductor inhalatory motion and to restore the normal respiratory pattern with vocal fold abduction. Depending on the patient profile, this behavioral treatment approach must be augmented with antireflux medication and psychological intervention as warranted.

Congenital Airway Anomalies: Subglottic Stenosis and Laryngomalacia

Voice pathologists who work with pediatric populations may see patients with congenital laryngeal disorders that affect respiration more than voice quality. Two of the most common varieties are congenital subglottic stenosis (Figure 4-27) and laryngomalacia[19,20,27,29] Subglottic stenosis occurs when maldevelopment of the cricoid cartilage or arrested embryonic development of the conus elasticus produces a narrowing of the larynx below the glottis, resulting in an airway obstruction that is accompanied by inhalatory stridor, even from birth. In some cases, as the cricoid cartilage continues to develop after birth, the problem is alleviated in infancy or early childhood. In more severe cases, surgical repair of the subglottic region is required.[95] Voice therapy often is necessary following surgery to aid the child in establishing normal phonation.

Laryngomalacia (congenital laryngeal stridor) is another pediatric congenital abnormality of the larynx that is of theoretical interest to the voice. This pathology occurs when the epiglottis fails to develop normally, remaining soft and pliable. As the

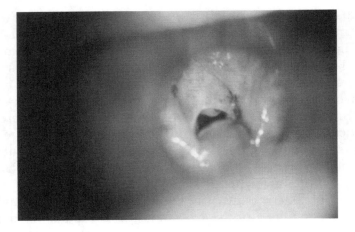

Figure 4-27. Laryngeal stenosis. From Abitbol[96(p367)] (See also Plate 24)

child breathes, the increased inspiratory and expiratory movements of the epiglottis offer considerable resistance to the air stream, causing stridor. Following diagnosis, no treatment is required for this condition, as the epiglottis will continue to develop and the condition will spontaneously clear by the third year with normal maturation.

Summary

This chapter has reviewed a large set of laryngeal pathologies that affect voice, speech, and respiration. Despite the broad range of potential etiologies, these pathologies will have similar effects on the quality, pitch, and loudness of voice production in many cases. Medical or organic contributors play a significant role in the voice-disordered patient population. By being familiar with the predisposing history, appearance, and common etiologic factors that may lead to their development, voice pathologists may plan appropriate management programs. The interaction between vocal function and laryngeal pathology, whether focal or systemic, has provided opportunity for development of new treatment approaches. Although medical diagnosis of the laryngeal pathology is the exclusive responsibility of the otolaryngologist, a voice pathologist who is well-informed about the process can increase the probability of an efficacious diagnostic voice evaluation and treatment plan. Options for medical treatments, voice rehabilitation, and phonosurgery have enhanced the opportunity for voice pathologists and otolaryngologists to apply a combined team approach to diagnosis, treatment planning, and rehabilitation of voice disorders.

References

1. Aronson A. *Clinical Voice Disorders: An Interdisciplinary Approach*. 3rd ed. New York, NY: Brian C. Decker; 1990.
2. Damste PH. Diagnostic behavior patterns with communicative abilities: In: Bless DM, Abbs J, eds. *Vocal Fold Physiology*. San Diego, Calif: College-Hill Press; 1987:435-444.
3. Verdolini K. *NCVS Guide to Vocology*. Iowa City, Ia: University of Iowa: National Center for Voice and Speech; 1998.
4. LaGuaite J. Adult voice screening. *J Speech Hear Disord*. 1972;37:147-151.
5. Herrington-Hall B, Lee L, Stemple J, Niemi K, McHone M. Description of laryngeal pathologies by age, gender, and occupation in a treatment seeking sample. *J Speech Hear Disord*. 1988;53:57-65.
6. Coyle S. *Incidence of Laryngeal Pathology in a Treatment-Seeking Population* [master's thesis]. Oxford, OH: Miami University.
7. Titze I, Lemke J, Montequin D. Populations in the US workforce who must rely on voice as a primary tool of trade: a preliminary report. *J Voice*. 1997;11:254-259.
8. Smith E, Lemke J, Taylor M, Kirchner H, Hoffman H. Frequency of voice problems among teachers and other occupations. *J Voice*. 1998;12:480-488.
9. Senturia B, Wilson F. Otorhinolaryngologic findings in children with voice deviations: preliminary report. *Ann Otol Rhinol Laryngol*. 1968;77:1027-1042.
10. Silverman E, Zimmer C. Incidence of chronic hoarseness among school-age children. *J Speech Hear Disord*. 1975;40:211-215.
11. Dobres R, Lee L, Stemple J, Kummer A, Kretchmer L. Description of laryngeal pathologies in children evaluated by otolaryngologists. *J Speech Hear Disord*. 1990;55:526-533.
12. Hirano M. Structure of the vocal fold in normal and disease states: anatomical and physical studies. In: Ludlow C, Hart M, eds. *Proceedings of the Conference on the Assessment of Vocal Pathology*. Rockville, Md: American Speech-Language-Hearing Association; 1981:11-30.
13. Bastian RW. Benign mucosal disorders. In: Cummings CW, Frederickson JM, Harker LA, Krause CJ, Schuller DE, eds. *Otolaryngology—Head and Neck Surgery*. St. Louis, Mo: CV Mosby Company; 1986:1965-1987.

14. Allen MS, Pettit JM, Sherblom JC. Management of vocal nodules: a regional survey of otolaryngologists and speech-language pathologists. *J Speech Hear Res*. 1991;34:229-235.
15. Colton R, Woo P, Brewer D, Griffin B, Casper J. Stroboscopic signs associated with benign lesions of the vocal folds. *J Voice*. 1995;9:312-325.
16. Goldman S, Hargrave J, Hillman R, Holmberg E, Gress C. Stress, anxiety, somatic complaints, and voice use in women with vocal nodules: preliminary findings. *Am J Speech Lang Pathol*. 1996;5:44-54.
17. Verdolini-Marston K, Burke MK, Lessac A, Glaze LE, Caldwell E. A preliminary study on two methods of treatment for laryngeal nodules. *J Voice*. 1995;9:74-85.
18. Sataloff R. *Professional Voice: The Science and Art of Clinical Care*. New York, NY: Raven Press; 1991.
19. Tucker HM. *The Larynx*. New York, NY: Thieme Medical Publishers; 1987.
20. Ballenger JJ. *Diseases of the Nose, Throat, Ear, Head, and Neck* 13th ed. Philadelphia, Pa: Lea and Febiger; 1985.
21. Yamaguchi H. Recent advances in the surgical treatment and development of laryngeal instruments for Reinke's edema. *Phonoscope*. 1998;1:27-34.
22. Koufman JA, Weiner GJ, Wu WC, Castell DO. Reflux laryngitis and its sequelae: the diagnostic role of ambulatory 24-hour pH monitoring. *J Voice*. 1988;2:78-89.
23. Crary M, Sapienza C, Cassissi N, Moore GP. *Am J Speech-Lang Pathol*. 1996;7(2): 92-96.
24. Kleinsasser O. Microlaryngoscopy and Endolaryngeal Microsurgery. Philadelphia, Pa: WB Saunders; 1968.
25. McGill T. Congenital abnormalities of the larynx. In: Fried M, ed. *The Larynx: A Multidisciplinary Approach*. Boston, Mass: Little Brown and Company; 1988:143-152.
26. Holinger P, Schild J, Mauriz D. Laryngeal papilloma: review of etiology and therapy. *Laryngoscope*. 1968;78:1462.
27. Holinger L. Congenital anomalies of the larynx. In: English G, ed. *Otolaryngology Vol 3*. Philadelphia, Pa: Harper and Row; 1979:1-15.
28. Jones S, Myers E, Barnes E. Benign neoplasms of the larynx. In: Fried M, ed. *The Larynx: A Multidisciplinary Approach*. Boston, Mass: Little Brown and Company; 1988:401-420.
29. Greene M, Mathieson L. *The Voice and Its Disorders*. 5th ed. London, England: Whurr Publishers; 1989.
30. Benjamin B. Congenital laryngeal webs. *Ann Otol Rhinol Laryngol*. 1983; 92:317-326.
31. Bouchayer M, Cornut G, Witzig E, et al. Epidermoid cysts, sulci and mucosal bridges of the true vocal cord: a report of 157 cases. *Laryngoscope*. 1985;95:1087-1094.
32. Tanaka S, Hirano M, Chijiwa K. Some aspects of vocal fold bowing. *Ann Otol Rhinol Laryngol*. 1994;103:357-362.
33. Pontes P, Belau M. Treatment of sulcus vocalis: auditory perceptual and acoustical analysis of the slicing mucosa surgical technique. *J Voice*. 1993;7:365-376.

34. Ringel R, Chodzko-Zaijko W. Vocal indices of biological age. *J Voice.* 1987;1:31-37.
35. Woo P, Casper J, Colton R. Dysphonia in the aging: physiology versus disease. *Laryngoscope.* 1993;102:139-144.
36. Blackwell KE, Calcterra YC, Fu, Y. Laryngeal dysplasia: epidemiology and treatment outcome. *Ann Otol Rhinol Laryngol.* 1995;104:596-602.
37. Pearson BW. Subtotal laryngectomy. *Laryngoscope.* 1981;91:1904-1912.
38. Lefebreve J. Laryngeal preservation: the discussion is not closed. *Otolaryngol Head Neck Surg.* 1999;118:389-393.
39. Wilatt D, Stell P. Vocal cord paralysis. In: Paparella M, Shumrick D, eds. *Otolaryngology.* 3rd ed. Philadelphia, Pa: WB Saunders; 1991.
40. Lawson G, Remacle M, Hamoir M, Jamart J. Posterior cordectomy and subtotal arytenoidectomy for the treatment of bilateral vocal fold immobility: functional results. *J Voice.* 1996;10:314-319.
41. Kelchner L, Stemple J, Gerdeman B, LeBorgne W, Adam, S. Etiology. Pathophysiology, treatment choices, and voice results for unilateral adductor vocal fold paralysis: a three-year retrospective. *J Voice.* In press.
42. Crumley R. Unilateral recurrent laryngeal nerve paralysis. *J Voice.* 1994; 8:79-83.
43. Dursum G, Sataloff R, Spiegel J, et al. Superior laryngeal nerve paralysis and paresis. *J Voice.* 1996;10:206-211.
44. Aronson A, Brown J, Litin E, Pearson J. Spastic dysphonia, I: Voice, neurologic, and psychiatric aspects. *J Speech Hear Disord.* 1968;33:203-218.
45. Brodnitz F. Spastic dysphonia. *Ann Otol Rhinol Laryngol.* 1976;85:210-214.
46. Aminoff M, Dedo H, Izdebski K. Clinical aspects of spasmodic dysphonia. *J Neurol Neurosurg Psychiatry.* 1978;41:361-365.
47. Cannito MP. Neurobiological interpretations of spasmodic dysphonia. In: Vogel D, Cannito MP, eds. *Treating Disordered Speech Motor Control: For Clinicians by Clinicians.* Austin, Tex: Pro-Ed; 1990:275-317.
48. Schaefer SD, Finitzo-Heiber T, Gerling IJ, Freeman, FJ. Brainstem conduction abnormalities in spasmodic dysphonia. In Bless DM, Abbs J, eds. *Vocal Fold Physiology.* San Diego, Calif: College-Hill Press; 1987:393-404.
49. Blitzer A, Brin MF. Laryngeal dystonia: a series with botulinum toxin therapy. *Ann Otol Rhinol Laryngol.* 1991;100:85-89.
50. Dedo H, Townsend J, Izdebski K. Current evidence for the organic etiology of spastic dysphonia. *Trans Otolaryngol.* 1978;86:875-880.
51. Heuer R. Behavioral therapy for spasmodic dysphonia. *J Voice.* 1992; 6:352-354.
52. Woodson GE, Zwirner P, Murry T, Swenson MR. Functional assessment of patients with spasmodic dysphonia. *J Voice.* 1992;6:338-343.
53. Larsson T, Sjögren T. Essential tremor: a clinical and genetic population study. *Acta Psychiatr Neurol (Scandinavia).* 1960;36(suppl 144):1-176.
54. Brown J, Simonson J. Organic voice tremor. *Neurology.* 1963;13:520-525.
55. Aronson A, Hartman D. Adductor spastic dysphonia as a sign of essential (voice) tremor. *J Speech Hear Disord.* 1981;33:52-58.
56. Darley F, Aronson AE, Brown J. *Motor Speech Disorders.* Philadelphia, Pa: WB Saunders; 1975.

57. Duffy J. *Motor Speech Disorders*. St. Louis, Mo: Mosby; 1995.
58. Sudarsky L, Feudo P, Zubick H. Vocal aberrations in dysarthria. In: Fried M, ed. *The Larynx: A Multidisciplinary Approach*. Boston, Mass: Little, Brown and Company; 1988:179-190.
59. Griffiths C, Bough ID Jr. Neurologic diseases and their effects on voice. *J Voice*. 1989;3:148-156.
60. Hartelius L, Buder E, Strand E. Long-term phonatory instability in individuals with multiple sclerosis. *J Speech Lang Hear Res*. 1997;40:1056-1072.
61. Ramig L, Countryman S, Thompson L, Horii Y. Comparison of two forms of intensive speech therapy for Parkinson disease. *J Speech Lang Hear Res*. 1995;38:1232-1251.
62. Kent J, Kent RD, Rosenbek J, et al. Quantitative description of the dysarthria in women with amyotrophic lateral sclerosis. *J Speech Hear Res*. 1992;35:723-733.
63. Ramig L, Scherer R, Klasner E, Titze IR, Horii Y. Acoustic analysis of voice in amyotrophic lateral sclerosis: a longitudinal case study. *J Speech Hear Disord*. 1990;55:2-14.
64. Silbergleit A, Johnson A, Jacobsen B. Acoustic analysis of voice in individuals with amyotrophic lateral sclerosis and perceptually normal voice quality. *J Voice*. 1997;11:222-231.
65. Roth C, Glaze L, David W, Goding G. Case report: amyotrophic lateral sclerosis presenting as signs of spasmodic dysphonia. *J Voice*. 1996;10:362-367.
66. Rubin W. Allergic, dietary, chemical, stress, and hormonal influences in voice abnormalities. *J Voice*. 1987;1:378-385.
67. Orlikoff RF. Vocal jitter at different fundamental frequencies: a cardiovascular-neuromuscular explanation. *J Voice*. 1989;3:104-112.
68. Orlikoff RF. Heartbeat-related fundamental frequency and amplitude variation in healthy young and elderly male voices. *J Voice*. 1990;4:322-328.
69. Abitbol J, de Brux J, Millot G, et al. Does a hormonal vocal cord cycle exist in women? *J Voice*. 1989;3:157-162.
70. Higgins M, Saxman J. Variations in vocal frequency perturbation across the menstrual cycle. *J Voice*. 1989;3:233-243.
71. Davis CB, Davis ML. The effects of premenstrual syndrome on the female singer. *J Voice*. 1993;7:337-353.
72. Martin FG. Drugs and vocal function. *J Voice*. 1988;2:333-344.
73. Dodd S, Longland J, Worrall L, Mitchell C, Yiu E. The prevalence and associated risk factors of dysphonia in inhaled corticosteroid users. *Phonoscope*. 1998;1:97-112.
74. Jafek BW, Esses BA. Manifestations of systemic disease. In: Cummings CW, Frederickson JM, Harker LA, Krause CJ, Schuller DE, eds. *Otolaryngology—Head and Neck Surgery*. St. Louis, Mo: CV Mosby Company; 1986:1933-1941.
75. Shemen L. Diseases of the thyroid as they affect the larynx. In: Fried M, ed. *The Larynx: A Multidisciplinary Approach*. Boston, Mass: Little, Brown and Company; 1988:223-233.
76. Bienenstock H, Ehrlich GE, Freyberg RH. Rheumatoid arthritis of the cricoarytenoid joint: a clinicopathologic study. *Arthritis Rheumat*. 1963;6:48-63.

77. Wolman L, Darke CS, Young A. The larynx in rheumatoid arthritis. *J Laryngol Otol.* 1965;79:403-434.
78. Shumrick K, Shumrick D. Inflammatory diseases of the larynx. In Fried M, ed. *The Larynx: A Multidisciplinary Approach.* Boston, Mass: Little, Brown and Company; 1988:249-278.
79. Pennover D, Shefer A. Immunologic disorders of the larynx. In: Fried M, ed. *The Larynx: A Multidisciplinary Approach.* Boston, Mass: Little, Brown and Company; 1988:279-290.
80. Jackson-Menalow C, Dzul AI, Holland R. Allergies and vocal fold edema: preliminary report. *J Voice.* 1999;13:113-122.
81. Pillsbury HC, Postma DS. Infections. In: Cummings CW, Frederickson JM, Harker LA, Krause CJ, Schuller DE, eds. *Otolaryngology—Head and Neck Surgery.* St. Louis, Mo: CV Mosby Company; 1986:1919-1931.
82. Vrabec DP. Fungal infections of the larynx. *Otolaryngol Clin North Am.* 1993;26:1091-1113.
83. Tashjian LS, Peacock JE. Laryngeal candidiasis. *Arch Otol.* 1984;110:806-809.
84. Jones NS, Lannigan FJ, McCullagh M, et al. Acid reflux and hoarseness. *J Voice.* 1990;4:355-358.
85. Koufman J, Sataloff R, Toohill R. Laryngopharyngeal reflux: consensus conference report. *J Voice.* 1996;10:215-216.
86. Lumpkin SMM, Bishop SG, Katz PO. Chronic dysphonia secondary to gastroesophageal reflux disease (GERD): diagnosis using simultaneous dual-probe prolonged pH monitoring. *J Voice.* 1989;3:351-355.
87. Morrison M, Rammage L. *The Management of Voice Disorders.* San Diego, Calif: Singular Publishing Group; 1994.
88. Morrison M. Pattern recognition in muscle misuse: how I do it. *J Voice.* 1997;11:108-114.
89. Stemple JC. *Voice Therapy: Clinical Studies.* St. Louis, Mo: Mosby-Year Book; 1993.
90. Stemple J, Stanley J, Lee L. Objective measures of voice production in normal subjects following prolonged voice use. *J Voice.* 1995;9:127-133.
91. Andrews ML, Schmidt CP. Gender presentation: perceptual and acoustic analysis of voice. *J Voice.* 1997;11:307-313.
92. Baker J. Psychogenic dysphonia: peeling back the layers. *J Voice.* 1998; 12:527-535.
93. Christopher K, Wood R, Eckert C, Blager F, Raney R, Souhrada J. Vocal cord dysfunction presenting as asthma. *New Engl J Med.* 1983;308:1566-1570.
94. Treole K, Trudeau M, Forrest LA. Endoscopic and stroboscopic description of adults with paradoxical vocal fold motion. *J Voice.* 1999;13:143-152.
95. Cotton R. Prevention and management of laryngeal stenosis in infants and children. *J Ped Surg.* 1985;20:845-851.
96. Abitbol J. *Atlas of Laser Voice Surgery.* San Diego, Calif: Singular Publishing Group; 1995: Figures reprinted with permission.

5

The Diagnostic Voice Evaluation

The previous chapters of this text have described the academic areas of knowledge from a clinical perspective, which are a necessary preparation for the evaluation and treatment of voice disorders. This chapter begins our concentration on the interpersonal skills that are necessary when we assume the responsibility of guiding and helping others. These skills include listening, hearing, feeling, connecting, empathizing, motivating, encouraging, reinforcing, and rewarding. Although one may study and learn academic information and then turn it into personal knowledge, communication skills develop over a lifetime of observation and interaction. The successful voice pathologist must possess an inherent "feel" for other people and combine vast academic knowledge with the ability to communicate at both a professional and personal level.

The primary objectives of the diagnostic voice evaluation are to discover the etiologic factors associated with the development of the voice disorder and to describe deviant vocal symptoms. In a systematic evaluation designed to determine specific causes of disorders, voice pathologists use their knowledge of laryngeal anatomy and physiology, pathologies of the laryngeal mechanism, and common etiologic factors. Once the causes are known and the symptoms are described, a vocal management plan tailored to the individual problems and needs of each patient may be developed.

G. Paul Moore, one of the pioneers in voice disorders said:

> Diagnosis is the process of discovering the cause of certain symptoms. Diagnosis of voice disorders ordinarily encompasses the recognition and description of individual vocal deviations and a systematic search for the factors that cause these deviations. [1]

The voice pathologist may also use the voice evaluation as a tool for patient education and motivation. Most individuals have little knowledge or understanding of voice production. Indeed, the majority of patients who present with voice disorders have little understanding of the problem. During the diagnostic evaluation, the voice pathologist will find it beneficial to explain in simple terms how voice is produced and the effect that the specific pathology plays on deviant voice production. With an understanding of voice production, patients can better respond to diagnostic questions specific to discovering the etiologies of the problem.

The patient who is well informed also will generally be more motivated to follow the necessary therapy regimen required to resolve the pathology. Patients who understand the causes of the disorder, are presented with a systematic management approach, and are given a reasonable estimate of the time needed for completion of the program usually develop a positive therapeutic attitude.

The Players

Many components comprise the diagnostic voice evaluation, including (1) the medical examination, (2) the patient interview, (3) the perceptual evaluation of voice, (4) the instrumental analysis of voice (including acoustic and aerodynamic analyses), and (5) the functional evaluation of vocal fold movement.

Members of our profession increasingly accomplish these diagnostic components through the teamwork of otolaryngologists, voice pathologists, and, when occasion dictates, other professionals such as vocal coaches, voice teachers, and other medical professionals. The otolaryngologist is trained to examine the laryngeal mechanism for pathology and to diagnose the voice disorder. Through the diagnosis, he or she determines whether to treat the disorder medically, surgically, or through referral for functional management. The voice pathologist is trained to identify the causes of the voice disorders, evaluate the vocal symptoms, and to establish improved vocal function through various therapeutic methods. The vocal coach or singing instructor evaluates the efficiency and correctness of performance technique and suggests modifications as needed. Other medical professionals, such as neurologists, allergists, and endocrinologists may be called upon in selected cases to aid in the evaluation process. These complementary professional relationships have significantly improved the care of patients with voice disorders.[2]

The teamwork model for evaluating and managing voice disorders has lead to the development of formal clinical voice laboratories. In these settings, patients have the opportunity to be evaluated by each of these core professionals during a single visit. In addition, modern instrumentation now permits reports of vocal function measures, as well as visual studies of vocal function. These more advanced laryngeal function studies are described in Chapter 6.

Patient Profile

Who are voice patients? They may be of any age, gender, race, or occupation. They may be professional voice users or Sunday morning choir members. Herrington-Hall et al[3] demonstrated this fact well in their review of patients who sought evaluation for voice disorders. The 10 most common patient occupations were retired, homemaker, factory worker, unemployed, executive or manager, teacher, student, secretary, singer, and nurse. In a more recent study that sought to compare current data to the Herrington-Hall et al[3] data, Coyle et al[4] reported that the 10 most common occupations among individuals seeking treatment were retired, executive or manager, homemaker, unemployed, student, teacher, clerical, factory, sales, and nurse. Cooper's[5] most frequently occurring occupations included housewives, teachers, students, salespeople, owners or managers, executives, singers, clerks, lawyers, and engineers. Koufman and Isaacson[6] suggested a useful four-level scale of vocal usage (Table 5-1). In reviewing this scale, however, the voice pathologist must not assume that a voice disorder classified as a Level IV is any less important or has any less functional or emotional impact on the patient than those classified as Level I. Although the financial implications of the voice disorder may not be as great, each patient dictates his or her own level of concern related to the effects of the voice problem.

Referral Sources

Voice pathologists receive the majority of voice referrals from the otolaryngologist. When the referral is from elsewhere, the voice pathologist must refer the patient for an otolaryngologic examination. The importance of this medical examination for both adults and children cannot be overstated. Although Sander[7] argued against aggressively pursuing voice treatment for children, we have unfortunately seen children who were treated unsuccessfully for "hoarseness" over long periods of time before they were referred for medical evaluation. Subsequent indirect laryngoscopy revealed a small anterior web in one child and papilloma in another. Even more dramatic was the discovery of

Table 5-1. Levels of Vocal Usage

	Description	*Examples*
Level I	Elite vocal performer	Singer, actor
Level II	Professional voice user	Clergyman, lecturer, broadcast journalist
Level III	Nonvocal professional	Teacher, lawyer
Level IV	Nonvocal nonprofessional	Laborer, clerk

a squamous cell laryngeal carcinoma in a 12-year-old girl that required a total laryngectomy. Certainly, the possibility of a life-threatening pathology is greater in the adult population, but these examples demonstrate the need and value of conducting the medical examination prior to the onset of voice therapy.

In more recent years, with the development of managed care insurance plans, the patient's primary care physician approves referrals to all medical specialists and therapy services. The voice pathologist must become educated about issues related to insurance and referral protocols to guarantee appropriate coverage for services provided to the patient. If the referral protocols are not followed, payment will be denied.

Initial identification of the voice problem may occur in several ways. From a management standpoint, it is optimal when the patient identifies the problem. Our definition in Chapter 1 established that a voice disorder may exist if the laryngeal mechanism's structure, function, or both no longer meets the patient's functional voice demands. Self-discovery and awareness of the problem often yield more motivated patients.

Friends or family members may also make an informal initial identification of vocal symptoms, or such identification may occur during a speech pathology screening in school or during a routine medical examination. When someone other than the patient identifies the symptoms, the patient may or may not consider them to be a problem. It then becomes the responsibility of the voice pathologist to educate the patient regarding the disorder and to point out potential problems associated with the disorder.[8] The ultimate decision for treatment or management remains the individual's or, in some cases, the caregiver's choice.

The voice pathologist must also remember that the patient is the "owner" of the voice problem, and he or she is ultimately responsible for resolving the problem. The history of the medical profession has traditionally placed the responsibility of our illness and wellness squarely on the shoulders of the physician. Too often, we hear statements such as "The doctor will take care of it. The doctor will make me better." Successful voice therapy is predicated on a motivated patient taking charge of a well-planned management program and following that program to the desired result: improved voice. The voice pathologist must not permit the patient to transfer ownership of the problem.

Medical Examination

A complete otolaryngologic examination involves taking a detailed history of the problem and examining the entire head and neck region. Pertinent medical history is also discussed. The examination includes otoscopic observation of the ears; examination of the oral and nasal cavities; palpation of the salivary glands, lymph nodes, and thyroid gland; and a visual examination of the larynx. The larynx is typically viewed utilizing indirect laryngoscopy (Figure 5-1). To perform this examination, the laryngologist grasps the tongue and gently pulls it forward and down while placing the laryngeal mirror in the pharynx. The

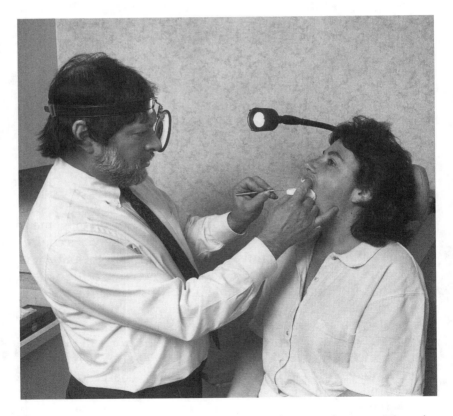

Figure 5-1. Indirect laryngoscopy using a laryngeal mirror. (Photo by Rick Berkey, Dayton, Ohio.)

head mirror directs artificial light to reflect off the laryngeal mirror, illuminating the pharynx. The larynx is then viewed on the laryngeal mirror with the image of the right and left vocal folds reversed. Patients are typically asked to produce the phoneme /i/ so that the vocal fold approximation may be easily viewed. The attempt to say /i/ draws the epiglottis forward to expose the interior of the larynx. Patients with a sensitive gag reflex may have the tongue and pharynx sprayed with a topical anesthesia to suppress the reflex.

Fiberoptic laryngoscopy is also available as a simple office procedure for examining the larynx directly. When using this technique, the physician introduces a fiberoptic laryngoscope into the patient's pharynx via the nasal cavity (Figure 5-2). This device is a long, flexible tube that contains fiberoptic light

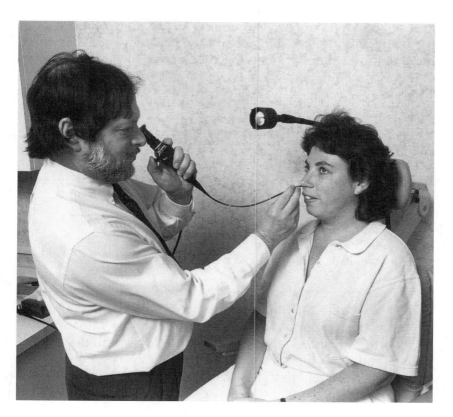

Figure 5-2. Flexible endoscopy. (Photo by Rick Berkey, Dayton, Ohio.)

bundles and a lens. A small hand control permits the physician to manipulate the flexible end of the scope. When the scope is attached to a light source, the larynx and surrounding structures may be viewed either through an eyepiece or on a video monitor when the eyepiece is attached to a video camera.[9] Fiberoptic laryngoscopy is often performed on patients who cannot tolerate indirect mirror laryngoscopy. A topical anesthesia may be used with this procedure.

The larynx may also be viewed through direct laryngoscopy. In this surgical procedure, the patient undergoes a general anesthesia, most often in outpatient surgery. A magnifying laryngoscope is then placed in the pharynx via the oral cavity to obtain a direct microscopic view of the larynx. Biopsies and surgical excisions may also be performed through the laryngoscope.

The medical examination also may include special radiographs of the head, chest, and neck, as well as blood analyses and swallowing studies. The final result of the medical examination and studies is a diagnosis of the problem and recommendations for treatment, including medical or surgical treatment, voice evaluation and therapy, or any combination of these choices.

Voice Pathology Evaluation

As previously stated, the three major objectives of the diagnostic voice evaluation are to

- identify the causes of the voice disorder,
- describe the present vocal components, and
- develop an individualized management plan.

Following referral from the otolaryngologist, the voice pathologist will begin this diagnostic process with the patient interview, the most important component of the voice evaluation.

During the interview, the voice pathologist will develop an understanding of the causes of the disorder and establish a rapport with the patient that permits the therapeutic process to proceed. The voice pathologist may use several formats to interview the patient. Some voice pathologists choose a questionnaire format that requires the patient to respond to prepared questions either prior to or during the evaluation. The answers to the prepared questions are then used to stimulate further understanding of the problem. Although helpful for the beginning clinician, we find prepared forms to be somewhat restrictive and prefer to use a less formal, yet systematic patient interview format. Goals have been established for each section of this format, and the voice pathologist makes every attempt to accomplish each goal during the interview. The suggested format that follows relates to the sample report (SR) located in Appendix 5-1.

Diagnostic Voice Evaluation

Referral

Goals: Establish the identity of the referral source.

The referral source should be clearly understood at the beginning of the evaluation. The major referral sources will be the otolaryngologist, other speech pathologists, physicians, voice teachers, vocal coaches, the patient's relatives and friends, or the patient may be self-referred. (See SR1.)

Reason for the Referral

Goals: (1) Establish exact reason for the patient referral; (2) establish patient's understanding for the referral; (3) develop patient knowledge of the voice disorder; (4) establish credibility of the examiner.

It is important that the voice pathologist have accurate information regarding the exact reason the patient was referred. When a physician refers the patient, the specific medical diagnosis should be reported along with the physician's expectations related to your contact with the patient. There are many reasons for patient referrals. These may include preoperative tape recording of the voice, laryngeal function studies (see Chapter 6), evaluation without management, preoperative trial voice therapy, postoperative evaluation and treatment, or a complete diagnostic voice evaluation with the appropriate management plan.

In our practice, patients often are referred only for a laryngeal videostroboscopic evaluation. Understanding the physician's expectations will avoid confusion and will help to maintain the necessary cooperative working relationships. (See SR2.)

It is also desirable to ensure that the patient understands the reason for the referral for "speech therapy." Quite often, the patient is confused about the purpose of being evaluated by a "speech therapist." This confusion may be addressed by simply asking the patient, "Do you understand why Dr A referred you here?" When confusion is evident, explain the voice pathologist's role along with the three major goals you intend to accomplish during the evaluation. As patients better understand the process and procedures, the more reliable they become in communicating pertinent information throughout the evaluation.

It is also helpful to educate the patient about the voice disorder before proceeding. This knowledge base may be developed by offering a brief description of how the normal laryngeal mechanism works and how the specific pathology affects it. With this information, patients will better understand where certain questions are leading and may be able to give more reliable information. Some patients even volunteer pertinent information following this discussion before questions are asked. A typical dialogue between a patient (Pt) and voice pathologist (VP) might be:

VP: Do you understand what vocal nodules are and how they might develop?

Pt: Dr A said that they're like bumps on my vocal cords and that I got them cause I holler too much.

VP: That may be, but there are many reasons why nodules may develop. Let's talk about it. When Dr A looked down your throat with his mirror, he was essentially looking at two solid shelves of muscle tissue, one on each side. (It is helpful to schematically draw the vocal folds or to show a picture so that patients may be able to visualize the anatomy. Use of the patient's own stroboscopic video is extremely helpful if available.) These shelves are the vocal cords, or folds, and we're looking straight down on top of them in this picture. The point where the two folds meet is inside the **V** of your Adam's Apple. Can you feel yours? Now, the space between the vocal folds is called the glottis, and the tube below the folds is the windpipe or trachea. This of course is the airway where air travels to the lungs as we breathe.

Attached to the back of each vocal fold, we have two cartilages, one here and one here. These cartilages serve as the points of attachment for the vocal folds and for other muscles responsible for opening and closing the vocal folds. When the vocal folds are approximated, air pressure from the lungs may build beneath the folds. When the pressure is great enough, the air will blow the folds apart and begin the vibration, which we hear as voice.

If the muscles pull too hard and the air pressure is too great, such as when we shout, talk loudly over noise, or even when we cough, this excessive tension and pressure will cause the vocal folds to bang and rub together. (Demonstrate with hand clapping movements.) If this banging and rubbing occurs frequently, the impact will eventually cause some swelling or edema of the vocal folds that will usually cause a temporary hoarseness. We have all experienced this kind of hoarseness, maybe at a party or a sporting event. In a day or two this hoarseness goes away. But if whatever caused the hoarseness persists, the folds may remain edemic and will eventually begin to try to protect themselves from further damage. In your case, they've done this by developing, layer by layer, small callouslike structures on the point of the vocal folds where they hit the hardest. These growths are called vocal nodules.

As you've experienced, the nodules have caused a change in your voice. Because of the edema and the presence of the nodules, your voice may have dropped in pitch; because the nodules cause gaps to occur on either side of them when the vocal folds close to vibrate, a greater amount of air escapes, causing you to sound breathy. You've also probably noticed that when you do a lot of talking, your voice weakens, and it becomes quite an effort just to talk. By the end of the day, some people report being worn out from the effort and simply don't feel like talking anymore.

One final point. Vocal nodules are not a cancerous type of growth and do not eventually lead to cancer. Many people do not understand this, so I think it's important to mention. Does this information help you to better understand what vocal nodules are and how they affect voice?

Pt: Yes, now I do. I am glad that you mentioned the part about cancer. I have to admit that I was worried about that. But, what do you think caused my nodules? I really don't raise my voice that much.

VP:That's what we're here today to try and find out. I'm going to ask you many questions. I need to get to know you and how you use your voice in all situations. From that information, we will try to determine specifically what caused your nodules and then develop a plan to attempt to resolve them. Any questions?

This type of discussion goes far in developing your credibility as the person who is qualified to help resolve this disorder. The voice pathologist will have managed to develop a high level of trust before the actual diagnostic questioning regarding the history of the problem begins.

History of the Problem

Goals: (1) Establish the chronological history of the problem; (2) seek etiologic factors associated with the history; (3) determine patient motivation for resolving the problem.

This section of the evaluation is designed to yield an exact history of the disorder from the onset of vocal difficulties, through the development of the problem over time, and ending with the patient's current vocal experiences. All questions are designed to yield information regarding the causes of vocal difficulties. Finally, the patient's motivation for seeking vocal improvement is determined. (Please refer to SR3.) A list of appropriate questions might include:

- Let's go way back. When did you first begin to notice some change or difficulty in your voice?
- Was that the first time that you ever experienced vocal difficulties?
- How did the problem progress from there?
- What finally made you decide to see your doctor about it?
- What did the doctor tell you?
- How did the doctor treat the problem?
- Did your family doctor refer you to the ear, nose, and throat doctor?
- Has anyone else in your family ever experienced a voice problem?
- Does your voice follow a pattern? For example, is it better in the morning than in the evening or vice versa?
- Do you get more hoarse simply by talking normally?
- Have you ever lost your voice totally?
- Do you have any occasion to raise your voice, to talk over noise, or to shout?
- Are you required to talk to anyone who is hard of hearing?
- Do you have a pet?
- Since I have never heard your voice before, I don't know what your normal voice sounds like. I have a 6-point scale where (0) represents perfectly normal voice and (5) repre-

sents as hoarse as you have ever been with this current problem. Where are you on that scale today?

■ How much does this problem actually bother you? Is it causing any daily problems at home or on your job?

■ What is your interest in pursuing voice therapy?

Questions similar to these will lead the voice pathologist along the trail of the development of the voice disorder. The answers will also provide the examiner with an idea of the severity level of the problem as perceived by the patient and the motivation to follow the course of treatment necessary for improvement. On rare occasions, patients have at this point expressed a disinterest in continuing with the diagnostic process. Usually, they have discovered that the problem is not of sufficient concern to them to proceed. A common example is patients who, once they understood that they did not have cancer, were not interested in the consequences of their dysphonia. Although it is the voice pathologist's responsibility to inform the patient and attempt to motivate the patient to seek positive change, the ultimate decision of following through with treatment rests with the individual.

Medical History

Goals: (1) Seek medically related etiologic factors; (2) establish awareness of patient's basic personality.

The medical history seeks out any medically related factors that may have contributed to the development of the present voice disorder. Utilizing our knowledge of medically related etiologies, the voice pathologist asks questions regarding past surgeries and hospitalizations. Chronic disorders are probed along with the use of medications. Smoking, alcohol, and drug use histories are also explored and the patient's current hydration habits are discussed.

The medical history also helps the voice pathologist establish how patients "feel" about their physical and emotional well-being. This may be accomplished by asking patients whether, on a day-to-day basis, they feel "excellent, good, fair, or poor." The response to this question will often offer this insight. For example, some patients report lengthy medical histories with many chronic disorders that would give them the right to feel "poor." Nonetheless, they may still indicate that on a day-to-day basis, they feel "good." Other patients, with unremarkable medical histories, may report feeling only "fair" or "poor."

The answer to this simple question helps the voice pathologist learn the basic personality of the patient. A negative response provides the voice pathologist with an excellent opportunity to pursue the line of questioning further. For example, your response may be, " Oh, why do you feel only fair?" This is often a pivotal moment in the evaluation process and, more often than not, patients share many important details related to their emotional well-being. These details may be related to marriage, family, job, or friends. Patients with voice disorders often share their emotions and concerns with voice pathologists because we are the first people to ask and show an interest. Handling this information and guiding the patient appropriately becomes a major responsibility. (See SR4.)

Social History

Goals: (1) Develop knowledge of the patient's home, work, social, and recreational environments; (2) discover emotional, social, and family difficulties; (3) seek additional etiologic factors.

The social history is the final opportunity to gather information about the patient and the patient's home, work, recreational and social environments, and lifestyle that may contribute to the development of the voice disorder. All questions probe for answers to possible etiologic factors. For example:

■ Are you married, single, divorced, or widowed?
■ How long have you been married, single, or divorced?
■ Do you live alone or with other people?
■ Do you have children? What are their ages? How many are still at home?
■ Does anyone else live in your home? Parents, aunts, friends?
■ Do you work outside of the home? Where? How long?
■ What kind of work do you do? Specifically, what do you do in your job?

- How much talking is required and how much is social?
- Does your husband/wife work? Where? How long? What shift?
- When you are not working, what do you enjoy doing (ie, clubs, hobbies, groups, organizations, sports, other social activities.)
- Are you involved in any hobbies or activities where you are in contact with dust, fumes, chemicals or paints?
- Sometimes stress and tension may contribute to the development of voice problems. In all of these activities and relationships that we've discussed, are there any issues that you think might contribute to this type of tension or stress?
- When you have a lot of stress or tensions, who helps you or takes care of you? (Persons who say "no one" are often at risk for emotional stress.)

As you begin the questioning related to the social history, you may find it helpful to explain to patients the need to get to know who they are and what they do in order to find the causes of their vocal difficulties. You want the patient to understand that, if some of the questions seem personal, they are necessary when trying to discover all possible causes. You should not be surprised when patients open up to you with many personal, family, social, marital, or work problems. When you develop credibility and gain the patient's trust, you often receive such important information. (See SR5.)

Oral-Peripheral Examination

Goals: (1) Determine the physical condition of the oral mechanism; (2) observe laryngeal area tension; (3) check for swallowing difficulties; (4) check for laryngeal sensations.

A routine oral-peripheral examination should be conducted to determine the condition of the oral mechanism in its relation to the patient's speech and voice production. The exam allows the voice pathologist to observe the patient's laryngeal area and whole body tension. This is accomplished through visually observing posture and neck muscle tension, as well as carefully digitally manipulating the thyroid cartilage. When tension is not present, the thyroid cartilage may be rocked gently back and forth in the neck. Laryngeal hyperfunction often contributes to laryngeal strap muscle tension, which precludes this rocking motion. The muscle tension often causes laryngeal area muscle aches or discomfort. Indeed, patients should be asked about laryngeal sensations because common symptoms associated with voice disorders include throat dryness, tickling, burning, aching, lump-in-the-throat, or thickness sensations. Finally, voice pathologists also should ask their patients whether any swallowing difficulties are present. This information will determine whether the swallowing function is affected by or is affecting vocal production. (See SR6.)

Evaluation of Voice Components

Goals: (1) Describe the present vocal components; (2) examine inappropriate use of vocal components.

The direct evaluation of voice is conducted to describe the present condition of voice production and to determine whether any vocal components are being used in a habitually inappropriate manner, contributing to the development or maintenance of the pathology. Each vocal component is examined separately following a general subjective description of voice quality.

Through the patient interview, the examiner has had an adequate sample of conversational voice to make a subjective description of the patient's voice quality. Several formal voice rating scales have been developed and utilized for perceptually judging voice quality.[10-13] One method used to report the degree of baseline dysphonia uses a 6-point, equal-appearing interval scale where (0) is normal, (1) mild, (2) mild to moderate, (3) moderate, (4) moderate to severe, and (5) severe dysphonia. This scaled description is followed, for the future reference of the examiner, by a descriptive characterization of the voice, including descriptive terms such as hoarseness, harshness, breathiness, raspiness, glottal fry, low pitch, and so on. (See SR7.)

A more formalized scale for evaluating hoarseness, "GRBAS," was developed by the Committee for Phonatory Function Tests of the Japan Society of Logopedics and Phoniatrics.[11] This scale evaluates five components of voice production: grade (G), rough (R), breathy (B), aesthenic (A), and strained (S). Each component is rated on a 4-point scale where "0" is normal, "1" is slight, "2" is moderate, and "3" is extreme.

Grade (G) represents the overall degree of hoarseness of voice abnormality. Rough (R) represents the perceptual impression of the irregularity of vocal fold vibrations. It corresponds to the irregular fluctuations in the fundamental frequency, the amplitude of vibration, or both. Breathy (B) represents the perceptual impression of the extent of air leakage through the glottis. Aesthenic (A) denotes weakness or lack of power in the voice. Strained (S) represents the perceptual impression of vocal hyperfunction.

As with all perceptual rating scales, "GRBAS" is subjective and depends on the trained clinical ear. Securing a tape recording of the pretreatment voice using a standard reading passage, such as *The Rainbow Passage*[14] (Appendix 5-2) for posttreatment comparison is advisable at this time. Following the perceptual description of voice production, each vocal property is then individually reviewed including:

■ **Respiration:** A description of conversational breathing patterns including supportive or nonsupportive thoracic or diaphragmatic breathing patterns. We have not observed the often-used term "clavicular" breathing in our patients. Use of limited breath support for phonation is determined through observation. The s/z ratio is formally tested in cases where vocal nodules are known to be present on the vocal folds.[15] The presence of laryngeal mass lesions will yield a longer voiceless /s/ than the voiced /z/ because of the inability of the folds to adequately approximate. Generally, ratios greater than 1:4 are considered abnormal. Several trials of each phoneme are conducted, and the patient is encouraged each time to give maximum effort in sustaining for as long as possible. In addition, they are coached to produce maximum inhalation. The usefulness of this method is most likely restricted to screening patients with vocal nodules.

Maximum phonation time (MPT) is also measured at a modal pitch level. MPT is often negatively affected by laryngeal pathology caused by inefficient vocal fold vibration. Therefore, pretest and posttest MPT measures may be used as a tool to demonstrate voice improvement.

However, phonatory airflow volume during MPT tasks is not well-correlated with actual measures of pulmonary function. For this reason, phonatory volume should not be accepted as an accurate estimate of lung volume. (See SR8.)

■ **Phonation:** Subjective observations regarding the actual voice onset, phonatory register, and strength of phonatory adduction may be made through critical listening. These observations may include the presence of hard glottal attacks, glottal fry, breathiness, or overly compressed adduction. These phonatory symptoms may be observed conversationally throughout the evaluation. The symptoms may also be rechecked by having the patient say the alphabet slowly and then more rapidly. (See SR9.)

■ **Resonance:** Observation regarding the type of resonance quality is made. When abnormal, the consistency and stimulability for normal production will be further tested. (See SR10.)

■ **Pitch:** The patient's present pitch range is tested by singing up and down the scale from mid-range voice in whole notes until the highest and lowest attainable notes have been identified. Usually, patients can benefit from both models and multiple trials to achieve best performance. Conversational inflection and pitch variability are also described. (See SR11.)

■ **Loudness:** The appropriateness of the patient's speaking loudness level and the variability of loudness, as observed during the interview, is described. It is also important to test the patient's ability to increase subglottic air pressure. This may be accomplished by asking the patient to shout *"Hey!"* We have found that the ability to produce a solid phonation during a shout, in the presence of a dysphonic conversational voice, is a positive prognostic sign. When the patient is able to override the dysphonia with increased intensity (which is determined by the ability of the folds to approximate tightly to increase subglottic air pressure), the disorder appears to respond more quickly to remediation methods. In contrast, determining the patient's ability to produce voice softly will demonstrate the efficiency or lack of efficiency of the vocal fold vibration. (See SR12.)

■ **Rate:** The rate of a patient's speech may contribute to the development of laryngeal pathology. This is especially true for the individual who speaks with an exceptionally fast rate of speech. As observed during the diagnostic workup, the speech rate may be described as normal, fast, or slow.

The rate may also be judged to be monotonous, and like pitch and loudness, rate may contribute to a lack of speech and voice variability. (See SR13 and Appendix 5-3.)

In reviewing each component of voice production, the voice pathologist must not only continually make note of the patient's current vocal behaviors, but must also probe for the best voice possible. Voice probing is a form of trial diagnostic therapy and can be done through reading, singing, chanting, or counting while shaping and experimenting with alternative methods of voice production. Habitual vocal habits and potential abilities are often not the same. The use of negative practice, even during this probing stage, can be revealing to the patient. In the end, the voice pathologist seeks to understand the performance gap between what the patient does habitually and what he or she potentially can do.

Impressions

Goal: To summarize the etiologic factors associated with the development and maintenance of the individual's voice disorder.

The impressions section of the diagnostic evaluation summarizes the causes of the voice disorder as determined through the evaluation. These causes are listed in order of perceived importance as they relate first to the initiation of the problem and second to the maintenance of the problem. Recall that the precipitating factor may not be the same as the maintenance factor. (See SR14.)

Prognosis

Goal: To analyze the probability of improvement through voice therapy.

The prognosis for improving many voice disorders through voice therapy is generally good. Nonetheless, many factors influence prognosis including the patient's motivation, interest, time available, ability to follow instructions, and physical and emotional status, to name a few. The prognosis statement permits the voice pathologist to give a subjective opinion regarding the chances for improved voice production based on the diagnostic information. A reasonable time frame for expected completion of the management program should also be stated. (See SR15.)

Recommendations

Goal: Outline the management plan.

The management plan is then briefly outlined based on the etiologic factors discovered during the evaluation and the medical examination. The outline will include the therapy approaches to be utilized and any additional referrals. (See SR16.)

Additional Considerations

The evaluation format we have presented is semistructured. The basic questions remain the same from patient to patient, but the answers given by individual patients dictate the direction in which the questions will proceed and the order in which each diagnostic section is reviewed. Although the beginning clinician may choose a more structured format, such as a questionnaire, the semistructured method is preferred because it allows a more patient-direct approach to diagnosis.

The diagnostic report should include only the information pertinent to the development and maintenance of the voice disorder, as well as the projected plan of care. Referring physicians are not interested in the patient's life history. Indeed, most physicians turn directly to the sections on impressions and recommendations, which justifies the need for a detailed explanation of the problem and the plan of care.

Some voice pathologists prefer to tape record the entire diagnostic session for later review. This review may help determine the exact vocal components produced during the evaluation and serves as a record of the baseline voice quality. Even when the entire diagnostic session is not recorded, recording of a standard speech sample is necessary for later reference. It is not unusual for the voice pathologist and the patient to forget the actual severity of the baseline voice quality. Tape recordings serve as an objective reminder and should be used liberally throughout the treatment course.

Finally, the American Speech-Language-Hearing Association mandates that patients who undergo speech, language, and voice evaluations must have a current hearing screening. Audiometric evaluation is important for the patient with a voice disorder. The inability to monitor voice well may result in the use of inappropriate vocal components. Severe voice disorders are often observed in the hard-of-hearing and deaf populations.

Patient Self-analysis of the Voice Disorder

This chapter has been designed to demonstrate to the voice pathologist the steps of the perceptual diagnostic voice evaluation. Another important aspect of the evaluation process is to gain an understanding of the functional impact of the voice disorder on the individual in daily life. Those in clinical practice know that different patients will perceive similar voice disorders differently. For example, a singer with a vocal nodule may be devastated by the effect that the nodule has on the voice, whereas a computer programmer may not consider the mild hoarseness to be a problem. One method of gaining this functional measure is through the use of the Voice Handicap Index (VHI), a test battery that has been statistically validated and is used in a wide variety of voice centers[16] (Appendix 5-4).

This instrument, completed before and after treatment by the patient, permits an understanding of the handicapping nature of the voice disorder as perceived by the patient. The 30-item VHI examines self-perceived voice severity as related to functional, physical, and emotional issues. The functional scale includes statements that describe the impact of the patient's voice disorder on daily activities. The physical scale contains statements representing self-perceptions of laryngeal discomfort and voice output characteristics. The emotional scale consists of statements representing the patient's affective responses to the voice disorder. A 5-point scale is used to rate each statement as it reflects the patient's experience with the voice disorder. The ratings of the 30 statements are totaled for both pretreatment and posttreatment scales. Any shift of 18 points or more represents a significant shift in the patient's psychosocial functioning, as related to the voice disorder.

We have found the use of the VHI to be an extremely valuable addition to the voice evaluation protocol. It provides great insight into the patient's perception of the voice disorder and serves as a natural point of departure in discussing the disorder and its impact on the patient.

Summary

Diagnosis is probably the most important single aspect of a remedial program.[1 (p108)]

A systematic diagnostic voice evaluation is important for all types of voice disorders, with minor modifications in the format made as needed to accommodate individual patients. The major goals are to

■ discover the causes of the voice disorder,
■ describe the present vocal components, and
■ determine the direction for intervention, if warranted.

Finally, the diagnostic voice evaluation teaches and educates the patient about the disorder. In this manner, the evaluation tool may be viewed in its own right as a primary therapy tool.

The goal of describing the vocal components has been greatly enhanced with the use of more objective procedures and techniques for assessing voice function. Chapter 6 introduces instrumental voice measurement techniques, including acoustic analysis, aerodynamic measurement, and laryngeal imaging. When combined with findings from the more subjective voice evaluation, these instrumental techniques have greatly enhanced the evaluation of voice disorders.

Appendix 5-1

Sample Report

Name: _____   Type of Case: Bilateral vocal fold nodules

Age: 44 years   Address: _____

Date of Birth: 2-14-50   Phone: _____

Date: 4-22-94   Examiner: JCS

SR1   **Referral:** The patient was referred by _____, MD, otolaryngologist, Dayton, Ohio.

SR2   **Reason for Referral:** The patient was referred for both evaluation and treatment with a diagnosis of small, bilateral vocal fold nodules and possible reflux laryngitis.

SR3   **History of the Problem:** The patient reported first experiencing vocal difficulties in April, 1993. At that time, she contracted a cold that created an excessive amount of coughing and throat clearing. She then experienced dysphonia, which persisted after the cold symptoms resolved. Another cold was experienced over the Labor Day weekend, at which time the patient became aphonic for two days. This motivated her to seek the medical examination. The patient reported that her voice quality is currently better in the morning and worsens with use as the day progresses. An increased amount of hoarseness has been noted following church choir rehearsals. Motivation for modifying these vocal difficulties appeared to be high because of the patient's vocal needs in her work setting.

SR4   **Medical History:** The patient was hospitalized in 1979 for a tonsillectomy and in 1981 for a complete hysterectomy. Chronic disorders reported by the patient included excessive sinus drainage, which creates coughing and throat clearing and nightly heartburn, which is exacerbated by stress and nervousness. The patient reported that she presently takes no medications and that she stopped smoking 3 weeks prior to this evaluation. Her liquid intake was poor and consisted of mostly caffeinated products. She previously smoked one package of cigarettes per day for 22 years. On a day-to-day basis, the patient reported that she generally felt "good."

SR5   **Social History:** Mrs. _____ was divorced in 1984 and has four children, ages 20, 21, 22, and 25 years. Three children still live at home. She is a civilian employee at Wright Patterson Air Force Base where she works as an Equal Employment Opportunity program manager. This position involves managing a federal woman's job program, career counseling of female employees, and the conduction of management relations seminars. Much speaking is required on a daily basis, which the patient continued during the initial cold and the onset of dysphonia.

Nonwork interests and activities include playing the piano, singing in the church choir, teaching Sunday School to pre-schoolers, conducting church youth meetings, sewing, and reading. The patient reported that singing, teaching Sunday school, and the youth meetings all tax her voice, creating increased dysphonia. Mrs. _____ also admitted to some shouting in the home environment. Other than job tension, no emotional difficulties were reported.

SR6   **Oral-Peripheral Examination:** The structure and function of the oral mechanism appeared to be well within normal limits for speech and voice production. Laryngeal sensations reported included dryness, burning, occasional pain, and a "lump-in-the-throat feeling." The patient reported having difficulty swallowing pills. Food and liquids were swallowed well. Laryngeal area muscle tension was not noted subjectively.

Voice Evaluation

SR7   **General Quality:** The patient demonstrated a mild dysphonia characterized by breathiness and intermittent glottal fry phonation. She further reported that the voice quality worsened with use and toward the end of every day.

SR8   **Respiration:** A supportive, thoracic breathing pattern was demonstrated. The patient was able to sustain the /a/ for 14 seconds, the /s/ for 27 seconds, and the /z/ for 22 seconds.

SR9   **Phonation:** Occasional glottal fry phonation and breathiness were noted. No hard glottal attacks were observed.

SR10   **Resonance:** Normal.

SR11   **Pitch:** The patient demonstrated an almost two-octave pitch range with good inflection and variability noted conversationally. Habitual pitch level was within normal limits for the patient's gender and age.

SR12   **Loudness:** Loudness was appropriate for the speaking situation. The patient was readily able to increase loudness to a shout.

SR13 **Rate:** Normal.

SR14 **Impressions:** It is my impression that this patient presents with a voice disorder with a primary etiology of voice abuse. These include the abusive behaviors of
  (1) coughing and throat clearing that have persisted since recovering from the April cold
  (2) straining the voice while singing and
  (3) raising the voice during youth meetings and in her home.

  Secondary precipitating factors include
  (1) the contribution of gastroesophageal reflux
  (2) poor hydration
  (3) the necessity to speak excessively on a daily basis in the presence of the current dysphonia
  (4) the use of breathy phonation and
  (5) general weakness and imbalance of the laryngeal musculature.

SR15 **Prognosis:** The prognosis for modifying these etiologic factors and resolving the laryngeal pathology is good. Based on the small size of the nodules, the continued fluctuation of the voice quality, and the patient's apparent desire to return to normal voicing. Estimated time for completion of the vocal management program is 8 to 10 weeks.

SR16 **Recommendations:** It is recommended that the patient enroll in a weekly voice therapy program with therapy focusing on:
  (1) vocal hygiene counseling
  (2) elimination of the abusive behavior of habit throat clearing
  (3) Vocal Function Exercises designed to balance respiration, phonation, and resonance
  (4) formal hydration program.

In addition, the patient will return to her family physician to discuss the possibility of being placed on an antireflux regimen.

Appendix 5-2

Rainbow Passage

When the sunlight strikes raindrops in the air, they act like a prism and form a rainbow. The rainbow is a division of white light into many beautiful colors. These take the shape of a long round arch, with its path high above, and its two ends apparently beyond the horizon. There is, according to legend, a boiling pot of gold at one end. People look, but no one ever finds it. When a man looks for something beyond his reach, his friends say he is looking for the pot of gold at the end of the rainbow.

Appendix 5-3

Vocal Component Checklist

Breathing Pattern

Clavicular ☐
Thoracic ☐
Abdominal-diaphragmatic ☐

Supportive ☐   Nonsupportive ☐
/s/ ☐   /z/ ☐

Phonation

Voice onset: hard glottal attack ☐
aspirate attack ☐
static attack ☐
Registration: glottal fry ☐
loft ☐
modal ☐

Resonance

Hypernasal ☐
Denasal ☐
Cul-de-sac ☐
Assimilative ☐
Normal ☐

Pitch

High ☐
Low ☐
Poor variability ☐
Normal ☐

Loudness

Too loud ☐
Too soft ☐
Poor variability ☐
Normal ☐
Ability to shout   yes ☐   no ☐

Rate

Too fast ☐
Too slow ☐
Poor variability ☐
Normal ☐

Appendix 5-4

Voice Handicap Index (VHI), Henry Ford Hospital

Instructions: These are statements that many people have used to describe their voices and the effects of their voices on their lives. Circle the response that indicates how frequently you have the same experience.

		Never	Almost Never	Sometimes	Almost Always	Always
Fl.	My voice makes it difficult for people to hear me.	1	2	3	4	5
P2.	I run out of air when I talk.	1	2	3	4	5
F3.	People have difficulty understanding me in a noisy room.	1	2	3	4	5
P4.	The sound of my voice varies throughout the day.	1	2	3	4	5
F5.	My family has difficulty hearing me when I call them throughout the house.	1	2	3	4	5
F6.	I use the phone less often than I would like.	1	2	3	4	5
E7.	I'm tense when talking with others because of my voice.	1	2	3	4	5
F8.	I tend to avoid groups of people because of my voice.	1	2	3	4	5
E9.	People seem irritated with my voice.	1	2	3	4	5
P10.	People ask, "What's wrong with your voice?"	1	2	3	4	5
F11.	I speak with friends, neighbors, or relatives less often because of my voice.	1	2	3	4	5
F12.	People ask me to repeat myself when speaking face-to-face.	1	2	3	4	5
P13.	My voice sounds creaky and dry.	1	2	3	4	5

	Never	Almost Never	Sometimes	Almost Always	Always
P14. I feel as though I have to strain to produce voice.	1	2	3	4	5
E15. I find other people don't understand my voice problem.	1	2	3	4	5
F16. My voice difficulties restrict my personal and social life.	1	2	3	4	5
P17. The clarity of my voice is unpredictable.	1	2	3	4	5
P18. I try to change my voice to sound different.	1	2	3	4	5
F19. I feel left out of conversations because of my voice.	1	2	3	4	5
P20. I use a great deal of effort to speak.	1	2	3	4	5
P21. My voice is worse in the evening.	1	2	3	4	5
F22. My voice problem causes me to lose income.	1	2	3	4	5
E23. My voice problem upsets me.	1	2	3	4	5
E24. I am less outgoing because of my voice problem.	1	2	3	4	5
E25. My voice makes me feel handicapped.	1	2	3	4	5
P26. My voice "gives out" on me in the middle of speaking.	1	2	3	4	5
E27. I feel annoyed when people ask me to repeat.	1	2	3	4	5
E28. I feel embarrassed when people ask me to repeat.	1	2	3	4	5
E29. My voice makes me feel incompetent.	1	2	3	4	5
E30. I'm ashamed of my voice problem.	1	2	3	4	5

Note: The letter preceding each item number corresponds to the subscale (E = emotional subscales, F = functional subscales, P = physical subscale).

Reprinted with permission from *American Journal of Speech-Language Pathology* (1997;6:66-70). Copyright 1997 by American Journal of Speech-Language Pathology.

References

1. Moore P. *Organic Voice Disorders*. Englewood Cliffs, NJ: Prentice-Hall; 1971.
2. Stemple J. *Voice Therapy: Clinical Studies*. St Louis, Mo: Mosby Year Book; 1993.
3. Herrington-Hall B, Lee L, Stemple J, Niemi K, McHone M. Description of laryngeal pathologies by age, sex, and occupation in a treatment seeking sample. *J Speech Hear Disord*. 1988;53:57-65.
4. Coyle S. *Incidence of Laryngeal Pathology in a Treatment Seeking Population* [master's thesis]. Oxford, Ohio: Miami University; 1999.
5. Cooper M. *Modern Techniques of Vocal Rehabilitation*. Springfield, Ill: Charles C Thomas; 1973.
6. Koufman J, Isaacson G. The spectrum of vocal dysfunction. *Otolaryngol Clin North Am: Voice Disorders*. 1991;24:985-988.
7. Sander E. Arguments against the aggressive pursuit of voice treatment for children. *Lang Speech Hear Serv Sch*. 1989;20:94-101.
8. Blood G, Mahan B, Hyman M. Judging personality and appearance from voice disorders. *Comm Disord*. 1979;12:63-67.
9. Yanagasawa E. Yanagasawa R. Laryngeal photography. *Otolaryngol Clin North Am: Voice Disorders*. 1991;24:999-1022.
10. Gelfer M. Perceptual attributes of voice: development and use of rating scales. *J Voice*. 1988;2:320-326.
11. Hirano M. *Clinical Examination of Voice*. New York, NY: Springer Verlag; 1981.
12. Wilson D. *Voice Problems of Children*. 2nd ed. Baltimore, Md: Williams and Wilkins; 1979.
13. Wilson F. The voice disordered child: a descriptive approach. *Lang Speech Hear Serv Sch*. 1970;4:14-22
14. Fairbanks G. *Voice and Articulation Handbook*. New York, NY: Harper & Row; 1960.
15. Eckel F, Boone D. The s/z ratio as an indicator of laryngeal pathology. *J Speech Hear Disord*. 1981;46:147-149.
16. Jacobson B, Johnson A, Grywalski C, Silbergleit A, Jacobson G, Benninger M, Newman C. The voice handicap index (VHI): development and validation. *Am J Speech Lang Pathol*. 1997;6:66-70.

6

Instrumental Measurement of Voice

No instrument can replace the clinical judgment required to integrate knowledge about case history, perceptual voice quality, and behavioral observation. Nonetheless, instrumental measures of voice production have made valuable contributions to voice evaluation protocols and augment the findings from traditional voice assessment methods. The most common instruments in a clinical voice laboratory assess voice production through one of three broad approaches: analyzing the acoustic signal, measuring aerodynamic changes in pressure or flow, or recording visual images of vocal fold vibration. All three of these approaches are indirect measures of voice production through which voice clinicians and researchers attempt to make accurate inferences about underlying laryngeal and vocal fold physiology and behavior. If used appropriately, clinical voice instrumentation may supply a critical contribution to diagnostic and treatment efforts by providing information about the respiratory, laryngeal, and acoustic contributions to voice production.

In the past two decades, voice clinicians and researchers have witnessed a rapid explosion of new technology designed to measure physiologic events related to voice production. As the speed, memory, and affordability of microprocessing capabilities have increased, research and development of clinically applicable voice measurement tools have expanded. The professional partnerships between voice pathologists and otolaryngologists have also contributed to the clinical utility of enhanced laryngeal imaging and video recording techniques.[1-6] The purpose of this chapter is to examine measurement instruments common to clinical voice laboratories and to discuss the scientific principles that underlie their development, application, and interpretation.

Unfortunately, the existence of a well-outfitted supply of speech and voice analysis tools does not necessarily mean better reliability or validity of so-called "objective" measures. Indeed, the utility and application of any tool is only as appropriate as the user's knowledge. Although product developers and vendors provide continual upgrades in the quality and accessibility of their devices, they necessarily maintain a marketing and business interest that may not always coincide with the best needs of the individual clinician or researcher. Because commercial and technological advances will continue to refine and broaden the range of tools available, this discussion addresses general principles, equipment, and measurement techniques without making specific reference to products in the marketplace.

If clinicians are to use instrumental voice measurements, the information provided must contribute to the diagnosis, etiology, severity, prognosis, or measurable change in the phonatory disorder.[2,3,6-8] The utility of instrumental measures can be assessed on four levels of clinical application: (1) detection, (2) severity, (3) diagnosis, and (4) treatment. Can the voice measurement validly and reliably:

- Identify the existence of a voice problem (detection)?
- Assess the severity or stage of progression of the voice problem (severity)?
- Identify the differential source of the voice problem (diagnosis)?
- Serve as a primary treatment tool, for behavioral modification, biofeedback, or patient education (treatment)?

The clinical validity of instrumental measures is essential to appropriate application of these measures. Nonetheless, evaluation of instrument efficacy is a complex task because clinical voice measurements represent a wide range of tools, analysis routines, and recording protocols. Furthermore, many vocal function measures have limited normative data available to ensure reasonable interpretations or comparisons across laboratories.[6,8,9] Finally, all equipment is subject to artifact and error, especially when calibration techniques are either unspecified or not adopted rigorously. A need for standardization of measurement techniques is recognized clearly among voice pathologists and scientists.[3-5,9-11]

Clinical Utility

The clinical voice pathologist is faced with many choices in vocal function measures, yet limited time and resources for testing, analysis, and interpretation(Table 6-1). To help determine the most useful tools and measures among the large array of options, Bless[8] offered several considerations for clinicians:

- Does the instrument pose restraints on the speech mechanism during the measurement process? Is the speech product sufficiently representative of typical behavior? For example, equipment or speech task artifacts (eg, tight-fitting face masks, rigid endoscopes in the mouth, sustained /i/ vowel) may limit or alter the voice production so that it is no longer representative of the voice pathology.
- Have the recording equipment, procedures, and analysis routines demonstrated reliability across time?
- Are there adequate normative references to allow useful comparison and interpretation of the resulting data?
- Are the protocols efficient and cost effective?

No measurement technique will satisfy all of these criteria. Clinicians must be aware of the limits of any particular measure to avoid inappropriate or misleading interpretations.

Often, voice laboratory equipment and measurements are described favorably as "objective," "documentable," "high resolution," and "noninvasive." Nonetheless, the user must always

Table 6-1. Instrumental Measures in the Voice Laboratory

Technique	Information
Stroboscopic imaging of the larynx	Gross structure
	Gross movements
	Vibratory characteristics
Acoustic recording and analysis	Fundamental frequency
	Intensity
	Signal/harmonics to noise ratio
	Perturbation measures
	Spectral features (spectrograms and line spectra)
Aerodynamic measurement	Airflow rate and volume
	Subglottal (intraoral) pressure
	Phonation threshold pressure
	Laryngeal resistance
Electroglottography (EGG)	Measure of vocal fold contact area
Electromyography (EMG)	Direct measures of muscle activity

recognize that all noninvasive voice laboratory measurements are indirect estimates of vocal function. The few direct measures of vocal function, such as direct measures of tracheal pressure or percutaneous laryngeal electromyography (muscle activity), are invasive and require needle placements and collaboration with an otolaryngologist or neurologist. Although clinicians can make judicious inferences about voice quality or laryngeal status from indirect measures, they must always interpret them with caution and cross validate them with a perceptual and visual monitor of speech and voice behaviors. Consider, for example, a patient who is referred for evaluation of incomplete glottic closure. The patient sounds severely breathy and has limited phonation time apparently caused by excessive glottal airflow leak. If airflow measurements are taken and fall within a normal range, then these findings should be viewed cautiously because the information is a complete mismatch with the other clinical impressions. Was the airflow mask applied securely? Is the airflow device calibrated accurately? Although instrumental measures will not always support our clinical and perceptual biases, they should not be accepted in exclusion of all clinical judgment.

Selecting acoustic equipment can be particularly confusing because of the broad range of analysis routines and measurement capabilities. Several key considerations may assist the clinician in defining the most important priorities for an individual setting:

- How is the system to be used? Will the overall purpose serve clinic, research, or teaching purposes?
- What specific analysis capabilities are desired?
- Are these measures to be integrated with other speech measurement signals, such as airflow, pressure, EGG signal, and kinematics?
- What equipment limits are posed by cost, technical support, and speed of the measures?
- Does the package include normative information specific to this equipment?
- Is there evidence of the comparability of data measures across laboratories to enhance the standardization and interpretability of findings?
- Are there particular clinical macros or test routines that can serve as a convenient framework for developing a user-friendly and standard clinical analysis protocol?

These and other considerations may all play a role in selecting specific acoustic measurement tools.[11-13]

Basics of Technical Instruments

Clinicians who first are learning about voice laboratory instrumentation will benefit from both coursework and many supportive textbook references that explain the general principles of electronics, physics, and mechanics underlying the process of signal measurement using voice laboratory tools.[4,14,15] These sources guide the reader in understanding the science and artifact of clinical voice laboratory instruments in greater detail than allowable in a clinical voice text. A basic introduction to general concepts and terms is included here.

Essentially, speech and voice measures rely on three events: signal detection, signal manipulation or conditioning, and signal reconversion.[14] In these three processes, the physical phenomenon is:

- detected and input by a device, such as a microphone, pressure transducer, flow meter, or electrode;
- manipulated in some form, such as filtering, amplification, or editing, for use with a specific type of equipment or analysis routine; and
- reconverted for output and display in some readable form, such as a numerical value, oscilloscope tracing, or speaker.

Because most voice measurement equipment relies on a series of inputs and outputs between electronic components (eg, microphone to computer to speaker), users must become familiar with some of the technical specifications of standard equipment. Each connection between components may potentially transmit error in signal accuracy. When individual electronic components are arranged, it is essential to attend to the proper sequence and technical requirements of each connection to ensure that error is not inadvertently transmitted along the component pathways.

Microphones

For acoustic measurement, signal detection generally begins with a microphone. Vibrating sound waves oscillate against an internal diaphragm or other sensing device that has electronic connections to an amplifier and, eventually, an output device, such as a monitor, oscilloscope, or speaker. The free-field, sound-pressure–level energy excites the microphone's internal diaphragm, changing acoustic sound energy into mechanical energy, then changing it again into electronic energy for transmission through the system. The process of changing energy from one form to another is called transduction, and any device that converts the energy is called a transducer. This electrical energy can then be connected to other clinical instruments for recording and subsequent analysis.[14]

When selecting a microphone for clinical recordings of voice quality, several technical specifications are useful to verify the capacity and limits of a microphone. Following a series of methodological studies, Titze and others have determined the optimal recommendations for microphone specifications to ensure reliable recording of the speech and voice signal, especially for subsequent acoustic analysis.[11,16] These recommendations suggest that a professional grade, condenser-type microphone with unidirectional or cardioid filtering characteristics is preferred. The microphone should be positioned off center from the mouth to avoid excessive aspirate noise from the mouth. Microphones should be positioned at a constant mouth-to-microphone distance of approximately 3 to 8 cm for sustained vowels, although longer distances may be acceptable for connected speech tasks. Recordings should be conducted in a controlled sound environment with ambient noise of less than 50 dB.[11,16] Finally, it has been shown that analog tape recorders of all varieties (cassette, reel-to-reel, and others) appear to introduce excessive mechanical error. Consequently, speech signals that are to be saved for subsequent acoustic analysis should be stored on a digital audio-tape (DAT) recorder or directly on computer files.[11,17-19]

Technical Specifications

Clinicians who are evaluating microphones and other electronic components for use in the voice laboratory will wish to have a basic understanding of various technical specifications that describe the equipment's signal processing capacity.

- **Amplification** means increasing the magnitude of a signal for capture and processing by a piece of equipment.
- **Gain** is the exact magnitude of the amplification, usually expressed as ratio of signal input to signal output (after amplification).
- The **linearity** of an amplifier is the degree to which gain is constant across all input magnitudes. For example, the amplifier gain across a speech signal should be equal across

all frequencies. If the amplifier characteristic is nonlinear, then distortions of the speech signal will be produced because some frequencies will be amplified disproportionally to others.

■ When the amount of amplification (gain) exceeds the linear limits of the microphone, a distortion called **peak clipping** occurs. In this situation, the amplitude peaks of the waveform are literally cut off or flattened, and the resulting acoustic signal is both incomplete and inaccurate.

■ The **frequency response** of a component refers to the range of frequencies that can be detected. If the frequency range is too small to accommodate the entire speech signal, then the signal will be distorted. Frequency response is commonly expressed as a range (eg, 20 to 20000 Hz) and can apply to microphones, recording devices, and speakers.

■ **Impedance** refers to the electronic current available at the output and input ports of different components. To avoid distortion, the input and output impedances must match. Without this interface matching, errors in the resolution and accuracy of the signal will be passed to the second component, resulting in inaccuracies in the final signal presented for analysis. A typical impedance standard for electronic components is 200 Ohms.[14]

Filters are used in speech signal processing to make certain that the frequency ranges of interest are "passed through" for analysis. Filtering characteristics define the process of reshaping the acoustic waveform to eliminate selected energy above or below a certain frequency range. Filtering is another form of signal conditioning that prepares it for subsequent analysis. While research applications may designate highly specific filtering needs, most clinical voice tools have a preselected (or recommended) filter designed for clinical voice analysis. Nonetheless, for filtering and for all other technical specifications, it is important for the clinician to understand what limits are established by various instrumental tools.[14,15]

■ **Low pass filters** allow energy in the lower frequencies to be passed through (high-frequency energy excluded).

■ **High pass filters** allow the high-frequency energy to pass through (excluding low-frequency energy).

▨ **Band pass filters** will only admit energy within a certain range (band) and excludes frequencies above and below that range.

Electrical Error and Safety

If possible, clinicians who are working in clinical voice laboratories should seek professional advice from biomedical technology services or other appropriate support personnel to assist with accurate equipment setup. These personnel can provide routine electronic and safety checks, recommend strategies to troubleshoot equipment problems, and ensure that both equipment and procedures meet safety standards appropriate for the voice laboratory site and equipment. Although facilities may have individual institutional requirements for electronic equipment control, some general recommendations for electronic setup and safety apply to all settings. Cables and wiring should be sufficiently strong and devoid of any breaks or weaknesses to allow accurate transmission of the current (signal) and should be checked periodically for line continuity. Usually, cables should be coaxial or triaxial and well insulated to avoid functioning as an antenna by picking up extraneous electrical signals or 60-cycle (60 Hz) noise from other electrical equipment in the room (eg, lights, lamps, heating units, etc). Cables should also be long enough to connect various components without stretching or bending the connections, but not overly long because the longer the cable, the greater the resistance along its path, and the greater the likelihood for increased error to be transmitted.[14]

Because clinical voice laboratories utilize electronic equipment, certain precautions are needed to protect the patient, the clinician, and the equipment in the voice laboratory. Always use grounded (three-prong) plugs for all electrical equipment. If old, ungrounded (two-prong) plugs or outlets are still present in the laboratory, have them replaced. Never use a two-prong adapter to override a three-prong plug in an ungrounded outlet. Fuses should be replaced carefully, using the exact size and strength recommended by the manufacturer. If a piece of equipment blows fuses repeatedly, the source of electrical overload must be examined and repaired. Fuses should never be replaced with a larger size to avoid blowout; this tactic only masks the real problem and can create dangerous electrical safety conditions. Patients must be protected from inappropriate grounding and low-resistance current. Equipment should be stored on nonmetal racks, if possible. If water is used in the laboratory, it should not be exposed to electrical wiring. Never use any equipment that shows signs of distressed wiring (cracks, taped connections, breaks in insulation seal). The wiring and electrical connections between the many components in a voice laboratory should be appropriately labeled and stored off the ground. Wires that are repeatedly pulled, stretched, stepped on, or rolled over will be easily damaged, which creates unnecessary repair expense and a potential electrical hazard.[4,14]

Hygienic Safety

All laboratory equipment that comes in contact with patients must be sterilized as recommended by the manufacturer. Whenever possible, disposable items should be used (eg, airflow tubes), despite the increased expense and waste. Most facilities have medical hygiene standards committees that can assist the voice laboratory in achieving compliance with the institutional requirements for safe precautions in clinical procedures and for equipment sterilization. The clinician, too, must practice stringent and rigid adherence to hygiene. Currently, voice laboratories are recommended to utilize Universal Precautions guidelines, as established by Occupational Safety and Health Administration (OSHA).[4,20] This includes thorough handwashing before and after having contact with a patient, and using gloves during any procedure that puts the clinician's hands or equipment (eg, endoscope) in contact with any mucous membrane of the mouth, nose, throat, or ears.[4] In some circumstances, additional guidelines are appropriate to protect patients or clinicians from infectious disease transmission by wearing eye shields or surgical masks. Whenever a patient is immunocompromised or otherwise at risk for transmission of airborne disease, it is appropriate to secure qualified advice from health care professionals to ensure patient safety.

Routine cleaning should be performed to maintain hygiene in the clinical voice laboratory, including equipment, racks, furniture, floors, and handwashing area. Sterilization of all equipment is required according to both institutional and product guidelines. Rigid and flexible endoscopes must be washed and soaked in an antimicrobial solution for prescribed periods after every use. Recommendations for antimicrobial sterilization do change as guidelines are updated and adopted by biomedical safety personnel. It is always essential to verify that the cleaning and sterilization procedures for a clinical voice laboratory are in maximum compliance with current recommended standards.

Digital Signal Processing

The basis for current acoustic analysis capabilities is digital processing of the speech signal, which has been described by Kent and Read.[15] Speech and voice signals travel in sound pressure waves that are composed of a series of compressions and rarefactions of air molecules, radiated from lips, teeth, and mouth. Sound waves are analog signals because they are continuous and time varying. These sound waves are registered by a microphone, which converts the sound pressure energy into an electrical signal. To then convert this continuous analog electrical signal into a digital (numeric) format for computer recording and digital speech processing, it must be divided up into small, discrete bits of information that can be represented numerically. This process is called digitization and is achieved by a hardware device called an analog-to-digital (A/D) board or converter. When a signal is digitized, it is divided up or "discretized" for numerical representation; the process must record the change in this continuous signal across time. Two important parameters are of interest. First, the time-varying component, as seen on the horizontal axis, represents the changes in signal characteristics across the duration of the signal. Second, the amplitude units, as displayed on the vertical axis, represent changes in signal height at any given moment. These components are converted from analog to digital form using two operations conducted simultaneously: **sampling rate** and **quantization level**. These processes will be described in greater detail in the next section. Together, sampling and quantization operations determine the adequacy of the conversion from a continuous analog signal to a digitized waveform. Fortunately, most computer-processing capabilities now have enough speed and memory to accurately digitize the speech signal according to minimum guidelines.

Kent and Read[15] described five steps in the analog-to-digital process. These steps incorporate both signal conditioning (filtering) and conversion (sampling and quantization).

Signal Conditioning

1. **Pre-emphasis**: In the speech signal, low-frequency energy is greater than high-frequency energy and can disproportionally dominate the acoustic analysis. To avoid this artifact, pre-emphasis is applied as a normalizing procedure, designed to equalize the strength of acoustic energy across all speech frequencies. In speech, the frequencies that need pre-emphasis usually fall between 100 and 1000 Hertz.

2. **Presampling filter**: The speech signal also contains a range of high frequencies, therefore, the digitizing process must be capable of sampling all of the frequencies of interest. To be certain that all of the frequencies are sampled accurately, a safeguard technique is used. This technique was first described by Nyquist, who determined that for valid sampling, the sampling rate must be *double the highest frequency of interest*. Thus, presampling is a low pass filter, designed to exclude high-frequency energy above the highest frequency of interest. Without this step, extraneous high frequencies could add unwanted error to the digitized acoustic waveform.

Digital Conservation

3. **Sampling**: Recall that to convert the analog speech signal to digital form, the continuous waveform must be divided into many discrete points, with each point assigned a numeric value. The intervals between points are eliminated, so it is critical that enough sampling points are included to faithfully reconstruct the analog waveform in digital format. The Nyquist theorem requires the sampling rate to be high enough to ensure that every frequency of interest is sam-

pled at least twice. In other words, the sampling rate must be twice the highest frequency of interest. An important source of error for digitization is in undersampling or "overwide" spacing between sampling points. This under-sampling can lead to an artifact known as *aliasing*, where high-frequency information is misrepresented because of too few sampling points. In other words, aliasing is an arti-fact created when high-frequency signals are misrepresent-ed as lower frequency events because of inadequate sam-pling rates. Current recommendations for sampling rates in acoustic analysis range from a minimum of 20 kHz (suffi-cient to sample frequencies of interest up to 10 kHz), but some digitizing routines adopt higher sampling rates up to 100 kHz. In other words, the original analog signal is "sam-pled" at least 20 000 times per second.

4. **Quantization**: This process converts amplitude height into discrete numerical values in a manner similar to the sam-pling process. The continuously varying amplitude wave-form is divided into small increments of amplitude height. These selected increments are converted to digital represen-tation. It is important that sufficient quantization levels (variations in height) are available to accurately reconstruct the amplitude heights. The greater number of quantization levels, the better representation of amplitude changes in the original analog signal. A similar type of error can occur if the quantization levels are too few and amplitude changes are insufficiently replicated in the digital signal. The num-ber of quantization levels available is determined by con-version "bits." Most computer systems are capable of the recommended level of 16 bits of amplitude quantization, which is equivalent to 65 456 different amplitude incre-ments or levels.

5. **Encoding**: This is the final process in the steps that convert, or digitize, the continuous analog signal to numerical repre-sentation so that it can be stored by computers for recall and a variety of acoustic analyses.

Although higher sampling rates and greater quantization levels improve the representation of the analog signal, they also require greater computer speed and memory. For this reason, the minimal standards for sampling rate and quantization level have increased as microprocessing capabilities have expanded. Once the analog signal has been successfully converted to digital format, it is prepared for subsequent acoustic analysis. An outstanding description of signal digitization is described by Kent and Read.[15]

Acoustic Measurements

Acoustic measures of voice production provide objective and noninvasive measures of vocal function. These measures are increasingly affordable, allowing more voice pathologists the opportunity to use them to document voice status across time. Figure 6-1 shows an acoustic analysis system for recording, storing, and analyzing the speech signal. Although normative information for acoustic measures is not complete, many acoustic measurement tools provide some guidelines for comparison so

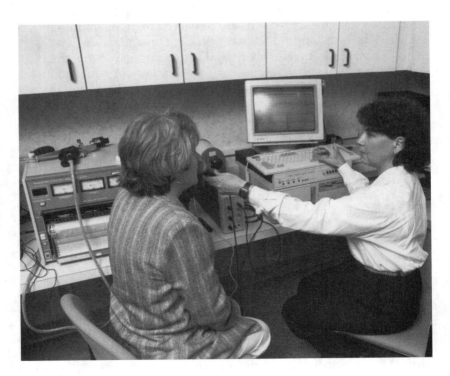

Figure 6-1. An acoustic analysis system for recording, storing, and analyzing the speech signal. (Rick Berkey, Dayton, Ohio)

that a user can discriminate normal performance from abnormal ranges based on that equipment. The validity of acoustic measures can be assessed on three levels:

■ Can the measure(s) discriminate a normal voice from a pathologic voice?
■ What association exists between acoustic measures and the clinical standard, audio-perceptual judgments of voice quality?
■ Are measures sufficiently stable to assess change in performance across time?

Before one can answer these questions, it is important to recognize that acoustic measures consist of a wide range of approaches to analyzing the voice signal. There is a large (and ever-increasing) number of acoustic measures, many of which are mathematical derivations of five common features. These measures are:

■ **fundamental frequency**, which is an acoustic measure of the perceptual judgment of pitch
■ **intensity**, which is an acoustic measure of the perceptual judgment of loudness
■ **perturbation measures**, which assess the cycle-to-cycle variation in the acoustic signal for either frequency or amplitude of the waveform
■ a **ratio of signal (or harmonic energy)-to-noise**, which is intended to reflect the relative contribution of periodic and aperiodic (noisy) components of the acoustic signal
■ various **spectral features**, which provide indications of the contribution of the supraglottic vocal tract to the voice signal.

Each of these measures will be described in greater detail in this chapter. Although some of these acoustic measures have been shown to successfully discriminate normal from disordered voice quality, the agreement between acoustic measures and audio-perceptual ratings of voice quality remains inconsistent.[21-32]

Another factor that has limited the standardization and interpretability of acoustic measures over the years is actually a sign of progress. The continual improvements in microprocessing speed and accuracy during the past 20 years have fostered the development of so many new mathematical algorithms and processing approaches to acoustic analysis that assessing new measures is difficult as older techniques become obsolete.[3,5,33-35] Other limits to clean interpretation of acoustic measures are common to all clinical assessment tools, for example:

- What are the optimal elicitation and recording tasks?
- How does one account for the known intrasubject variability and achieve stable baseline data?
- How many samples are needed for reliability?
- What lengths of speech or voice segment are required?

Nonetheless, the largest contribution of acoustic measures to the clinical process appears to be their success in measuring change in vocal productions *across time* within a patient's course of evaluation and treatment.[36-39] Comparison of pretreatment and posttreatment acoustic measures may serve two purposes. At diagnosis, they may allow an indirect inference about the severity of the voice pathology and reflect the status of vocal function generally, even if they do not relate specifically to various etiologies.[40] To date, no acoustic measure purports to differentially diagnose the source of the voice pathology. Secondly, these measures help evaluate the effects of the rehabilitation plan across time.

Pitch Detection Algorithm

A starting point for acoustic analysis is to determine the fundamental frequency of a given signal. This process is known commonly as "pitch detection." In normal speakers, the digitized acoustic waveform reveals a complex, but quasi-periodic repetition of pitch periods across time. The purpose of pitch detection is to identify and extract the pitch of an acoustic signal. Various mathematical schemes have been used, but historically, two approaches prevailed: **peak-picking** and **zero-crossing.** The peak-picking method identifies the highest point of amplitude excursion in successive periods and calculates the period distance between "peaks" to reveal the pitch period (Figure 6-2). Zero-crossing uses a similar technique by identifying the point of waveform crossing on the horizontal axis. When the waveform pattern is noisy or deteriorated, as in a severely dysphonic

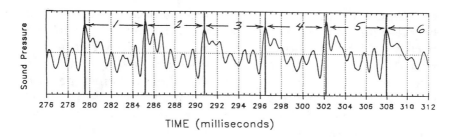

Figure 6-2. Fundamental frequency. Detecting fundamental period using the "peak picking method" (From *Clinical Speech and Voice Measurement*, by R. Orlikoff and R. Baken, 1993, p. 157. Copyright 1993 by Singular Publishing Group. Reprinted with permission.)

voice, the amplitude peaks and axis crossing points can be highly irregular or difficult to detect. No pitch detection algorithm can account for extreme acoustic distortion, but zero-crossing and peak-picking algorithms are particularly susceptible to error if multiple peaks or axis crossings occur within a pitch period, thus masking the true distance between waveform periods.[21,33]

A more recent technique[41] utilizes many points along a waveform to identify the shape of a whole pitch period. This method has been termed **waveform matching**, because it tracks the entire shape of successive waveforms and uses a mathematical cross-comparison (autocorrelation) of the shape and length of successive waveforms across cycles, with interpolation between samples to detect variability or waveform deviations. This pitch detection algorithm appears to be more valid because it is resistant to error from fluctuations in peak amplitude or axis crossing.[11,33,34,41]

Fundamental Frequency

Once the pitch period (T) is detected, then fundamental frequency (Fo) can be calculated from the reciprocal (Fo = 1/T). Fundamental frequency is the rate of vibration of the vocal folds and is expressed in Hertz (Hz) or cycles per second. Recall that fundamental frequency is the acoustic measure of an audio-perceptual correlate, pitch. Several frequency measures are useful in assessing vocal function. The mean fundamental frequency can be measured during sustained vowels or extracted from connected speech. Variation in fundamental frequency during connected speech can be used to reflect changes in intonation. Fundamental frequency range, also called phonation range, measures the highest and lowest pitch a patient can produce. Voice clinicians often find change in habitual frequency or frequency range an important indicator of increased vocal flexibility, a loss of mass on the vocal folds, or more appropriate pitch placement. For example, patients with vocal nodules often exhibit increased fundamental frequency following successful rehabilitation.

If fundamental frequencies are used to compare change across time, it is important to understand that the numeric values of fundamental frequency are nonlinear. For example, the perceptual difference in pitch between 200 and 400 Hz is far greater than the perceptual difference between 600 and 800 Hertz. Therefore, statements about the absolute change in the number of frequencies are virtually meaningless unless they are compared as pretreatment and posttreatment values. Usually, a better approach is to convert the Hertz value to notes on the musical scale. This conversion essentially "normalizes" the values so they can be expressed as a number of notes, or semitones.[7] Finally, it is important to understand that fundamental frequency does covary with intensity, so clinicians should always control, or at least document, the intensity level at which the frequency production was measured. Besides intensity, other aspects of a clinical protocol that will affect fundamental frequency include the speech sample (sustained vowel or connected speech) and the vowel type (high or low). Most protocols recommend multiple trials to ascertain the stability of repeated productions of the sample and to establish a stable baseline for fundamental frequency measurement.

Intensity

Vocal intensity (Io) is the acoustic correlate of another perceptual attribute, loudness. It is referenced to sound pressure level (SPL) and measured on the logarithmic decibel (dB) scale, and is represented on the acoustic waveform by amplitude height (Figure 6-

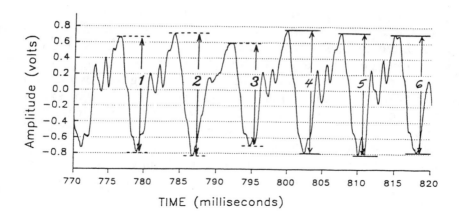

Figure 6-3. Intensity. Examining amplitude height from an acoustic waveform. (From *Clinical Speech and Voice Measurement, by R. Orlikoff and R. Baken, 1993, p. 205.* Copyright 1993 by Singular Publishing Group. Reprinted with permission.)

3). Both habitual intensity and intensity range (maximum and minimum) are useful clinical measures of vocal function. Intensity measurements can be made with a number of different instruments, including sound level meters, acoustic analysis programs, and some aerodynamic measurement devices. Intensity measures are subject to several artifacts, however, including influence of ambient or background noise; variations with changes in speech task, vowel production or fundamental frequency; and inconsistencies in mouth-to-microphone distance. A constant mouth-to-microphone distance must be maintained each time intensity is recorded because the intensity measure will vary with changes in distance from the mouth to the microphone or sound level meter. Recall the inverse square law that applies to this concept, meaning that intensity will drop 6 dB for every doubling of distance.[11,14]

As for all acoustic measures, clinicians who assess intensity should adopt a standard, well-monitored elicitation protocol to minimize the potential sources of error in intensity measures. The speech sample used for recording intensity can (and should) vary to reflect a variety of both habitual and maximal speech tasks. Common intensity tasks include sustained vowels at softest possible loudness, shouting "Hey!" at maximal loudness, and connected speech samples at habitual loudness levels. Intensity measures tend to be influenced highly by both environmental noise and by the clinician's model, so it is critical that patients receive the appropriate cueing to provide both habitual and maximal performance on these tasks. For example, most patients require at least two trials to achieve a true "minimum" or "maximum" loudness. By providing an excellent model (even of a loud "Hey!"), the clinician can encourage improved performance on these tasks. Usually, a patient will feel more comfortable when they are given the incentive to match a model.

Voice Range Profile, Phonetogram, and Physiological Frequency Range of Phonation

The voice range profile (VRP), phonetogram, and physiological frequency range of phonation (PFRP) are three names given to a similar clinical task that assesses both fundamental frequency and intensity across an individual's absolute minimum and maximum capabilities of voice production. Specifically, these techniques ask a patient to produce his or her lowest fundamental frequency at minimum loudness, followed by the same frequency at maximum loudness. The patient then continues up the frequency range semitone by semitone to the absolute highest production. At each note, the patient must produce the tone at his or her minimum and maximum intensity. The frequency and intensity data are plotted on a matrix with fundamental frequency in the horizontal axis, and intensity on the vertical axis (Figure 6-4). The resulting plot is an ellipse-shaped frequency-intensity profile, and its dimensions are expressed in semitones. This profile is a thorough description of the physiologic limits of voice production and the covariation of fundamental frequency and intensity for an individual.[7,8,42-45]

Clinically, this technique can be somewhat time consuming and fatiguing for some patients. Occasionally, only intermittent probe samples of certain frequencies are used to abbreviate the format. The task also demands careful monitoring of fundamental frequency matching during the many trials to ensure that

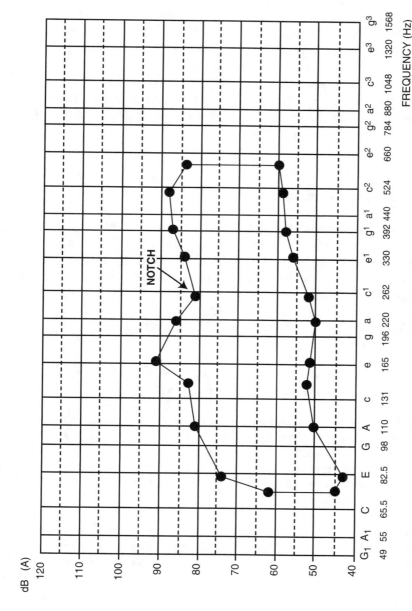

Figure 6-4. Voice range profile. Vowel produced at minimum and maximum intensity (dB) across minimum and maximum frequency range (Hz and musical notes). (From *Clinical Speech and Voice Measurement*, by R. Orlikoff and R. Baken, 1993, p. 179. Copyright 1993 by Singular Publishing Group. Reprinted with permission.)

accurate data are achieved. Some computer programs provide semiautomatic elicitation and recording routines to present appropriate cue tones in succession. Despite its technical rigor, this clinical assessment paradigm has been used by voice pedagogues and phoniatricians in Europe for many years and has gained recent attention for its wide application to functional changes in voice production. This comprehensive assessment is an especially useful measure for monitoring changes in vocal range for professional voice users.[5,7]

Perturbation Measures

Most acoustic analysis programs offer measures of voice perturbation. Perturbation is defined as the cycle-to-cycle variability in a signal and can only be applied to sustained vowel or extracted vowel segments. Two common expressions of this term are **jitter** (frequency perturbation) and **shimmer** (amplitude perturbation). There is a range of mathematical calculations for these terms, which are usually specified by three general parameters.[4,6,11,14]

- **Length of the voice analysis window**, as perturbation measures can be calculated in either short-term or long-term averages.
- **Absolute or relative measurement units**, as perturbation measures can be reported as an absolute amount, a ratio, or a percentage of the whole voice segment.
- **Statistical emphasis**, as perturbation measures are reported as means (eg, central tendency) and coefficients of variation (eg, variability).

There is poor agreement among voice laboratory users, including speech scientists, clinicians, and vendors who develop these tools as to the preference of one measure over another. This lack of comparable measures has limited the development of a coherent normative base of acoustic measures and has impeded cross-comparison of studies conducted in different sites with different measurement tools.[19,23,25,35] Another point of confusion in assessing the validity of derived values of perturbation measures is the independent variable of technology advancement. Titze[3] observed that so-called "normal" measures of jitter values have dropped across 4 decades of analysis as the increased fidelity of microphones and increased speech and memory of signal processing continues to provide better waveform resolution in the acoustic analysis. Technical capabilities continue to improve, and optimal recording standards and equipment specifications may lead to increased stability and validity of acoustic measures in the future.[5,16,17] Finally, perturbation measures can be difficult to interpret because of the variable potential contributors to vocal instability. Just as aerodynamic, neurologic, biomechanical, source-filter, and other systemic factors can all influence voice quality perceptually, so can these variables affect the cycle-to-cycle variability of acoustic frequency and amplitude.[17,46-50] Certainly, improvements in perturbation values across a pretreatment and posttreatment period are viewed favorably, but it is virtually impossible to assign a direct association between any single contributor and the decrease in perturbation. For this reason, acoustic perturbation measures, as with all other clinical instrumental data, should be interpreted in combination with other clinical impressions and cross-validating data.

Signal (or Harmonic)-to-Noise Ratios

Acoustic analysis programs often produce a ratio measure of the periodic or harmonic signal energy to the aperiodic or noise energy in the voice waveform. As with perturbation measures, signal-to-noise ratios are derived from different algorithms and expressed in various units, limiting comparison across laboratories. Nonetheless, the general principle is retained; greater signal or harmonic energy in the voice is thought to reflect better voice quality. Large noise energy (random aperiodicity in the voice signal) represents more abnormal vocal function.[42] As with other acoustic measurements, signal-to-noise ratio can supply a useful comparative value across pretreatment and posttreatment measures.

Sound Spectography

Sound spectrography and spectral analysis are acoustic techniques that create visual displays that provide information about the fundamental frequency and the higher harmonic energies in the sound. By displaying influences of both the glottal sound source and the vocal tract (supraglottic), clinicians can learn more about the relationship between vocal fold vibration represented by the fundamental frequency and vocal tract features, such as vowel type, coarticulatory factors, or other speech variables. Two common forms of sound spectrography that have been used clinically are the **sound spectrogram** and the **spectral analysis**.[15]

The sound spectrogram, which can be displayed as wide- or narrow-bandwidth, displays the glottal sound source and filtering characteristics of the speech signal across time. Both formant frequency energy (concentrations of resonant energy in the vocal tract) and noise components (aperiodicity, transient or turbulent noise) of the speech production are presented in a three-dimensional scale. The horizontal axis is time. The vertical axis is frequency. A third scale is the darkness or "gray" scale (or color difference) that represents intensity change among these various spectral energies (Figure 6-5). The lowest energy band always represents the fundamental, with formant energies in the higher frequencies above. In wide-band spectrograms (which include most of the harmonic spectrum), however, the fundamental and first formant may be so close that it is difficult to separate them visually. Narrow-band spectrograms (which exclude higher frequencies) are useful for observing the spectral energy of the fundamental in detail. When the spectral energies are easily visualized by dark bands (gray scale concentration), the formant energy is strong, in contrast to lighter or diffuse gray bands, which suggest a noisier signal and poorly identified formant energies. In this manner, visual inspection of the spectrogram can provide an estimate of the harmonic-to-noise ratio of a speech production.[10,14,15]

The second form of spectral analysis is the line spectrum. Unlike the sound spectrogram, which displays the acoustic spectrum across time, the line spectrum only plots all harmonic

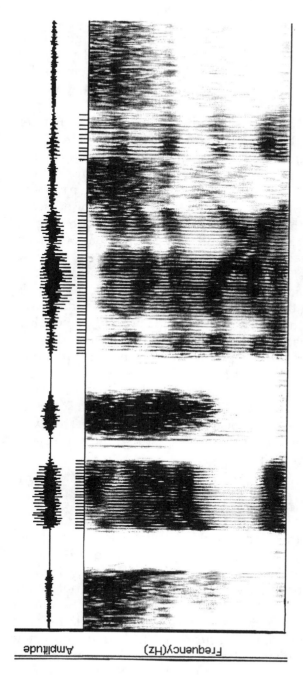

Amplitude

Frequency(Hz)

Figure 6-5. Wide band spectrogram. Upper waveform displays the acoustic signal for the sample phrase "speech analysis," with the spectrogram displayed below. Note the formant concentrations (darker horizontal bands) produced during the vowel segments.

203

energies at a single time point. Frequencies are plotted on the horizontal axis; amplitude is on the vertical axis (Figure 6-6). Because a line spectrum is confined to harmonic display at only one moment in time, it is common to use a series of temporally adjacent line spectra to observe changes in formant patterns within a time-varying speech sample.[10,14,15]

Advanced spectral analysis routines, such as Fast Fourier Transform (FFT) and Linear Predictive Coding (LPC), have been applied to line spectra to identify formant characteristics of the vocal tract. FFT analysis achieves this formant analysis by dividing up the complex speech waveform into individual harmonics. These harmonic amplitudes are plotted in a series of adjacent peaks that indicate the individual harmonic amplitude heights across all resonant frequencies in that single moment of speech production. LPC analysis produces a smoothed trajectory line above the FFT peaks that identifies the vocal tract formants created by the sum of individual harmonics. The LPC analysis is useful in identifying the major formant energy concentrations at any given point in the speech sample. For both FFT and LPC, microprocessing capabilities have increased the speed and accessibility of spectral processing greatly. Nonetheless, as with other forms of acoustic analysis, FFT and LPC routines are highly sensitive to noise and other signal artifacts. To avoid error, care must be taken to ensure that a clean, undistorted signal is presented to the system for analysis. For voice pathologists, spectral analysis is useful to assess the interaction between the sound source and vocal tract (supraglottic) influences.[10,14,15]

Acoustic Recording Considerations

To further consider the special problems associated with acoustic analysis of voice, the National Center for Voice and Speech held a consensus conference in 1995. Voice scientists, acoustic engineers, product developers, and clinicians met to determine the acceptable standards for acoustic analysis. A Summary Statement from that conference provides recommendations for methods in pitch detection, measuring perturbation, and using equipment.[11] Because acoustic analysis routines are written based on assumptions of a quasi-periodic, stable sound source, recording protocols must accommodate this underlying princi-

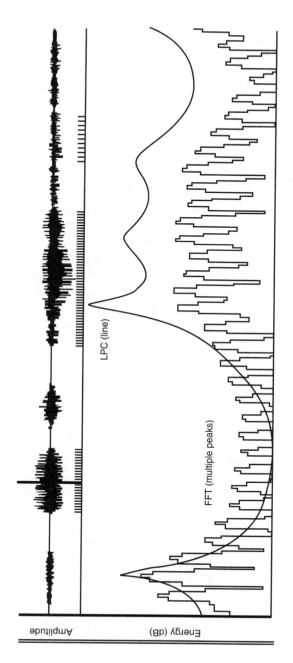

Figure 6-6. Same acoustic waveform as Figure 6-5, with a line spectrum displayed below. LPC and FFT formant tracings correspond to a single spectral moment extracted from the midpoint of the /i/ vowel (see vertical cursor bar on acoustic waveform).

205

ple. To ensure valid acoustic measurements, a new concept was proposed, suggesting that all voice waveforms be inspected visually and classified as Type I (quasiperiodic), Type II (modulating and variable), or Type III (random and chaotic) signals. The classification of Type I, II, and III voice can be made from visual displays of the acoustic waveform or spectral representations. Type I voice is essentially quasi-periodic and continuous and contains a single cluster of dominant fundamental frequency values. Clinically, Type I voice is usually represented by normal voice or a mild impairment that does not include obvious perceptual deviations or distortions. Perturbation analysis of Type I voice is acceptable, based on the consistency and reliability of the fundamental frequency.[11]

Type II voice may contain identifiable periodic segments, but across time, there is sufficient modulation in the signal that no "obvious **single** fundamental frequency" emerges. These modulations in the continuity and consistency of the signal result in either multiple or intermittent fundamental frequencies. Clinically, this Type II signal can arise from both disordered productions (such as glottal fry, vocal tremor, intermittent aphonia, or roughness), or it may result from other intentional modulations (such as vibrato). Type II voice is usually degraded in quality because of excessive noise, variations, and aperiodicity, which ultimately preclude reliable acoustic analysis using pitch detection and perturbation analysis. The NCVS Summary Statement recommends the acoustic analysis of Type II voice be limited to spectral analysis or other visual displays.[11]

Finally, Type III voice represents random, aperiodic signals that have no identifiable fundamental frequency pattern whatsoever. Clinically, these voices are considered to be severely impaired and contain large noisy components caused by breathiness, roughness, or a combination of perceptual distortions. Type III voices are not suitable for instrumental acoustic analysis and can only be assessed using audio-perceptual judgments.

In summary, then, only Type I voices are eligible for valid acoustic perturbation analysis, but Type II voice signals may be evaluated using visual spectral display. Whenever the disordered sound source is so aphonic (as in Type III voice) or so intermittent (eg, spasmodic dysphonia) that the patient cannot produce sustained voice, acoustic analysis cannot be used with confidence for that speaker.[11]

Other guidelines for acoustic recording protocols also emerged from that consensus conference and from methodologic research. For example, acoustic assessment should include recommendations for multiple trials (tokens) to consider individual variability and establish a stable baseline performance. The number of trials must be adequate to represent the speech behavior. Occasionally, patients will offer an unrepresentative first trial production (eg, too loud, too high pitched) because of some form of uncertainty with the task or because of test anxiety. It is crucial that the voice pathologist observe the patient's production carefully to elicit the most representative production.[11]

Clinicians must be aware of the interactions between fundamental frequency, intensity, and perturbation values. Each is known to influence the others. For example, frequency rises with increased intensity. Perturbation values are known to decrease with increased fundamental frequency. Variations in fundamental frequency, intensity, and perturbation will also vary with the vowel selection.[38,40,46-50] Realistically, the clinician cannot hold frequency and intensity constant in all clinical measures, but these values should always be documented to help account for differences in pretreatment and posttreatment comparisons. Sustained or extracted vowel samples are the most reliable speech tasks for acoustic analysis, and the segment length must be sufficient to preserve the validity of acoustic measurement.[33,36] A sample recording protocol for acoustic measures is contained in Appendix 6-4.

Aerodynamic Measurements

Aerodynamic measurements are another common and highly useful clinical method available to achieve objective and noninvasive information about vocal function. Two principle aerodynamic components, subglottic pressure and transglottic flow, reveal indirect information about the underlying valving activity of the larynx. The interchange of pressure and flow are an essential component of vocal fold vibration, and aerodynamic measures are sometimes called "physiologic" measures because they tend to relate more closely to the vocal fold valving capabilities than do acoustic analysis data.[7-9,51-56] A number of airflow and pressure measures are available clinically. Additional derived (combination) measures that integrate pressure and flow in mathematic ratios (single measure) have also been examined, such as laryngeal resistance or glottal power.[7,57-60] Other aerodynamic measures are specific to clinical tasks such as phonation threshold pressure, which is the minimum subglottal pressure needed to initiate vocal fold vibration,[10,60,61] or average transglottal flow, which is assessed under sustained vowel conditions.[62,63]

In speech production, pressure and flow variations are both dynamic and transient because of rapid sequencing of speech and voice sounds. Momentary changes in oral pressure measured during production of plosive or fricative consonants are examples of transient or short-term aerodynamic measures.[52,55,64] Clinically, however, it is often useful to measure average airflow rate or flow volume during sustained productions, reflecting long-term or average aerodynamic measures. Figure 6-7 displays an aerodynamic recording system for measurement of airflow during voice production.

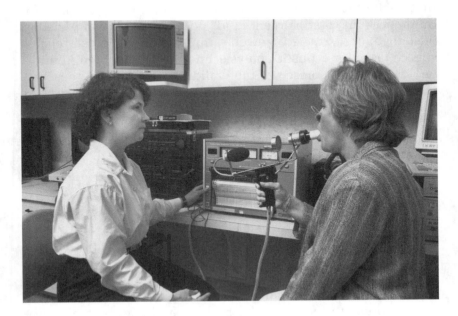

Figure 6-7. An aerodynamic recording system for measurement of airflow during voice production. (Rick Berkey, Dayton, Ohio)

Constraints that limit the clinical application of other instrumental measures also limit the utility of aerodynamic measures. These constraints include technological error,[53] type of speech sample,[62] and intrasubject variability.[65] Nonetheless, measures of intraoral pressure, transglottal flow, and derived measures (eg, laryngeal resistance) have been used to discriminate normal and pathologic vocal function, to assess disorder severity, and, in some cases, suggest implications for the diagnostic source of the voice pathology. For example, an excessive average flow rate usually indicates and underlying glottal incompetence. Increased subglottic pressure measures often are associated with hyperfunctional voice use patterns.[51,63] When aerodynamic measures provide a real-time visual display, clinicians can use these readings as primary treatment feedback tools to offer support for behavioral changes in vocal fold valving during voice production. An emerging normative database for aerodynamics expands the clinical utility of these measures and allows some comparison across clinical sites.[54,65-67]

Calibrating Equipment

For speech and voice analysis, one should be able to measure pressure and flow events under dynamic (real speech) conditions. Although it may be interesting to note the maximal intraoral pressure one can build up to overcome resistance and blow up a balloon, for example, this nonspeech task has less relevance to clinical voice than a connected speech utterance that assesses intraoral pressure peaks during plosive production. Nonetheless, static pressure and flow measures are occasionally useful clinically to verify the potential to build up intraoral pressure or flow. Furthermore, direct measures of static or stable pressure and flow are useful for calibrating pressure flow equipment.

Two simple instruments can be used to measure static pressure and static flow directly. The pressure meter is called a **U tube manometer** and consists of a glass tube shaped into a long U standing upright with a calibrated index along the tube. The tube is filled with water or mercury, depending on the type of pressure measurement needed. Pressure is applied to one side of the U, and the displaced amount of liquid is read directly off the contralateral side in appropriate units (cm H_2O or mm Hg).[4,14]

Airflow rate can be similarly measured, using a **rotameter**, which is a tall glass tube with a small float inside and a calibrated index along the side. When airflow is blown into a port at the base of the tube, the float rises to the level that corresponds with the rate of flow. Again, the measure is read directly (ml or cc per second). As indicated previously, the significant limit to these two measurement devices is that they can only measure static (or long-term), sustained pressure and flow. Because many pressure and flow measurements in speech production are short-term and rapidly varying, the manometer and rotameter cannot be used conveniently. When combined with a compressed air source, however, they are useful as external measures for calibrating other devices used to measure pressure and flow.[4,14]

Pressure, Flow, and Resistance

The instrumentation used for aerodynamic measurement exploits the integral relationship between pressure, flow, and resistance. These physical events behave in predictable ways, and it is useful for the clinician to understand how their interactions are applied to aerodynamic equipment and measures. Recall that molecules in fluid (air or water) will always flow from a region of higher density (tight, compressed) to lower density (more space). As a schematic demonstration, imagine 100 people crowded together in a small room. Suddenly, a small door opens to the outside. Feeling crowded, the people start pushing toward the door, trying to get outside. The flow of people spreading out into a wider space mimics the activity of compressed molecules or electrons; if given an outlet, no matter how small, molecules will dissipate into regions of lesser concentration (crowding). This molecular movement from regions of higher to lower density is flow; when electrons do the same, it is called current. Current (electrons) and flow (molecules) are analogous. Resistance is simply the impediment to flow, whether molecular or electronic. In the crowded room, the flow of people out the door is limited by the physical constraints of the walls and small door, which pose a restriction or constriction on the natural tendency of people who wish to spread out.

So, asymmetries in the concentration of molecules (or electrons) result in flow. The difference in concentration between two points creates a driving pressure and a potential for molecular flow. In aerodynamic terms, this asymmetry is represented as differential pressure, which is defined as the difference in pressure between two points, and thus the potential to do work. In the electronic form, this potential is called voltage. Consider again the image of crowded people pushing up against the door jam, trying to ease through the small opening. The pressure just inside the doorway is far greater than the pressure just outside of it, where newly unconstrained people wander about freely. The relative pressure inside (p1) versus outside (p2) is different. This differential pressure represents the flow asymmetry on either side of the constriction.

Ohm's Law

The relationship between differential pressure, flow, and resistance has been clarified in the electrical principle known as Ohm's Law, which states that voltage (E) is equal to current (I) times the resistance (R): $E = IR$. In the analogy with aerodynamic processes, differential pressure (p1 vs. p2) is equal to flow (V) times the impediment to flow (R): $[p1 - p2] = VR$. This means that two separate pressure points, measured on either side of a known resistance, can be used to calculate the magnitude of flow (Figure 6-8).[14] This same principle is used to calculate airflow.

Airflow Equipment

The most common airflow device is the **pneumotachograph,** which uses the principle of differential pressure across a known resistance to estimate flow rate. A pneumotachograph is essentially a metal tube, with a mechanical resistance (usually a wire mesh screen or a series of small tubes) inside. As airflow is blown through the tube and its resistance, differential pressures are measured at sites directly upstream and downstream to the resistance. Recall that with Ohm's law, flow is calculated using the differential pressure divided by the resistance. The amount of flow divided over the amount of time equals flow rate. Another device used to measure airflow is the **warm wire**

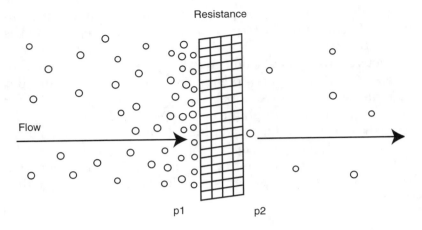

Figure 6-8. Flow, resistance and differential pressure. As flow passes through a known resistance, it creates a pressure change (p1 vs p2).

anemometer. When flow passes over a warm wire within this instrument, the wire is cooled, changing the electrical resistance of the wire with the change in temperature. The change in resistance in the wire is proportional to the flow, and flow rate can be calculated from that change.[14,55]

When airflow is measured, the transducer must be coupled to the face through some form of airflow mask or mouthpiece. Flow masks must be airtight to avoid measurement error, but this creates some artifact because of a sensation of "backpressure," which may cause the patient to perform differently. Occasionally, patients will need coaching to produce a natural and comfortable voice sample. Coaching will ensure that performance is representative of free speech conditions. Rothenberg[68] developed a mask with screen vents, which gives acoustic feedback to the speaker and alleviates the problem of excess backpressure. For this device, the wire mesh screens serve as the resistance, and the pressure drop is calculated from pressure inside the mask relative to atmospheric pressure (outside the mask).

Pulmonary function testing requires the use of a **spirometer**, which is a respiratory measurement device that records volume measures. Two forms of this instrument are available: wet and dry. The wet spirometer has two chambers with known volumes of air and water contained within them. As the patient blows air into the upper chamber, the volume of water displaced by the flow is measured directly. A dry spirometer is an alternate respiratory function measurement device that utilizes a turbine mechanism. As air passes across the turbine, the number of rotations is calibrated with a specific volume amount.[4,14]

Flow Measurement

There are two basic measurements of airflow used in speech production: **average flow rate** and **flow volume**. To measure average transglottal flow, the airflow mask or mouthpiece is placed firmly on the patient's face or in the mouth. Following a comfortable breath, the patient is instructed to produce a steady vowel at normal pitch and loudness for at least 5 to 10 seconds. If a real-time display is available, the clinicians can inspect the pattern of average flow, whether stable, falling, or irregular. In normal speakers, average flow rates are approximately 80 to 200 cc/s. In patients with respiratory compromise or neurologic disease, unstable or irregular patterns of average flow can be seen. Patients with severely hyperfunctional voice or glottal fry will demonstrate markedly reduced airflow rates, as low as 10 to 15 cc/s. Conversely, patients with primary glottal incompetence, such as vocal fold paralysis, may generate average airflow rates as high as 400 to 600 cc/s, accompanied by short vowel durations.

Volume is the total amount of flow used during a certain production, in a task similar to a maximum phonation time. Volume is generally measured in liter or milliliter units. When total volume of airflow is measured during a maximum sustained vowel production, the resulting measure is usually called phonatory volume. To measure phonatory volume, a patient must take the largest possible breath and hold out a steady vowel as long as possible. For adults, phonatory volume amounts range from 1500 mL to nearly 4000 mL, depending on the patient's gender and body size. This technique allows a gross estimate of a patient's breath supply for voice and speech, but it is not an accurate estimate of pulmonary function or other respiratory measures, such as tidal volume (the amount of air in an average breath) or vital capacity (the maximum amount of air that can be exhaled after a maximum inhalation).[67] Because the amount of air needed for connected speech and voice is small relative to total lung capacity, most voice patients will not need comprehensive pulmonary function testing to determine sufficient breath support for speech. Nonetheless, patients who have respiratory compromise or obvious shortness of breath should be referred for qualified pulmonary function testing.

Subglottal Air Pressure Measurement

Pressure is defined as the force per unit area, acting perpendicular to the area. In voice production, respiratory (subglottal) pressure acts as a force building up below the adducted vocal folds, rising until the folds overcome resistance and set the closed folds into oscillation. Subglottal air pressure is essentially the power supply, and variables such as vocal fold stiffness, hyperfunctional compression, and incomplete glottic closure will influence the amount of subglottal effort needed to initiate phonation. Thus, voice pathologists use measures of subglottal pressure as one indicator of the valving characteristics of the vocal folds. Subglottal pressure can only be measured directly through an invasive procedure that requires a needle puncture into the trachea directly below the vocal folds. The needle is attached to a catheter and pressure transducer, which sense the change in force and calculate the units of pressure. With this puncture technique, tracheal (subglottic) pressure can be measured directly, but this method is not used clinically.[14,69]

Estimating Subglottal Pressure

A noninvasive, indirect approach has been used to estimate subglottal pressure clinically. This method measures the intraoral pressure during production of the unvoiced bilabial plosive consonant /p/. Theoretically, this intraoral pressure is a feasible estimate of the subglottal pressure if the following assumptions are met:

■ The oral plosive constriction creates a momentary airtight seal, with a continuous opening from the lungs to the lips. (Note that velopharyngeal incompetence (leak) would violate this assumption.)

■ The vocal folds are open so that the oral pressure produced in the plosive production is equivalent to the tracheal driving pressure that would be available to set the vocal folds in oscillation.[56,64]

Although the relationship between indirect estimates of oral pressure and direct tracheal pressure are not identical under all circumstances, this indirect method is our most clinically viable approach to assessing tracheal pressure at present. In this indirect method, subglottic pressure is estimated from repeated production of an unvoiced plosive + vowel syllable (eg, /pi/). An oral tube is placed between the closed lips and connected to a pressure transducer, which will record the intraoral pressure. Usually, dual channel recorders will allow simultaneous airflow recording, which are used to verify that during pressure peaks, airflow is at zero (Figure 6-9).

Procedures for recording intraoral pressure are specific and must be followed carefully. The oral catheter must be placed carefully in the mouth, sealed by the lips, and not occluded by the tongue or by saliva. The length, diameter, and angle of the tube can influence the pressure measurement. Some clinicians recommend that the end of the intraoral catheter be occluded (crimped or sealed) and that air pressure be detected through a series of small holes placed in the distal sides of the catheter, where they will not be affected by excessive aspirate pressure peaks. The velum must be closed, and if nasal air leak is suspected, it is appropriate to use nose clips. It is also important for clinicians to control the rate and loudness of the /pi/ syllable repetitions, to keep elicitation cues stable and constant. If the syllable train is produced too quickly, pressure peaks may be artificially lower than actual driving pressure. Clinicians can pace the patient's productions by modeling, tapping, patting a shoulder, or using other external pacing cues. Under these careful elicitation and production procedures, the peak intraoral pressure recorded during the plosive /p/ production should be a reasonable estimate of tracheal pressure.[56]

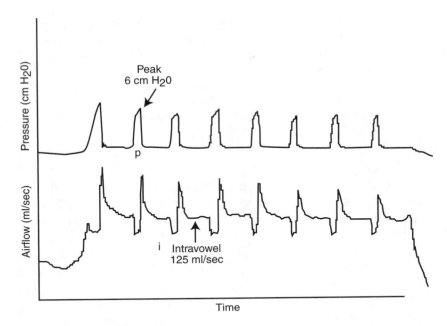

Figure 6-9. Simultaneous pressure (upper trace) and airflow (lower trace) recordings in a repeated /pi/ task. Note the reciprocal timing of pressure and flow peaks. Pressure peaks just before the aspirate airflow peak for /p/. During vocalic /i/, pressure is zero, whereas mean flow rate is quasi-level. (Courtesy of the Speech Physiology Laboratory, University of Minnesota, Minneapolis, Minn.)

Phonation Threshold Pressure

A special application of indirect pressure estimates has gained increasing attention in clinical voice pathology. Titze[10,60] first defined the concept of **phonation threshold pressure (PTP)**, which is the minimal pressure required to set the vocal folds into oscillation. PTP is thought to be a potentially important predictor of the structure and function of the vocal fold vibratory capabilities. The measure has been estimated indirectly using intraoral pressures (described above) during a repeated syllable task that is the minimal loudness level for phonation.[70] Titze[60] has defined the theoretical relationship between phonation threshold pressure and the presumed vocal fold tissue properties that affect PTP. To summarize, phonation threshold pressure is affected by,

- prephonatory glottal width
- thickness of the vocal fold edge
- amount of tissue damping (gradual loss of oscillation amplitude)
- mucosal wave velocity.

Under favorable conditions for decreased PTP, the prephonatory glottal width is small, the vocal fold edge is relaxed and rounded, tissue damping is minimal (vocal fold flexibility is greater), and mucosal wave velocity is decreased. For most speakers, these conditions for lower PTP are met when the fundamental frequency drops. In general terms, PTP can be interpreted as a measure of the effort needed to begin phonation. Because speakers with vocal pathologies frequently report greater effort in "turning on the voice," this newer measure may prove highly useful for assessing effects of treatment or phonosurgical results. Additional PTP research has shown that at high frequencies, PTP increases when subjects have undergone "dehydrating" conditions, but decreases again when the vocal folds have been well hydrated.[70]

Laryngeal Resistance

Derived measures that utilize measures of pressure and flow in a ratio or product have also been examined.[7,10] Laryngeal resistance is the quotient of peak intraoral pressure (estimated from production of an unvoiced plosive /p/) divided by the peak flow rate (measured from production of a vowel /i/) as produced in a repeated train of /pi/ syllables. This measurement is intended to reflect the overall resistance of the glottis and, by extension, serves as an estimate of the valving characteristic, whether too tight (hyperfunctional), too loose (hypofunctional), or normal.[56-58] Laryngeal resistance and other derived ratios (eg, glottal power) have been used in experimental settings to further analyze the covarying relationship between pressure and flow in vocal fold vibration. A word of caution is useful, however, because derived measures pose some limits to interpretability. The magnitude of a particular derived value is not meaningful without examining the separate contributions of pressure and flow. For example, a measure of increased laryngeal resistance values might be attributable to excessive subglottal pressure, insufficient transglottal flow, or both.

Aerodynamic Recording Considerations

Like all instrumental measures, aerodynamic assessment must be observed carefully to avoid equipment or task artifact. Airflow masks, oral pressure sensing tubes, and oral coupling tubes for spirometry all require an airtight seal with the face or lips. The clinician will need to monitor the patient's comfort and compliance to elicit as natural a speech production task as possible. Multiple trials are always useful to secure a stable baseline. Finally, the clinician should verify the validity of aerodynamic measures by conducting a standard calibration routine prior to each examination session. A sample recording protocol for aerodynamic measures is contained in Appendix 6-4.

Inverse Filter

Inverse filtering is a special analysis technique that can be applied to either acoustic or aerodynamic signals for specialized analysis of the glottal waveform (Figure 6-10). Because all speech signals (acoustic and aerodynamic) are measured at the mouth, the resulting waveform is a product of two components, the glottal sound source and the resonance characteristic from the vocal tract. Inverse filtering is a technique that theoretically isolates these two components. Through a series of special computer filtering processes, the effects of the supraglottic (vocal tract) influences can be removed. The remaining waveform will reflect only the glottal contributions to the sound source or to flow. Thus, inverse filtering allows the clinician to observe real-time patterns of the glottal acoustic source or glottal airflow source. The inverse filtered signal usually is described by the opening and closing slopes of the waveform. Typical measures include timing features, such as ratios of opening or closing time to the total period, and shape changing features, such as waveform minima or peaks.[71,72] When inverse filtering techniques are used clinically, they usually are combined with other real-time measures of glottal function, such as electroglottography.

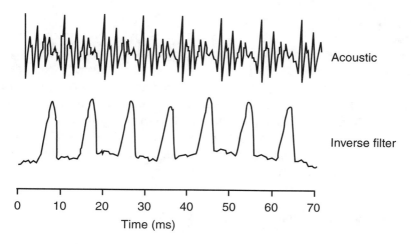

Figure 6-10. Sample acoustic waveform (upper trace) with inverse filter waveform (lower trace) below. (From Kent R., Read C. *The Acoustic Analysis of Speech.* Copyright 1992 by Singular Publishing Group. Reprinted with permission.)

Laryngeal Imaging

Laryngeal imaging offers the greatest potential for detection, severity assessment, and diagnosis in patients with voice disorders. Historically, the voice pathologist relied on the otolaryngologist's verbal description of gross laryngeal structure and function and on audio-perceptual judgments of voice quality to assess, diagnose, and plan remediation for a voice disorder. Current video processing and laryngeal imaging capabilities allow the clinician to view and record images from flexible and rigid endoscopes on a monitor to provide a bigger, brighter, and longer look at the larynx. Attaching the endoscope to a strobe generator allows clinicians to make visual judgments about the estimated vibratory pattern of the vocal folds during phonation.[1,8,9,14,20,73] These visual imaging techniques allow the clinician to consider vocal fold appearance and movement and its potential contribution to voice production.

Speech-language pathologists never make medical diagnoses, but for the purposes of interpreting the impact that visual features may have on voice production and rehabilitation, imaging has provided our profession a critical advantage. Increasingly, clinicians have used the technique of endoscopy with a stroboscopic light source to augment the indirect examination. Stroboscopy has been shown to contribute significantly to accurate medical diagnosis of laryngeal lesions and voice disorders.[20,73-75] Clearly, the endoscopic examination is never a substitute for the otolaryngologist's indirect examination, but the two procedures offer complementary information. Figure 6-11 shows a rigid endoscopic examination using the stroboscopic unit for laryngeal imaging.

Professional Ethics in Endoscopy

The important role that speech-language pathologists serve in the performance of laryngeal endoscopy was clarified in a joint position statement approved by the American Speech Language Hearing Association (ASHA) and the American Academy of Otolaryngology—Head and Neck Surgery.[76] Using rigid and

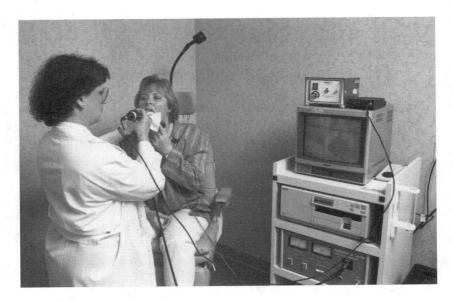

Figure 6-11. The stroboscopic unit used for laryngeal imaging. (Rick Berkey, Dayton, Ohio)

flexible endoscopy is part of the speech-language pathology scope of practice and is considered a critical component of the Preferred Practice Patterns for Voice Assessment and Voice Treatment.[77] (Both the joint statement and the Preferred Practice Patterns are contained in Appendixes; 6-1, 6-2, and 6-3.) However, with this practice comes professional responsibilities and issues that require clinicians to seek appropriate academic preparation and clinical competence, including mentorship from an experienced clinician, before using these procedures independently with patients. The ASHA Special Interest Division 3 (Voice and Voice Disorders) prepared a comprehensive set of recommendations for Training Guidelines for the Performance of Endoscopy and Stroboscopy.[78] These guidelines provide a thorough overview of both the knowledge base and the skill required to perform these procedures safely.

This chapter will provide general guidelines to assess patients using a rigid 70° endoscope, which is the most common approach to video endoscopy with strobe lighting. Regardless of the endoscope type (flexible or rigid), however, it is recommended that clinicians achieve mentored training with at least 20 normal subjects to develop both confidence and competence before attempting rigid examination of a patient. It is the responsibility of the clinician and his or her mentor to establish skill-based criteria to determine when independent endoscopy can be performed competently.[20] State licensure guidelines, institutional endoscopy boards, and individual practice patterns may contribute to decisions about who conducts endoscopy and when, and how it is conducted in a given setting. Overall, patient safety and professional standards must take precedence over other concerns.

Endoscopy Using Steady Light

Rigid or flexible endoscopy of the vocal mechanism allows the clinician to observe anatomical structures and vocal fold function. Steady light observation of the larynx and vocal folds is a beneficial imaging technique, similar to the otolaryngolgist's indirect examination. Nonetheless, steady light imaging does not allow the clinician to make any inferences about the vocal fold vibratory pattern. Steady light is produced by a halogen bulb, which is a filament bulb.

The selection of endoscope type will depend on the needs of the examination and the patient's age and compliance. Rigid endoscopy allows a close view of the larynx and vocal folds and generally supplies better lighting to the image because of larger fiberoptic bundles. Flexible endoscopy allows observation of the velopharynx, vocal tract, and larynx from a macroscopic view. Patients who undergo flexible endoscopy can often make use of the onscreen image of the velum or vocal folds in a biofeedback protocol to alter position of the speech structures, the vocal tract posture, or vocal fold closure patterns.[20,73] Using steady light, various treatment targets can be specified and successfully modified using visual biofeedback, even in children. Some relevant examples include increased velopharyngeal closure, relaxed vocal tract and supraglottis, and modified glottic closure to either close gaps or relax excessive medial compression.

Stroboscopy

The science of stroboscopy is founded on the principle of Talbot's Law, which defines an optical phenomenon called "persistence of vision" of the human retina. This law describes the limits of the retina, which can only perceive a maximum of five separate images per second, at a rate not faster than .2 seconds per image. If separate images are presented at this speed, then the eye will perceive each image independently. However, if images are presented to the eye at faster rates, they will be perceived visually as "fused" or connected images. When a strobe light illuminates the larynx at a pulse rate faster than five images per second, the result is a visual-perceptual composite of the images, perceived as continuous motion.[14,20]

Human vocal folds vibrate at rates from approximately 60 (low bass) to greater than 1400 (whistle register) Hz. Therefore, the vocal folds repeat these rapidly oscillating vibratory cycles at rates far faster than could be perceived by the naked eye. Stroboscopy light pulses achieve a systematic sampling of these quasi-periodic waveforms to allow a composite vibratory cycle, sampled from many single points along multiple waveforms, and fused together based on Talbot's Law of optics. Thus, the stroboscopy image, although representative of the general pattern of vocal fold vibration, is actually a composite of separate points sampled across many repetitions.

Mechanics of the Stroboscope

The lighting of the strobe unit is usually achieved by two separate sources: a steady halogen light, as described previously, and a flashing xenon light. (Note that one strobe manufacturer offers a unit with only a xenon light source.) The strobe pulse light is achieved by the xenon light, which is composed of a xenon gas, and the brightness of the light source dissipates over time instead of burning out at one moment.[20] The timing of the xenon strobe flash is triggered by the fundamental frequency of the voice, as detected by a contact microphone placed tightly over the neck (usually near the thyroid lamina). The strobe flash pulses are short (<40 microseconds) and are triggered under two operating modes to create either a still or traveling image of the vocal folds:

- In the still mode, the strobe flashes occur at exactly the same point within the vibratory cycle, and the resulting image appears stable or "locked" (Figure 6-12).
- In the traveling mode, the strobe flashes occur at different points within the vibratory cycle, and the resulting image appears as a moving or "walking" wave of vibration (Figure 6-13). Most strobe units achieve this slow-motion effect by strobing at a rate that is slightly slower than the fundamental frequency (–1 to –2 Hz).

The fundamental frequency for most speakers is between 90 to 300 Hz. Current video technology only allows 50 to 60 separate images (video fields) per second, however. Therefore, strobing at or near the fundamental frequency results in multiple exposures per video field. If the fundamental frequency is 120 Hz, for example, then approximately two strobe flashes will occur in each video field. These multiple exposures per frame create a "blinky" and sometimes blurred image. Note that one strobe manufacturer provides the ability to strobe at the variable fundamental frequency rate or at a constant rate consistent with the video field rate (VHS: 60 Hz). The resulting strobe image is clearer than it would be under traditional flashing rates because

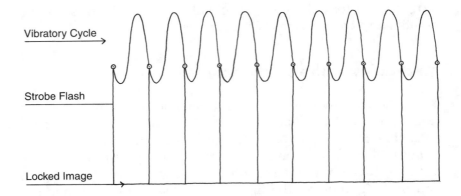

Figure 6-12. Strobe flash at the same point in the vibratory cycle: still image.

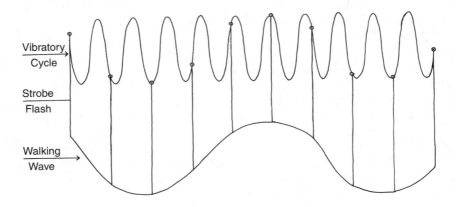

Figure 6-13. Strobe flashing at different points in the vibratory cycle: traveling image.

only one strobe flash is generated in each video field. When the clinician desires frame-by-frame video playback, each frame will supply only one clean image (flash) at a time. Fundamental frequency information is still relevant, however, because the contact microphone is used to trigger the strobe pulse at the appropriate moment within the glottic cycle phase (John Crump, Kay Elemetrics, personal communication, June 1993).

Similar cautions apply to stroboscopy as were pertinent to our discussion of acoustic waveforms. Because the strobe flash is triggered in direct response to the fundamental frequency, highly periodic fundamental frequencies will produce a more regular and evenly triggered strobe pulse that will faithfully represent the underlying vocal fold vibration. Unfortunately, clinical voice pathologists often examine patients whose voices are incapable of stable fundamental frequencies. Under those conditions, the resulting stroboscopic image is likely to result from strobe flash points triggered aperiodically at various places in the glottic cycle because of the irregular fundamental frequency. Obviously, the composite vibratory image may be substantially different from the real-time vocal fold vibration, and clinicians have reason to be less confident of any visual perceptual judgments for those images.

Endoscopes

Both flexible and rigid endoscopes may be coupled to a strobe generator for the examination (Figures 6-14, 6-15, and 6-16). In

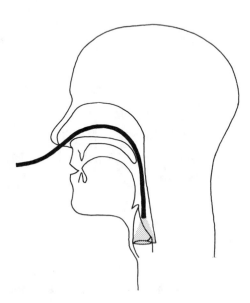

Figure 6-14. Flexible endoscope position.

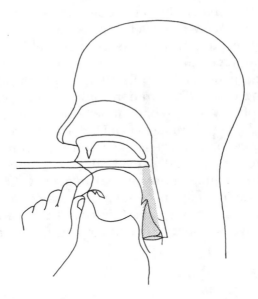

Figure 6-15. Ninety-degree endoscope position.

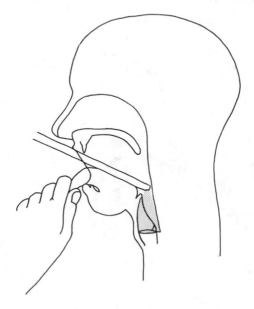

Figure 6-16. Seventy-degree endoscope position.

general, the flexible endoscope offers a more natural production, allowing the patient to perform multiple speech tasks and the clinician to observe the vocal tract and supraglottic region. Flexible endoscopy is slightly more invasive than the rigid endoscopy, however, and is subject to disruptive vertical movements as the patient alters position of the velum, base of tongue, and swallows. It is consequently more difficult to achieve a stable image, especially during connected speech. Because of the smaller diameter of the fiberoptic light bundle, the image may also be darker, although some camera peripherals may improve the lighting.[20,73,79,80] Nonetheless, the fiberoptic scope is ideal whenever:

■ Rigid endoscopy is not possible because of anatomic limits or patient tolerance.
■ Connected speech samples must be observed, as for patients with a motor speech disorder.
■ The vocal tract movements are important to assess, such as for professional voice users.
■ Velopharyngeal function is of interest.

Rigid endoscopes offer larger, more stable, and often brighter images of the vocal folds but require a sustained vowel /i/ to draw the epiglottis forward and view the larynx. Rigid endoscopy has many advantages because it is easier for clinicians to see a larger view of the vocal folds and it avoids some of the optical artifacts common in flexible imaging because of its brighter light illumination and a stable lens to object distance.[20,73,80]. Both 90° and 70° scopes offer similar views but require different positioning in the oral cavity (see Figures 6-15 and 6-16). Rigid endoscopy is advantageous whenever:

■ Close views of the vocal folds or lesion detail is needed.
■ Patients can tolerate the rigid scope and a full view of the vocal folds (from anterior commissure to arytenoid cartilage) can be seen.
■ Vocal fold vibratory patterns are important to observe.

If the patient has a hypersensitive gag reflex, then the rigid endoscope may be more difficult to tolerate. Although most patients can be relaxed through coaching, approximately 5% to 10% of all patients may require intraoral topical anesthesia to suppress the gag reflex to tolerate the rigid examination.

Peppard and Bless[81] have demonstrated that the use of topical anesthesia does not alter the resulting visual image of the larynx. Topical anesthesia should not be administered without a standing order from a physician and only in a medical setting that is prepared to handle the remote possibility of complications.[20]

Levels of Error

At this point, it is useful to consider four levels of error that underlie the stroboscopic images[20]:

- **Stroboscopy is not real time.** The vibratory image achieved is a result of flashes that are triggered at various phases of the glottic cycle, across many waveforms. The resulting image does not represent a true, continuous waveform "slowed down," but rather a composite group of single flashes across time.
- **Image is seen through optic devices.** The resulting image seen on the monitor screen has been projected through optic devices, including an endoscope, a camera lens (sometimes magnified), and pixels on a monitor screen. Consequently, variables such as lighting, lens focus, lens-to-object distance, uneven angle of lens, color, and video-system resolution all contribute to the adequacy and accuracy of the resulting image. The possibility for visual artifacts and distortions from these optic devices must be considered critically as possible limits to the interpretation.
- **Speech sample may not be representative.** If stroboscopy is conducted using rigid endoscopy, then the speech sample is limited to sustained vowel productions (usually /i/), sometimes at pitches higher than conversational connected speech and certainly in a posture unnatural for speech (eg, mouth open, tongue and neck extended). The resulting vibratory image may not be fully representative of vocal fold patterns during uninhibited speech. Even the use of a flexible fiberscope can alter the patient's voice performance sufficiently to pose a level of error in the recording and interpretation process. Thus, task-based artifacts do exist and must be explored with caution.
- **Individual subject variability is large.** Many patient factors can influence the success and interpretability of the image, including anatomical limits to full visualization, the levels of comfort and compliance with the tasks, and the

severity of the voice disorder. Because the accuracy of the strobe flashing rate is dependent on stable pitch tracking from the contact microphone, a very aperiodic or aphonic voice may not trigger the strobe light accurately. When this occurs, the image will flicker in a rapid, irregular fashion and is not representative of the vocal fold vibratory pattern. Consequently, individual variability may influence the interpretability of the resulting image.

Criteria for Videostroboscopic Examination

Is a videostroboscopic examination warranted for every patient with a voice disorder? The answer to this question will depend on the medical delivery model and ultimately must be decided by the professionals who use and interpret this technique. Certainly, permanent documentation of the vocal pathology or status of vocal fold function is worthwhile. However, more critical rationales for using this diagnostic tool are essential if stroboscopy is to be justified to both patients and insurers. The central questions to be addressed include:

- What information does stroboscopy provide that is not available in the otolaryngologist's indirect examination? Voice pathologists have recognized the unique importance of assessing the vibratory pattern of phonation, an event that cannot be seen without this special lighting technique.
- How might the stroboscopic image influence (in fact, change) either the diagnosis or the treatment plan (whether medical or rehabilitative)? If the diagnosis or treatment plan is not affected by findings on stroboscopy, then the utility of the procedure is limited to documentation and may not be seen as essential to case reviewers.

One set of conservative indications criteria includes the following profiles:

- Patients with **persistent dysphonia** (greater than 3 weeks' duration) unexplained by findings on indirect exam (normal or inconclusive).
- Patients who are **professional voice users** and have noted changes or deterioration in voice performance (eg, range, quality, stability, or endurance).

■ Whenever **phonosurgery** is planned, to allow adequate preoperative examination of the vocal fold status and post-operatively, to assess recovery from the procedure.

■ To **clarify the etiology** of the voice disorder, when organic or functional contributors are unclear.

■ To determine an **optimal management plan**, whether medical, surgical, or rehabilitative.

These criteria are far from all-inclusive but address the questions posed above and provide justifiable utilization criteria for using stroboscopic imaging to make decisions in the assessment and treatment process.

Imaging Techniques Using a Rigid Endoscope

The patient is seated comfortably in a supportive chair, with hips back into the seat and leaning slightly forward. The patient is instructed to open the mouth, relax the tongue, and begin saying a prolonged /i/ sound. With a 70° endoscope, the clinician inserts the scope directly in the center of the mouth, pressing firmly down on the tongue and angling the endoscope backward until the larynx comes into view on the monitor. The endoscope does not need to go very far back; in most patients, the angle of insertion will bring the vocal folds into viewing range easily. Care should be taken to avoid touching the back of the pharynx or faucial pillars with the endoscope, which may elicit a gag reflex. The endoscope position should be stable and firm because light and inconsistent pressure on the tongue may also trigger a gag.

Some "tips of the trade" can assist clinicians in achieving a full view of the larynx and vocal folds, and ensure patient comfort:

■ The patient should breathe gently through the mouth during the examination. It is usually helpful to have the patient keep his or her eyes open during the exam. If possible, ask the patient to observe the imaging simultaneously (via second monitor or a well-placed mirror). Otherwise, an interesting photograph or other visual attraction may help the patient remain relaxed and focused during endoscopy.

■ Warm the endoscope tip to reduce fogging. During the exam, intermittent fogging can be removed by touching the endoscope to the buccal mucosa.

■ The endoscope can be rotated forward and back, angled upward and down; the tip can be rotated laterally in either direction. An optimal view is one in which the vocal folds are large enough to be clearly visible and centered on the screen. When the image is angled or otherwise distorted on the monitor, it may be impossible to judge movement patterns accurately, and an artifactual left-right imbalance may appear. Clinicians should learn to rotate the scope in any of these three planes to obtain the optimal view.

■ Adjust the endoscope to achieve a stable vertical level (lens-to-object distance) on the left versus right side, working toward achieving a full image (anterior commissure to posterior rim of the glottis), as well as a clear, well-lit and well-focused image.

■ The recorded sample should be long enough (5 seconds or longer) to allow sufficient successive strobe images for recording. If the images are fleeting and cannot be sustained, the vibratory pattern cannot be assessed reliably.

■ If mucus is obscuring the image of the vocal folds, have the patient perform a gentle glottal stop or throat clear. Mucus seems to settle on lesions site, so it is important to clear it to appreciate the underlying vocal fold mucosa.

For imaging with steady or stroboscopic light, the recording protocol is according to individual patient needs, but generally includes:

■ full face recording with a connected speech sample (eg, counting, standard passage, and sustained vowels). This allows the clinician to assess overall perceptual quality and free-field speech and voice behaviors. It also heps match a "face" to the "larynx."

■ sustained /i/ vowel productions, which will bring the epiglottis forward and allow the clinician to view the vocal folds during vibration. In early trials, a full view is easier to achieve during higher pitched /i/ productions. The patient can be cued to decrease pitch once the clinician obtains a satisfactory view. The sustained vowels should include habitual and range tasks of pitch and loudness capabilities.

■ laryngeal diadochokinesis, using repeated /i i i i/ and /hi hi hi hi/ to observe the glottic closure pattern and rapid abduction and adduction of the vocal folds.

■ vegetative maneuvers (including inhalation, rest breathing, coughing, laughing, and throat clearing). These allow the clinician to observe the laryngeal valve function and help identify any structural or movement problems.

■ multiple trials of all speech tasks are necessary. These maneuvers are necessary, if possible, to assess individual variability. Occasionally, the patient's tolerance for scoping will not allow for repeated trials.

Visual Perceptual Judgments

Both steady (halogen) light and strobe (xenon) light observations will be made from the recorded image. Although a variety of rating scales and schemes exist, some consensus has been achieved about the salient features for visual perceptual judgments (see Table 6-2).[20] Steady light observations include:

■ **glottic closure pattern**, which can be categorized according to appearance. If glottic closure is incomplete, the gaps are noted as irregular, hourglass, posterior, anterior, or spindle-shaped (bowing). Note that glottic closure judgments must also be made during vibratory samples, for comparison with steady light image; often, slight gaps that are apparent during vibratory closure patterns are not seen in steady light.

■ **supraglottic hyperfunction**, including medial compression of the lateral ventricular folds, and the anterior-to-posterior "squeeze" of the epiglottis and arytenoids. This tension may be accompanied by a general lowering of the larynx during phonation but will then relax during rest breathing. Supraglottic hyperfunction can also be seen under stroboscopic light.

■ **mucus** presence on the vocal folds. This may signal a lesion or irritation of the mucosa and should be noted by location and appearance (eg, tacky, pooling, etc).

■ **structural appearance** of the entire larynx, including vocal folds, epiglottis, posterior glottic rim, ventricular folds, and pyriform sinuses. These features should be explored under steady light along with movement (abduction and adduction) of the vocal folds to reveal any gross asymmetry or abnormality.

Vibratory features for visual perceptual judgments include ratings for shape-changing and timing factors. The following are the most common vibratory observations under stroboscopic light:

Table 6-2. Visual Perceptual Judgments of Stroboscopic Image

Steady light	Glottic closure (static)
	Supraglottic hyperfunction
	Mucus
	General appearance and movement
Strobe light	Glottic closure (vibratory)
	Phase closure
	Symmetry
	Amplitude
	Mucosal wave
	Stiffness/nonvibrating portion/adynamic segment
	Periodicity
Other observations	Patient tolerance
	Endoscope type
	Topical anesthesia
	Perceptual quality
	Fundamental frequency and intensity: range and habitual
Drawing/sketch	Adduction and Abduction Pattern
	Midline closure pattern (adduction)
	Lateral excursion of the vocal folds (abduction)
	Sites of notable features (eg, hemorrhage, lesions, mucus, etc)

■ **Glottic closure pattern** under vibratory conditions is compared with steady light impressions. Phase closure is the relative ratio of glottis-open to glottis-closed within a single vibratory cycle.

■ **Mucosal wave** reflects the longitudinal flexibility of the vocal fold during vibration. Absence of mucosal wave, called nonvibrating portion, stiffness, or adynamic segment, can be described in terms of its location and extent of the vocal fold.

■ **Amplitude** reflects the medial to lateral excursion of the vocal fold from midline.

■ **Symmetry** refers to the shape-changing relationship between left and right vocal folds. For example, do they move in the same manner at the same time?

■ **Periodicity** or **regularity** is a timing characteristic and refers to the cycle-to-cycle stability of the vocal fold oscillation. This judgment is difficult to make unless the strobe image can be set to "locked" phase. In this setting, the image will appear to be very still if the vibratory pattern is regular (periodic). If not, the image is "jumpy" or unstable, revealing an aperiodic vibratory waveform.

As for all perceptual ratings, it is difficult to achieve reliability in visual perceptual judgments of laryngeal images under steady and stroboscopic lighting. Nonetheless, the observations and judgments made by clinicians who have used the technique will continue to be refined in individual settings. One approach to increasing intrajudge and interjudge familiarity and reliability in assessing these images is to schedule frequent "strobe review" meetings. These sessions are especially beneficial when voice pathologists and otolaryngologists can share impressions of the laryngeal images. Although rating schemes should be tailored to individual needs and settings, a sample rating form for stroboscopy judgments is contained in Appendix 6-5.

Finally, general comments related to the adequacy, compliance, and tolerance of the examination are useful and help ensure test-retest reliability for reexaminations. If the pretest fundamental frequency, intensity, and audio-perceptual judgments of voice quality are noted at the initial endoscopy, then these factors may be considered and monitored in subsequent exams. Peppard and Bless[82] described a technique for increasing reliability of repeated stroboscopic examinations. A plastic transparency is placed over the still video image on the monitor, and anatomical landmark boundaries are traced to form a "template." This transparency record is affixed to the monitor in follow-up exams to line up the retest image for comparable size and angle of view.

Laryngeal imaging offers extraordinary diagnostic and rehabilitative potential for voice clinicians. Although laryngeal imaging requires greater academic preparation, a commitment to skill-based competencies, and additional professional responsibilities, clinicians who use this technique consistently reap the benefits of this visual information.

Electroglottography (EGG)

Electroglottography is a noninvasive technique that uses electrical current passing through the neck to measure vocal fold contact across time. Two electrodes are placed on either side of the thyroid alae, with a small electrical current passing through as the vocal folds vibrate. The electrodes measure the variable resistance as the vocal folds vibrate. Because tissue conducts the electrical current better than air does, the resistance increases when the vocal folds are opening or opened and decreases during the closing or closed phase. The EGG waveform displays this variable resistance and serves as a real-time analog of the vocal fold vibratory pattern, with peaks and troughs representing maximum points of open and closed phases.[83-85] The technique is subject to artifact, however, because variations in tissue thickness, electrode placement, mucous interference, and laryngeal movements can produce errors in this measure. Using a dual channel EGG can reduce some of this error.[68] This device positions two electrodes vertically on each side of the thyroid to achieve better representation of the upper and lower dimensions of vocal fold contact during the vibratory cycle. Nonetheless, EGG has been used in combination with other physiologic measures of glottal function, such as inverse filtering, to cross-validate the simultaneous glottal measures.[86] A most useful application of EGG was suggested by Karnell,[87] who synchronized an EGG signal with stroboscopy flash pulses to offer a real-time monitor of the vibratory phase points across the stroboscopic image. Since that time, stroboscopy manufacturers have incorporated an EGG signal in most computer integrated strobe units.

Electromyography (EMG)

Electromyography is a direct measure of laryngeal muscle activity and function and because it is an invasive procedure, it must be performed by a neurologist or otolaryngologist. Needle electrodes are inserted percutaneously into the laryngeal muscles, and the pattern of electrical activity is studied.[7,88-91] Because the placement of the electrodes cannot be seen directly in laryngeal muscles, insertions are essentially "blind." A series of vocal tasks are used to confirm electrode placement in the correct muscles.[91] To verify correct placement in the cricothyroid muscle, for example, the EMG activity should be active as soon as the patient produces a high pitch but should be entirely "quiet" (inactive) during rest breathing. On the other hand, electrical activity for the thyroarytenoid muscle is stronger during firm glottal stop productions. EMG recordings are used to assess the onset, timing, and amplitude patterns of muscle activity and can be used to discriminate normal function from neurologic impairment (eg, paralysis) or mechanical fixation (eg, ankylosis).[90,91] The electrical signals recorded from the muscles are interpreted as normal or pathologic based on four basic features: timing (onset and offset) of muscle activity, and the pattern, number, and amplitude of muscle action potentials.[90] The widest clinical application of laryngeal EMG is in providing diagnosis and prognosis for suspected vocal fold neuropathy, including paralysis, dystonia, and other neuromuscular disorders and for discriminating vocal fold paralysis from mechanical fixation of the cricoarytenoid joint. A more recent clinical use for percutaneous EMG is to confirm the correct muscle placement for BOTOX injections to treat spasmodic dysphonia.[89-92]

Normative Information

Normative information is essential to establish the clinical utility of instrumental measures of voice. Without reliable normative standards, it is impossible to compare individual measures to normal and pathologic groups. Normative information also gives information about the range and variability of performance in speakers with and without voice complaints. Ideally, the collection of a normal database for clinical comparisons should account for many factors that might influence the instrumental results. For example, the demographic groups of speakers, including different gender, age, health history, and local dialect should be reported. Elicitation techniques and sample tasks may vary across studies, as well as equipment and analysis routines. These factors limit the ability to compare findings across studies or sites.

A practical solution to the problem of collecting normative data is available to any voice pathologist. "Local norms" can provide an opportunity to run a large group of normal speakers through the voice laboratory. Then clinicians can construct a normative database that is easily referenced for demographics (age, gender, vocal behaviors, and health history). More important, the findings can be interpreted with confidence because data are collected on the same equipment using the exact elicitation methods and recording techniques applied to pathologic speakers in that clinical laboratory.

A summary of some of the published normative information available for fundamental frequency, intensity, aerodynamics, and stroboscopy is presented below. Unfortunately, no well-accepted normative standards are available for perturbation measures and signal/harmonic-to-noise ratios because of differences in recording techniques, analyses, units of measurement, and equipment variables. Recently, acoustic analysis programs have begun to include normal and disordered speaker databanks specific to their technology and equipment as part of the system package. Nonetheless, the emerging normal database for instrumental measures of voice must continue to expand with cooperative contributions across laboratories.

Fundamental Frequency

Many studies have examined the speaking fundamental frequency sampled from spontaneous speech or reading passages. Because variables in speech utterance, loudness, and intonational patterns may influence the resulting fundamental frequency, other researchers have used a stable, sustained vowel at comfortable pitch and loudness to minimize variability in findings. The data in Table 6-3 were collected during production of a sustained neutral /a/ vowel and are commensurate with other reported fundamental frequency data.

Table 6-3. Normative Fundamental Frequency

	Mean	*Minimum*	*Maximum*
Children (6-10 years)*			
Boys (N = 59)	226 Hz	179 Hz	272 Hz
Girls (N = 62)	238 Hz	193 Hz	294 Hz
Adults**			
Males (N = 58)	106 Hz	77 Hz	482 Hz
Females (N = 61)	193 Hz	137 Hz	634 Hz

*Data from Glaze, Bless, Milenkovic, and Susser.[48]
**Data from Bless, Glaze, Biever-Lowery, Campos, and Peppard.[9]

Intensity Range

Recording considerations for intensity measurements are both task and equipment based. Measures are known to vary based on the vowel or speech utterance, mouth-to-microphone distance, and filtering characteristics of the sound level meter. The data in Table 6-4 were collected on vowel /a/, using a sound level meter with C scale weighting held a constant 12 inches from the mouth.

Airflow Rate

Airflow rate is affected by the speech sample measured. Sentence productions yielded greater intrasubject variability in airflow than sustained vowels in 11 male and 10 female speakers measured within and across sessions.[65] The data in Table 6-5 were collected using a Nagashima Phonatory Function Analyzer and sampled during production of a sustained /a/ vowel at comfortable pitch and loudness.

Intraoral Pressure Estimates

Holmberg, Hillman, and Perkell[62] reported intraoral estimates of subglottal air pressure for normal adult speakers under

Table 6-4. Normative Intensity

	Mean	Range
Children 6-10 years (N = 97)*	70 dB	60-99 dB
Adults**		
Males (N = 58)	70 dB	<60-110 dB
Females (N = 61)	68 dB	<60-106 dB

*Data from Glaze, Bless, and Sussex.[49]
**Data from Bless, Glaze, Biever-Lowery, Campos, and Peppard.[9]

Table 6-5. Normative Airflow Rate

	Mean	Range
Adults		
Males (N = 67)	119 cc/s	40-320 cc/s
Females (N = 78)	115 cc/s	50-220 cc/s

Data from Bless, Glaze, Biever-Lowery, Campos, and Peppard.[9]

three conditions: normal, soft, and loud productions, and find-ings confirmed the covarying proportional relationship between subglottic pressure and loudness. In a follow-up study using low, normal, and high pitch conditions, the authors found increased pressure in both low and high pitch (see Table 6-6).[63]

Stroboscopic Judgments

Bless, Glaze, Biever-Lowery, Campos, and Peppard[9] examined visual-perceptual ratings of stroboscopic vibratory features in a study of 121 normal speakers ranging in age from 16 to 92 years. The vibratory features that regressed significantly with increased age were supraglottic activity, amplitude, and mucosal wave. Older female speakers also displayed significantly less regularity in vocal fold vibration with increased age.

Table 6-6. Normative Intraoral Pressure Estimates

	Normal	Soft	Loud
Adults*			
Males (N = 25)	5.91 cmH$_2$O	4.79 cmH$_2$O	8.39 cmH$_2$O
Females (N = 25)	6.09 cmH$_2$O	4.79 cmH$_2$O	8.46 cmH$_2$O
	Normal	**Low Pitch**	**High Pitch**
Adults**			
Males (N = 25)	6.3 cmH$_2$O	7.0 cmH$_2$O	7.5 cmH$_2$O
Females (N = 20)	5.8 cmH$_2$O	6.7 cmH$_2$O	6.1 cmH$_2$O

*Data from Holmberg, Hillman, and Perkell.[62]
**Data from Holmberg, Hillman, and Perkell.[63]

The Clinical Voice Laboratory

The data generated by instrumental measures of voice have contributed greatly to our understanding of vocal function and the seemingly infinite variability and flexibility of human voice production. Instrumental data must be paired with clinical impressions and audio-perceptual judgments of voice quality to be used meaningfully. Nonetheless, instruments have provided the first step toward understanding the complex relationship between voice quality, laryngeal anatomy and physiology, and objective measures of vocal function. Multiple sources of complementary information improve our ability to observe and monitor vocal capabilities in normal and professional speakers and voice production limits in disordered patients.

The clinical utility of the voice laboratory is still emerging. Even as new and better tools are refined, as normative information continues to accrue, and as equipment becomes increasingly accessible, these instrumental measures are valid tools for detecting pathology, assessing vocal severity, and contributing to accurate diagnoses. Currently, instrumental measures offer varying success at each of these levels. In the rehabilitation process, however, voice pathologists use instrumental measures as a primary treatment tool to display, instruct, motivate, and justify treatment needs. For example, instrumental feed-back may assist a patient in achieving target behaviors. Re-peated pretest and posttest measurements may reinforce the patient's progress. Finally, vocal function measures offer a means to document the pathology that may be far more con-vincing than perceptual judgments of voice quality alone. Ultimately, the goal of the clinical voice laboratory is to inform patients, clinicians, and scientists about the nature and limits of human voice production.

Summary

Instrumental measures of voice have expanded greatly over the past decades. Better recording devices have enhanced acoustic, aerodynamic, imaging, and other physiologic measures of vocal function, signal processing techniques, and analysis routines. Voice pathologists have recognized the clinical applications of these measurement tools and integrated instrumental measure-ments in the diagnosis and treatment of patients with voice dis-orders. Nonetheless, interpretation must always be done with care, and users must be knowledgeable about the risks of artifact and error to ensure valid application of these measures. Norm-ative information is still insufficient in most areas but continues to improve.

Glossary

Acoustics

Acoustic Waveform

Frequency: The rate of vibration, represented by a number of wave-form periods per unit time, for example, Hertz (Hz) as the number of cycles per second.

Fundamental frequency: The lowest periodic waveform of vocal fold vibration. Fundamental frequency is the reciprocal of the pitch period $(Fo = 1/T)$.

Intensity: Sound energy present in a signal, represented by waveform amplitude.

Perturbation: Measures of variability or instability in a quasi-periodic waveform.

Jitter: Also known as pitch perturbation; a measure of cycle-to-cycle variability in fundamental frequency. Can be expressed in absolute measures or as a percentage referenced to the fundamental frequency.

Shimmer: Also known as amplitude perturbation; a measure of the cycle-to-cycle variability in waveform amplitude.

Pitch: The perceptual correlate of the fundamental frequency, based on a judgmental rating from low to high.

Pitch detection algorithm (PDA): A mathematical equation designed to detect the fundamental frequency of a speech waveform. Several methods are used commonly: zero-crossing, peak-picking, and waveform matching with autocorrelation.

Pitch period: The length of time for one waveform of vocal fold vibration. The pitch period is the reciprocal of fundamental frequency ($T = 1/F$).

Semitone: A unit devised for comparison of frequencies (eg, 200 Hertz to 400 Hertz represents a 12-semitone range). The semitone scale includes all of the notes (sharps and flats included) on the musical scale and is logarithmic. The semitone scale reflects perceptual attributes of the human ear because the difference in hertz between semitones lower on the musical scale is smaller than the interval for semitones in higher frequencies.

Signal (or harmonic)-to-noise ratio: The mathematical ratio of periodic energy (signal) to random or aperiodic energy (noise) in a given signal.

Spectrogram: A visual display of a speech signal across time (horizontal axis), giving information about frequency (vertical axis) and intensity (gray or color variation) in the display.

Spectrum: A plot of signal energy (intensity) by frequency at a single point in time.

Signal Processing

Amplification: Increasing the amplitude of a signal to increase the "gain" (measurable or detectable changes) in time-variation for purposes of recording, playback, data measurement, or signal processing.

Analog-to-digital (A/D) processing: Conversion of an analog signal to digital form using a computer hardware device (A/D board or converter). An analog signal is time- and amplitude-varying and continuous. Digital processing, or digitization, divides the signal into discrete bits of information which are encoded numerically.

Filters: A method of including (passing) and excluding (filtering) specified levels of energy in the signal, usually in the course of signal processing. A "low pass" filter excludes energy at high frequencies; a "high pass" filter excludes energy at low frequencies; and a "band-pass" filter excludes energies higher or lower than a specified band of frequencies.

Quantization: The division of amplitude in an analog signal into discrete numeric values. The greater the quantization levels, the more adequately the amplitude waveform is represented.

Sampling rate: The number of samples per second of a digital signal. The greater the sampling rate, the more information obtained for signal processing.

Transducer: A device that converts energy from one form to another, for example, flow or pressure into an electrical signal.

Aerodynamics

Pressure

Differential pressure: Referenced to some other pressure (eg, between two measured sites, such as left and right nares).

Driving pressure: Flow of a gas from higher to lower regions of molecular concentration.

Intraoral pressure: Obtained from the closed oral cavity when the vocal folds are abducted, as in an unvoiced plosive consonant; an indirect estimate of subglottal pressure.[56]

Phonation threshold pressure: The minimal pressure needed to set the vocal folds into oscillation, considering variables of tissue damping, mucosal wave, vocal fold thickness, prephonatory glottal width, and transglottal pressure.[10]

Pressure: Force per unit area acting perpendicular to the area.

Subglottal pressure: Measured directly from the lung pressures below the glottis, when the vocal folds are adducted. Subglottic pressure: estimated clinically using intraoral pressure peaks produced during an unvoiced plosive consonant; a measure of the tracheal (respiratory) driving pressure used during phonation.

Airflow and Volume

Flow: The movement of a quantity of gas through an area.

Flow rate (volume velocity): Speed (and direction) of flow per unit time.

Flow volume: Quantity of flow.

Pneumotachograph: A differential pressure-sensing device that measures the drop in pressure when airflow passes across a known mechanical resistance (eg, wire-mesh screen or narrow tubes).

Rotameter (flow meter): Airflow measurement device; a cylindrical tube with a ball "float" within and an external measurement index. As flow passes through the bottom of the tube, the float rises to a level corresponding to the flow rate.

Spirometer: Flow volume measurement device (wet and dry varieties); records the total amount of air blown across a sensing device (dry) or volume of water displaced (wet) during exhalation.

U-tube manometer: Pressure measurement device; a bent glass tube with external measurement index, filled with liquid (usually water or mercury). As pressure is applied to one side of the U, the direct reading can be taken from the liquid displacement on the other side.

Warm-wire anemometer: Flow measurement device; as airflow passes over (and cools) the warm metal wire, its electrical resistance changes, and flow magnitude can be predicted from the change in resistance of the wire.

Stroboscopy

Talbot's Law: Persistence of vision on the retina; the human retina cannot perceive more than five separate images per second (each image "rests" 0.2 seconds on the retina) and, when presented in succession, are fused into one apparent continuous image. Thus, a series of still images presented at this rate (or faster) will be perceived visually as a connected, moving image.

Vibratory Features

Amplitude: The lateral excursion of the vocal folds.

Mucosal wave: The movement of the vocal fold cover in lateral, longitudinal, and vertical waveform motion.

Periodicity: Regularity of the timing of successive cycles.

Phase closure: Ratio of open-to-close phase of the glottis during one full vibratory cycle.

Stiffness / nonvibrating portion / adynamic segment: Commonly expressed as a percentage of the full length of the membranous portion of the vocal fold.

Symmetry: The extent to which the left and right vocal folds appear to move as mirror images; changes in phase are identical.

Appendix 6-1*

The Roles of Otolaryngologists and Speech-Language Pathologists in the Performance and Interpretation of Strobovideolaryngoscopy

American Academy of Otolaryngology Voice and Swallow Committee and the ASHA Special Interest Division on Voice and Voice Disorders

This joint statement regarding the use of strobovideolaryngoscopy has been developed by the American Academy of Otolaryngology Voice and Swallow Committee and the Special Interest Division on Voice and Voice Disorders of the American Speech-Language-Hearing Association.

Strobovideolaryngoscopy (including rigid and flexible endoscopy) is a laryngeal imaging procedure that may be used by otolaryngologists and other voice professionals as a diagnostic procedure. Physicians are the only professionals qualified and licensed to render medical diagnoses related to the identification of laryngeal pathology as it affects voice. Consequently, when used for medical diagnostic purposes, strobovideolaryngoscopy examinations should be viewed and interpreted by an otolaryngologist with training in this procedure. Speech-language pathologists with expertise in voice disorders and with specialized training in strobovideolaryngoscopy are professionals qualified to use this procedure for the purpose of assessing voice production and vocal function. Within interdisciplinary settings, these diagnostic and vocal function assessment procedures may be accomplished through the combined efforts of these related professionals. Strobovideolaryngoscopy may also be used as a therapeutic aid and biofeedback tool during the conduct of voice treatment. Care should be taken to use this examination only in settings that assure patient safety.

*Reprinted with permission from American Speech-Language-Hearing Association (*Asha.* 1998; 40 (suppl 18): 32).

Appendix 6-2*
ASHA Preferred Practice Patterns for Voice: Assessment

12.7 Voice Assessment

> *Procedures to assess vocal structure and function, identifying strengths, deficits, contributing factors, and implications for functional communication.*
>
> Voice assessment is conducted according to the Guiding Principles, p. 7, and Fundamental Components of Preferred Practice Patterns, p. 9.

Professionals Who Perform the Procedure(s)
- Speech-language pathologists.

Expected Outcome(s)
- Assessment is conducted to diagnose a voice disorder or a laryngeal disorder affecting respiration, describe perceptual phonatory characteristics, measure aspects of vocal function, and examine phonatory behavior.
- Assessment may result in recommendations for treatment or follow-up, or in referral for other examinations or services.

Clinical Indications
- Individuals of all ages are assessed as needed, requested, or mandated; when their vocal function is altered, impaired, or inadequate to meet their communication, educational, emotional, vocational, social, and health needs; or when the impairment has implications beyond vocal status (e.g., neurological dysfunction, inadequate airway, laryngeal dysfunction).
- Assessment is prompted by referral, by the patient's/client's medical status, or by failure of a speech screening (see Procedure 02.0).

Clinical Process
- All patients/clients with voice disorders must be examined by a physician, preferably in a discipline appropriate to the presenting complaint. The physician's examination may occur before or after the voice evaluation by the speech-language pathologist.
- Assessment includes:
  - Case history and vocal use history
  - Perceptual aspects of vocal production/behavior
  - Acoustic parameters of vocal production/behavior
  - Physiological aspects of phonatory behavior
  - Patient's/client's ability to modify vocal behavior
  - Emotional/psychological status
  - Medical history and associated conditions
  - Review of auditory, visual, motoric, and cognitive status
  - Observation or review of articulation, fluency, and language
  - Functional consequences of the voice disorder

- Assessment includes use of perceptual and/or instrumental measures. Procedures include:
  - Perceptual ratings
  - Acoustic analysis
  - Aerodynamic measures
  - Electroglottography
  - Imaging techniques such as endoscopy and stroboscopy. (These procedures may be conducted and interpreted in collaboration with other professionals.)
- Patients/clients with identified voice disorders receive follow-up services to monitor voice status and to ensure appropriate treatment.

Setting/Equipment Specifications

- Assessment is conducted in a clinical or natural environment conducive to eliciting a representative sample of the patient's/client's voice production.

Safety and Health Precautions

- All procedures ensure the safety of the patient/client and clinician and adhere to universal health precautions (e.g., prevention of bodily injury and transmission of infectious disease).
- Decontamination, cleaning, disinfection, and sterilization of multiple-use equipment before reuse are carried out according to facility-specific infection control policies and procedures and according to manufacturer's instructions.

Documentation

- Documentation includes pertinent background information, results and interpretation, prognosis, and recommendations. Recommendations may include the need for further assessment, follow-up, or referral. When treatment is recommended, information is provided concerning frequency, estimated duration, and type of service (e.g., individual group, home program) required.

ASHA Policy and Related References

In addition to the references on p. 6, the following references apply specifically to these procedures:

American Speech-Language-Hearing Association. (1992). Position statement and guidelines for evaluation and treatment for tracheoesophageal fistulization/puncture. *Asha, 34* (Suppl. 7), 17-21.

American Speech-Language-Hearing Association. (1992). Position statement and guidelines for vocal tract visualization and imaging. *Asha, 34* (Suppl. 7), 31-40.

American Speech-Language-Hearing Association. (1992). Sedation and topical anesthesia in speech- language pathology and audiology. *Asha, 34* (Suppl. 7), 41-42.

American Speech-Language-Hearing Association. (1993). Position statement and guidelines for oral and oropharyngeal prostheses. *Asha, 35* (Suppl. 10), 14-16.

American Speech-Language-Hearing Association. (1993). Position statement and guidelines on the use of voice prostheses in tracheotomized persons with or without ventilatory dependence. *Asha, 35* (Suppl. 10), 17-20.

Appendix 6-3
ASHA Preferred Practice Patterns for Voice: Treatment*

15.6 Voice Treatment

> *Procedures for addressing disorders of voice production, including possible organic, neurologic, behavioral, and psychosocial etiologies, and alaryngeal speech disorders.*
>
> Voice treatment is conducted according to the Guiding Principles, p. 7, and the Fundamental Components of Preferred Practice Patterns, p. 9.

Professionals Who Perform the Procedure(s)
- Speech-language pathologists

Support Personnel Who Perform the Procedure(s)
- Speech-language pathology assistants under the supervision of a certified speech-language pathologist (in accordance with the ASHA Guidelines for the Training, Credentialing, Use, and Supervision of Speech-Language Pathology Assistants).

Expected Outcomes
- Treatment is conducted to achieve improved voice production, coordination of respiration and laryngeal valving, and/or acquisition of alaryngeal speech sufficient to allow for functional oral communication
- Treatment may result in recommendations for reassessment or follow-up, or in referral for other examinations or services.

Clinical Indications
- Individuals of all ages receive treatment when their ability to communicate effectively is impaired and there is reason to believe that treatment will reduce the degree of impairment or disability and lead to improved communication behaviors.

Clinical Process
- Treatment of voice disorders, alaryngeal speech, and/or laryngeal disorders affecting respiration should be long enough for effective change, but should not be continued when there is no longer any further benefit.
- Treatment should provide information and guidance to patients/clients, families, and significant persons about the nature of voice disorders, alaryngeal speech, and/or laryngeal disorders affecting respiration, the goals, procedures, respective responsibilities, and the likely outcome of treatment.
- Treatment plans should address the patient's unique concerns, abilities, or priorities, and be individualized to meet the needs of special populations, including pediatrics, geriatrics, professional voice users, and diverse racial and cultural groups.
- Depending on the assessment results, treatment addresses the following:
  - Appropriate voice care and conservation guidelines, including strategies that promote healthy laryngeal tissues and voice production and reduce laryngeal trauma or strain.
  - Proper use of respiratory, phonatory, and resonatory processes to achieve improved voice production, coordination of respiration and laryngeal valving, with appropriate treatment to enhance these behaviors.
- Patient/client-directed selection of preferred alaryngeal speech communication means, including development of one or more of the following alaryngeal alternatives: esophageal speech, artificial larynx speech, or tracheoesophageal prosthesis speech.

*Reprinted with permission from *Preferred Practice Patterns: Voice Assessment; Voice Treatment*. Rockville, Md: American Speech-Language-Hearing Association; 1998

- Assisting the person with a voice disorder, alaryngeal speech, and/or laryngeal disorder that affects respiration to maintain treatment targets in oral communication in occupational and social situations in everyday living.
- Development of plans, including interdisciplinary referrals, for other speech and health problems that may accompany the voice disorder, alaryngeal speech, and/or laryngeal disorder affecting respiration including medical concerns, dysarthria, swallowing difficulty, psycho-emotional disturbance, and other problems.

Setting/Equipment Specifications

- Treatment is conducted in a clinical or natural environment conducive to observing, modifying, and monitoring the patient's/client's voice, alaryngeal speech, and/or laryngeal disorder affecting respiration.
- When available, instrumental measures may be used in treatment to monitor progress and to provide appropriate patient/client feedback of voice production and/or laryngeal function. Instrumental techniques should ensure validity of signal processing, analysis routines, and elimination of task or signal artifacts.
- Laryngeal imaging techniques and selection/placement of tracheoesophageal prostheses must be conducted in settings that have access to emergency medical treatment, if needed.

Safety and Health Precautions

- All procedures ensure the safety of the patient/client and clinician and adhere to universal health precautions (e.g., prevention of bodily injury and transmission of infectious disease).
- Decontamination, cleaning, disinfection, and sterilization of multiple-use equipment before reuse are carried out according to facility-specific infection control policies and procedures and according to manufacturer's instructions.

Documentation

- Documentation includes pertinent background information, treatment goals, results, prognosis, and specific recommendations. Recommendations may include the need for further treatment, follow-up, or interdisciplinary referral. When further treatment is recommended, information is provided concerning the frequency, estimated duration, and type of service (e.g., individual, group, home program) required.
- Documentation includes evaluating treatment outcomes and effectiveness.

ASHA Policy and Related References

In addition to the references on p. 6, the following references apply specifically to these procedures:

American Speech-Language-Hearing Association. (1992). Position statement and guidelines for evaluation and treatment for tracheoesophageal fistulization/puncture. *Asha, 34* (Suppl. 7), 17-21.

American Speech-Language-Hearing Association. (1992). Position statement and guidelines for vocal tract visualization and imaging. *Asha, 34* (Suppl. 7), 31-40.

American Speech-Language-Hearing Association. (1993). Position statement and guidelines for oral and oropharyngeal prostheses. *Asha, 35* (Suppl. 10), 14-16.

American Speech-Language-Hearing Association. (1993). Position statement and guidelines on the use of voice prostheses in tracheotomized persons with or without ventilatory dependence. *Asha, 35* (Suppl. 10), 17-20.

Appendix 6-4
Phonatory Function Test
(Acoustic and Aerodynamic Analysis)

**Institute for Voice Analysis
and Rehabilitation**
369 West First Street
Suite 408
Dayton Ohio 45402-3065
(513) 496-2622 FAX (513) 496-2610

Joseph C. Stemple, Ph.D.
Bernice K. Gerdeman, Ph.D.
Lisa N. Kelchner, M.S.

Name: _____   Date: _____   Age: _____

Occupation: _____   Physician: _____

Type: _____

PHONATORY FUNCTION TEST

ACOUSTIC ANALYSIS

SUSTAINED VOWEL /a/	f_0 (Hz)	jitter (%)	shimmer (dB)	N/H (dB)
Comfort				
Avg				
High				
Avg				
Low				
Avg				

FREQUENCY RANGE	Glide from mid-voice to as **low** as possible	Glide from the mid-voice to as **high** as possible
	_____ (Hz)	_____ (Hz)

SPEAKING FUNDAMENTAL FREQ	Reading	Conversation
	_____ (Hz)	_____ (Hz)

INTENSITY	Habitual level	Loudest tone level	Softest tone level
	_____ (dBSPL)	_____ (dBSPL)	_____ (dBSPL)

Comments:

_____

_____

_____

AERODYNAMIC ANALYSIS

SUSTAINED VOWEL /a/	Phonation Flow Volume (mL)	f0 (Hz)	Mean Air Flow Rate (mL/s)	Maximum Air Flow Rate (mL/s)	Intensity (dBSPL)	Maximum Phonation Time (sec)
Comfort	___	__	___	___	___	___
	___	__	___	___	___	___
	___	__	___	___	___	___
Avg	___	__	___	___	___	___
High	___	__	___	___	___	___
	___	__	___	___	___	___
	___	__	___	___	___	___
Avg	___	__	___	___	___	___
Low	___	__	___	___	___	___
	___	__	___	___	___	___
	___	__	___	___	___	___
Avg	___	__	___	___	___	___

SUBGLOTTIC PRESSURE   Repeat Ipipi (cm H_2O)

Comfort	___
	___
	___
Avg	___
	___

Perceptual Quality:

_____

_____

Comments & Recommendations:

_____

_____

_____

_____

Appendix 6-5
Stroboscopic Evaluation

Institute for Voice Analysis and Rehabilitation
369 West First Street
Suite 408
Dayton Ohio 45402-3065
(513) 496-2622 FAX (513) 496-2610

Joseph C. Stemple, Ph.D.
Bernice K. Gerdeman, Ph.D.
Lisa N. Kelchner, M.S.

Name: _____ Date: _____ Age: _____

Occupation: _____ Physician: _____

Type: _____

STROBOSCOPIC EVALUATION

VOICE QUALITY	Normal	Mildly Dysphonic	Mild-Mod Dysphonic	Moderately Dysphonic	Mod-Severely Dysphonic	Severely Dysphonic	Aphonic

GLOTTIC CLOSURE	Cannot Rate	Complete	Anterior	Irregular	Spindle	Posterior	Hourglass	Incomplete

SUPRAGLOTTIC ACTIVITY Latero-Medial Compression	(0) None	(1) Mild compression of vent. folds	(2) Mild-Mod	(3) Moderate	(4) Mod-severe	(5) Severe	(6) Dysphonia Plica Ventricularis TVF not visible

Antero-Post Compression	(0) None	(1) Mild	(2) Mild-Mod	(3) Moderate	(4) Mod-Severe	(5) Severe

VERTICAL LEVEL APPROX.	(0) Cannot Rate	(1) Equal	(2) Right Lower	(3) Left Lower	(4) Questionable

VOCAL FOLD EDGE	LEFT	(0) Cannot Rate	(1) Smooth Straight	(2)	(3)	(4)	(5)	(6) Rough Irregular
	RIGHT	(0)	(1)	(2)	(3)	(4)	(5)	(6)

VOCAL FOLD MOBILITY	LEFT	(0) Cannot Rate	(1) Normal	(2) Limited Adduction (mild) (mod) (sev)	(3) Limited Abduction (mild) (mod) (sev)	(4) Fixed (mild) (mod) (sev)
	RIGHT	(0)	(1)	(2)	(3)	(4)

AMPLITUDE	LEFT	(0) Cannot Rate	(1) Normal	(2) Mildly Decreased	(3) Mild-Mod Decreased	(4) Mod Decreased	(5) Mod-Sev Decreased	(6) Severely Decreased	(7) No Visible Movement
	RIGHT	(0)	(1)	(2)	(3)	(4)	(5)	(6)	(7)

MUCOSAL WAVE	LEFT	(0) Cannot Rate	(1) Normal	(2) Mildly Decreased	(3) Mild-Mod Decreased	(4) Mod Decreased	(5) Mod-Sev Decreased	(6) Severely Decreased	(7) Absent
	RIGHT	(0)	(1)	(2)	(3)	(4)	(5)	(6)	(7)

NON-VIBRATING PORTION	LEFT	(0) None	(1) 20%	(2) 40%	(3) 60%	(4) 80%	(5) 100%
	RIGHT	(0)	(1)	(2)	(3)	(4)	(5)

PHASE CLOSURE	Cannot Rate	(-5) Open Phase Predominates (Whisper dysphonia)	(-4)	(-3) (-2) (-1)	(0) Normal	(1) (2)	(3) (4)	(5) Closed Phase Predominates (Glottal fry-extreme hyperadduction)

PHASE SYMMETRY	Cannot Rate	(0) Regular always symmetrical	(1) Irregular during end or begin tasks	(2) Irregular during extremes pitch or loud	(3) 50% asymmetrical	(4) 75% asymmetrical	(5) always asymmetrical

OVERALL LARYNGEAL FUNCTION	(0) Normal	(1) Hypofunction	(2) Hyperfunction	(3) Laryngeal tremors (sust. v) (speech) (mild) (mod) (severe)	(4) Phonatory spasms (add) (abd) (mild) (mod) (severe)

Strobe Comments and Interpretations:

References

1. Sataloff RT, Spiegel JR, Carroll LM, Darby KS, Hawkshaw MJ, Rulnick RK. The clinical voice laboratory: practical design and clinical application. *J Voice.* 1990;4:264-279.
2. Hicks DM. Functional voice assessment: what to measure and why. In: *Assessment of Speech and Voice Production: Research and Clinical Applications.* Bethesda, Md: National Institute on Deafness and Other Communicative Disorders; 1991:204-209.
3. Titze IR. Measurements for assessment of voice disorders. In: *Assessment of Speech and Voice Production: Research and Clinical Applications.* Bethesda, Md: National Institute on Deafness and Other Communicative Disorders; 1991:42-49.
4. Orlikoff RF, Baken RJ. *Clinical Voice and Speech Measurement.* San Diego, Calif: Singular Publishing Group; 1993.
5. Titze IR. Towards standards in acoustic analysis of voice. In: Titze IR, ed. *Progress Report 4.* Iowa City, Iowa: National Center for Voice and Speech; 1993:271-280.
6. Behrman A, Orlikoff R. Instrumentation in voice assessment and treatment: what's the use? *Am J Speech-Lang Pathol.* 1997:6(4) 9-16.
7. Hirano M. *Clinical Examination of Voice.* New York, NY: Springer-Verlag; 1981.
8. Bless DM. Assessment of laryngeal function. In: Ford CN, Bless DM, eds. *Phonosurgery.* New York, NY: Raven Press; 1991:91-122.
9. Bless DM, Glaze LE, Biever-Lowery D, Campos G, Peppard RC. Stroboscopic, acoustic, aerodynamic, and perceptual attributes of voice production in normal speaking adults. In: Titze IR, ed. *Progress Report 4.* Iowa City, Iowa: National Center for Voice and Speech; 1993:121-134.
10. Titze IR. *Principles of Voice Production.* Englewood Cliffs, NJ: Prentice-Hall; 1994.
11. Titze I. *Workshop on Acoustic Voice Analysis: Summary Statement.* Denver, Colo: National Center for Voice and Speech, Wilbur James Gould Research Center; February 17, 1995.
12. Read C, Buder EH, Kent RD. Speech analysis systems: a survey. *J Speech Hear Res.* 1990;33:363-374.
13. Read C, Buder EH, Kent RD. Speech analysis systems: an evaluation. *J Speech Hear Res.* 1992;35:314-332.
14. Baken RJ. *Clinical Measurement of Speech and Voice.* Boston, Mass: College-Hill Press; 1997.
15. Kent RD, Read C. *The Acoustic Analysis of Speech.* San Diego, Calif: Singular Publishing Group; 1992.
16. Titze IR, Winholtz WS. Effect of microphone type and placement on voice perturbation measurements. *J Speech Hear Res.* 1993;36:1177-1190.
17. Titze IR, Horii Y, Scherer RC. Some technical considerations in voice perturbation measurements. *J Speech Hear Res.* 1987;30:252-260.
18. Jiang J, Lin E, Hanson D. Effect of tape recording on perturbation measures. *J Speech Lang Hear Res.* 1998;40:1031-1041.

19. Perry C, Ingrisano D, Blair, B. The influence of recording systems on jitter and shimmer estimates. *Am J Speech-Lang Pathol.* 1996;5(2):86-90.

20. Hirano M, Bless DM. *Videostroboscopic Examination of the Larynx.* San Diego, Calif: Singular Publishing Group; 1993.

21. Davis S. Acoustic characteristics of normal and pathologic voices. *ASHA Reports.* 1981;11:97-115.

22. Horii Y. Jitter and shimmer differences among sustained vowel phonations. *J Speech Hear Res.* 1982;25:12-14.

23. Askenfelt A, Hammarberg B. Speech waveform perturbation analysis: a perceptual-acoustic comparison of seven measures. *J Speech Hear Res.* 1986;29:50-64.

24. Ludlow CL, Bassich CJ, Connor NP, Coulter DC, Lee YJ. The validity of using phonatory jitter and shimmer to detect laryngeal pathology. In: Baer T, Sasaki C, Harris K, eds. *Laryngeal Function in Phonation and Respiration.* Boston, Mass: College-Hill Press; 1987:492-508.

25. Hill DP, Meyers AD, Scherer RC. A comparison of four clinical techniques in the analysis of phonation. *J Voice.* 1990;4:198-204.

26. Hillman RE, Holmberg EB, Perkell JS, Walsh M, Vaughn C. Phonatory function associated with hyperfunctionally related vocal fold lesions. *J Voice.* 1990;4:52-63.

27. Kempster G, Kistler DJ, Hillenbrand J. Multidimensional scaling analysis of dysphonia in two speaker groups. *J Speech Hear Res.* 1991;34:534-543.

28. Wolfe V, Cornell R, Palmer C. Acoustic correlates of pathologic voice types. *J Speech Hear Res.* 1991;34:509-516.

29. Wolfe V, Fitch J, Cornell R. Acoustic prediction of severity in commonly occurring voice problems. *J Speech Lang Hear Res.* 1995;38:273-279.

30. Martin D, Fitch J, Wolfe V. Pathologic voice type and the acoustic prediction of severity. *J Speech Lang Hear Res.* 1995;38:765-771.

31. Rabinov C, Kreiman J, Gerratt B, Bielamowicz S. Comparing reliability of perceptual ratings of roughness and acoustic measures of jitter. *J Speech Lang Hear Res.* 1995;38:26-32.

32. Hillenbrand J, Houde R. Acoustic correlates of breathy voice quality: dysphonic voices and continuous speech. *J Speech Lang Hear Res.* 1996;39:311-321.

33. Karnell MP. Laryngeal perturbation analysis: minimum length of analysis window. *J Speech Hear Res.* 1993;34:544-548.

34. Titze IR, Liang H. Comparison of Fo extraction methods for high-precision voice perturbation measurements. *J Speech Hear Res.* 1993;36:1120-1133.

35. Bielamowicz S, Kreiman J, Gerratt B, Dauer M, Berke G. Comparison of voice analysis systems for perturbation measurement. *J Speech Lang Hear Res.* 1996;39:126-134.

36. Scherer R, Vail V, Guo C. Required number of tokens to determine representative voice perturbation values. *Journal Speech Lang Hear Res.* 1995;38:1260-1269.

37. Garrett KL, Healey EC. An acoustic analysis of the fluctuations in the voices of normal adult speakers across three times of day. *J Acoust Soc Am.* 1987;82:58-62.

38. Nittrouer S, McGowan RS, Milenkovic PH, Beehler D. Acoustic measurements of men's and women's voice: a study of context effects and covariation. *J Speech Hear Res.* 1990;33:761-775.
39. Stone RE, Rainey CL. Intra- and intersubject variability in acoustic measures of normal voice. *J Voice.* 1991;5:189-196.
40. Pausewang Gelfer M. Fundamental frequency, intensity, and vowel selection: effects on measures of phonatory stability. *J Speech Lang Hear Res.* 1995;38:1189-1198.
41. Milenkovic PH. Least mean squares of waveform perturbation. *J Speech Hear Res,* 1987;29:529-538.
42. Titze IR. Acoustic interpretation of the voice-range profile (phonetogram). *J Speech Hear Res.* 1992;34:21-35.
43. McAllister A, Sederholm A, Sundberg J, Gramming P. Relations between voice range profile and physiological and perceptual voice characteristics in ten-year old children. *J Voice.* 1994:8:230-239.
44. Heylen L, Wuyts F, Mertens F, DeBodt M, Pattyn J, Croux C, Van de Heyning P. Evaluation of the vocal performance of children using a voice range profile index. *J Speech Lang Hear Res.* 1998:40:232-238.
45. Orlikoff RF, Kahane JC. Influence of mean sound pressure level on jitter and shimmer measures. *J Voice.* 1991;5:113-119.
46. Laver J, Hiller S, Beck JM. Acoustic waveform perturbations and voice disorders. *J Voice.* 1992;6:115-126.
47. Higgins M, Netsell R, Schulte L. Vowel-related differences in laryngeal articulatory and phonatory function. *J Speech Lang Hear Res.* 1998;41:712-724.
48. Glaze LE, Bless DM, Milenkovic P, Susser RD. Acoustic characteristics of children's voice. *J Voice.* 1988;2:312-319.
49. Glaze LE, Bless DM, Susser RD. Acoustic analysis of vowel and loudness differences in children's voice. *J Voice.* 1990;4:37-44.
50. Rothenberg M. Measurement of air flow during speech. *J Speech Hear Res.* 1977;2:155-176.
51. Iwata S. Aerodynamic aspects for phonation in normal and pathologic larynges. In: Fujimura O, ed. *Vocal Physiology.* New York, NY: Raven Press: 1988:423-432.
52. Scherer RC. Aerodynamic assessment in voice production. In: *Assessment of Speech and Voice Production: Research and Clinical Applications.* Bethesda, Md: National Institute on Deafness and Other Communicative Disorders; 1991:12-49.
53. Schutte HK. Integrated aerodynamic measurements. *J Voice.* 1992;6:127-134.
54. Kitajima K, Fujita F. Clinical report on preliminary data on intraoral pressure in the evaluation of laryngeal pathology. *J Voice.* 1992;6:79-85.
55. Miller CJ, Daniloff R. Airflow measurements: theory and utility of findings. *J Voice.* 1993;7:38-46.
56. Smitheran J, Hixon YJ. A clinical method for estimating laryngeal airway resistance during vowel production. *J Speech Hear Disord.* 1981;46:138-146.

57. Melcon M, Hoit JD, Hixon TJ. Age and laryngeal airway resistance during vowel production. *J Speech Hear Disord.* 1989;54:282-286.

58. Hoit JD, Hixon TJ. Age and laryngeal airway resistance during vowel production in women. *J Speech Hear Res.* 1995;35:309-313.

59. Finnegan E, Luschei E, Barkmeier J, Hoffman H. Sources of error in estimation of laryngeal airway resistance in persons with spasmodic dysphonia. *J Speech Lang Hear Res.* 1996;39:105-113.

60. Titze IR. Phonation threshold pressure: a missing link for glottal aerodynamics. In: Titze IR, ed. *Progress Report 1.* Iowa City, Iowa: National Center for Voice and Speech; 1991:1-14.

61. Fisher K, Swank P. Estimating phonation threshold pressure. *J Speech Lang Hear Res.* 1997;40:1122-1129.

62. Holmberg EB, Hillman RE, Perkell JS. Glottal airflow and transglottal air pressure measurements for male and female speakers in soft, normal and loud voice. *J Acoust Soc Am.* 1988;84:511-529.

63. Holmberg EB, Hillman RE, Perkell JS. Glottal airflow and transglottal air pressure measurements for male and female speakers in low, normal and high pitch. *J Voice.* 1989;3:294-305.

64. Netsell R. Subglottal and intraoral air pressures during intervocalic contrast of /t/ and /d/. *Phonetica.* 1969;20:68-73.

65. Higgins MB, Netsell R, Schulte L. Aerodynamic and electroglottographic measures of normal voice production: intrasubject variability within and across sessions. *J Speech Hear Res.* 1994;37:38-45.

66. Higgins MB, Saxman JH. A comparison of selected phonatory behaviors of healthy aged and young adults. *J Speech Hear Res.* 1991;34:1000-1010.

67. Sawashima M, Niimi S, Horiguchi S, Yamaguchi H. Expiratory lung pressure, airflow rate, and vocal intensity: data on normal subjects. In: Fujimura O, ed. *Vocal Physiology.* New York, NY: Raven Press; 1988:415-422.

68. Rothenberg M. A multichannel electroglottograph. *J Voice.* 1992;6:36-43.

69. Plant R, Hillel A. Direct measurement of subglottic pressure and laryngeal resistance in normal subjects and spasmodic dysphonia. *J Voice.* 1998;12:300-314.

70. Verdolini-Marston K, Titze IR, Drucker DG. Changes in phonation threshold pressure with induced conditions of hydration. *J Voice.* 1990;4:141-151.

71. Fritzell B. Inverse filtering. *J Voice.* 1992;6:111-114.

72. Sapienza C, Stathopoulos E. Comparison of maximum flow declination rate: children versus adults. *J Voice.* 1994;8:240-247.

73. Yanagisawa E. Fiberoptic and telescopic videolaryngoscopy—a comparative study. In: Baer T, Sasaki C, Harris K, eds. *Laryngeal Function in Phonation and Respiration.* Boston, Mass: College-Hill Press; 1987:475-484.

74. Woo P, Colton R, Casper J, Brewer D. Diagnostic value of stroboscopic examination in hoarse patients. *J Voice.* 1991;5:231-238.

75. Colton R, Woo P, Brewer D, Griffin B, Casper J. Stroboscopic signs associated with benign lesions of the vocal folds. *J Voice.* 1995;9:312-325.

76. American Speech-Language-Hearing Association. The role of otolaryngologists and speech-language pathologists in the performance and interpretation of endoscopy with stroboscopy. *Asha.* 1998; Suppl.

77. American Speech-Language-Hearing Association. *Preferred Practice Patterns: Voice Assessment; Voice Treatment.* Rockville, Md: ASHA; 1998.

78. Karnell MP, Silbergleit AK, Adams LR, Skwarecki RM, Perlman AL, Stone RE Jr, Savage HE. Training guidelines for the performance of laryngeal endoscopy and stroboscopy. *Special Interest Division 3 Newsletter.* October 1996.

79. Casper JK, Brewer DW, Colton RH. Pitfalls and problems in flexible fiberoptic videolaryngoscopy. *J Voice.* 1988;2:347-352.

80. Hibi SR, Bless DM, Hirano M, Yoshida T. Distortions of videofiberoscopy imaging: reconsideration and correction. *J Voice.* 1988;2:168-175.

81. Peppard RC, Bless DM. The use of topical anesthesia in videostroboscopic examination of the larynx. *J Voice.* 1991;5:57-63.

82. Peppard RC, Bless DM. A method for improving measurement reliability in laryngeal videostroboscopy. *J Voice.* 1990;4:280-285.

83. Childers DG, Alsaka YA, Hicks DM, Moore GP. Vocal fold vibrations: an EGG model. In: Baer T, Sasaki C, Harris S, eds. *Laryngeal Function in Phonation and Respiration.* Boston, Mass: College-Hill Press; 1987:11-202.

84. Colton RH, Contour EG. Problems and pitfalls of electroglottography. *J Voice.* 1990;4:10-24.

85. Orlikoff R. Scrambled EGG: the uses and abuses of electroglottography. *Phonoscope.* 1998;1:37-53.

86. Vieira M, McInnes F, Jack M. Comparative assessment of electroglottographic and acoustic measures of jitter in pathological voices. *J Speech Lang Hear Res.* 1997;40:170-182.

87. Karnell MP. Synchronized videostroboscopy and electroglottography. *J Voice.* 1989;3:68-75.

88. Harris K. Electromyography as a technique for laryngeal investigation. *ASHA Reports.* 1981;11:70-87.

89. Hirose H. Electromyography of the laryngeal and pharyngeal muscles. In: Cummings CW, Frederickson JM, Harker LA, Krause CJ, Schuller DE, eds. *Otolaryngology—Head and Neck Surgery.* St. Louis, Mo: CV Mosby Company; 1986:1823-1828.

90. Ludlow CL. Neurophysiological assessment of patients with vocal motor control disorders. In: *Assessment of Speech and Voice Production: Research and Clinical Applications.* Bethesda, Md: National Institute on Deafness and Other Communicative Disorders; 1991:161-171.

91. Kotby M, Fadly E, Madkour O, Barakah M, Khidr A, Alloush T, Saleh M. Electromyography and neurography in neurolaryngology. *J Voice.* 1992; 6:159-187.

92. Koufman J, Walker F. Laryngeal electromyography in clinical practice: indications, techniques, and interpretation. *Phonoscope.* 1998;1:57-70.

7

Survey of Voice Management

The extensive diagnostic voice evaluation has provided the voice pathologist with answers to what has caused the voice disorder and a description of the current vocal symptoms. The answers to the etiologic questions include primary causes as well as secondary etiologic factors. In addition, an understanding of the present vocal physiology and the relationship of respiration, phonation, and resonance has been established. A systematic management approach must now be initiated with the purpose of modifying or eliminating the etiologic factors and improving voice by rebalancing the three subsystems of voice production. This chapter is designed to survey the basic philosophies of voice treatment and to introduce the reader to some specific voice therapy techniques. Although the information contained in this chapter is by no means an exhaustive presentation of all voice therapy approaches, the survey is a useful point of departure for the study of voice management.

Voice Therapy Orientations

As stated in Chapter 1, the management of voice disorders by "speech correctionists" began in the 1930s. Since that time, a rich and interesting history of voice therapy approaches has evolved leading to several philosophical orientations of therapy. These orientations include **hygienic, symptomatic, psychogenic, physiologic,** and **eclectic** voice therapies.[1]

Hygienic Voice Therapy

Hygienic voice therapy is often the first step in many voice therapy programs. As discussed in Chapter 3, there are many etiological factors that contribute to the development of voice disorders. Poor vocal hygiene may be a major developmental factor. Some examples of behaviors that constitute poor vocal hygiene include shouting, talking loudly over noise, screaming, vocal noises, coughing, throat clearing, and poor hydration. When the inappropriate hygienic behaviors are identified, appropriate treatments can be devised for modifying or eliminating those behaviors. Once modified, voice production has the opportunity to improve or return to normal.

When poor vocal hygiene behaviors are modified, vocal symptoms often improve without direct manipulation of the voice subsystems (respiration, phonation, resonance). A common example is the reduction of the abusive behavior of shouting in children who have nodules. By eliminating the shouting behavior, the nodules are given an opportunity to resolve, and the voice improves. This improvement results without any need for direct modification of the voice components, such as inappropriate pitch, breathiness, glottal attacks, and so on, which may have resulted from the presence of the nodules.

Poor vocal hygiene may also include the habitual use of voice components in an inappropriate manner. Changes in these components often are the compensatory results of the vocal pathology. In the case of poor vocal hygiene, use of an inappropriate pitch or loudness, reduced respiratory support, poor phonatory habits (glottal attacks, fry), or inappropriate resonance are simply functional vocal behaviors. We recently evaluated a patient who attempted to sound more authoritative by using a pitch that was too low with intermittent glottal fry phonation, for example. The use of this inappropriate pitch created the patient's laryngeal fatigue and dysphonia. These poor hygienic voice behaviors were modified, and his vocal complaints resolved.

Hygienic voice therapy presumes that many voice disorders have a direct behavioral cause. This therapy strives to instill healthy vocal behaviors in the patient's habitual speech patterns. Good vocal hygiene also focuses on maintaining the health of the vocal fold cover through adequate internal hydration and diet. Once identified, poor vocal hygiene habits can be modified or eliminated leading to improved voice production.

Symptomatic Voice Therapy

The focus of symptomatic voice therapy is on the modification of the deviant vocal symptoms or perceptual voice components that were identified during the diagnostic voice evaluation. Aberrant symptoms include a pitch that is too high or low, voice that is too soft or loud, breathy phonation, or the use of hard glottal attacks or glottal fry. Daniel Boone[2] was the first voice pathologist to organize previous literature and introduce this symptomatic therapy orientation to our profession. Symptomatic voice therapy is based on his premise that most voice disorders are caused by the functional misuse or abuse of the voice components including respiration, phonation, resonance, pitch, loudness, and rate. When identified through the diagnostic process, the misuses are eliminated or reduced through various voice therapy facilitating techniques. Boone[2(p11)] stated:

> In the voice clinician's attempt to aid the patient in finding and using his best voice production, it is necessary to probe continually within the patient's repertoire to find that one voice that sounds "good" and which he is able to produce with relatively little effort. A voice therapy facilitating technique is that technique which, when used by a

particular patient, enables him easily to produce a good voice. Once discovered, the facilitating technique and resulting phonation become the symptomatic focus of therapy . . . This use of a facilitating technique to produce a good phonation is the core of what we do in symptomatic voice therapy for the reduction of hyperfunctional voice disorders.

Boone's original facilitating techniques included:

- altering tongue position
- change of loudness
- chewing exercises
- digital manipulation
- ear training
- elimination of abuses
- elimination of hard glottal attack
- establish new pitch
- explanation of the problem
- feedback
- hierarchy analysis
- negative practice
- open-mouth exercises
- pitch inflections
- pushing approach
- relaxation
- respiration training
- target voice models
- voice rest
- yawn-sigh approach.

As you read through this chapter, many of these approaches are described in detail, as they continue to be well utilized in the treatment of voice disorders. To summarize symptomatic voice therapy, we conclude that:

- the voice pathologist evaluates the presence of deviant voice components,
- the voice pathologist constantly probes for the "best" voice in the presence of the disorder, and
- when the best voice is found, facilitating techniques are used to stabilize the improved voice production.

Symptomatic voice therapy assumes voice improvement through direct symptom modification.

Psychogenic Voice Therapy

Psychogenic voice therapy is based on the assumption of under-lying emotional or psychosocial behavioral causes for the voice disturbance. The relationship of emotions to voice production has been well documented in the literature starting as early as the middle 1800s to the present[3-5] West, Kennedy, and Carr[6] and Van Riper[7] discussed the need for emotional retraining in voice therapy, whereas Murphy[8] and Brodnitz[9] presented excellent information related to the psychodynamics of voice production. In her comprehensive discussion of voice therapy and children, Moya Andrews[10] presented a compelling argument for examining the psychodynamics of the child's speaking environment when treating voice disorders in this population.

Aronson[11(p131)] first articulated his description of a psychogenic voice disorder when he stated that:

> A psychogenic voice disorder is broadly synonymous with a functional one but has the advantage of stating positively, based on the explanation of its causes, that the voice disorder is a manifestation of one or more types of psychological disequilibrium, such as anxiety, depression, conversion reaction, or personality disorder, which interfere with normal volitional control over phonation.

Aronson,[12] Case,[13] and Colton and Casper[14] further discussed the need for determining the emotional dynamics of the voice disturbance from the interactive perspectives of emotions as a cause for voice disorders and voice disorders as the cause of emotional disequilibrium.

In other words, psychogenic voice therapy focuses on identification and modification of the emotional and psychosocial disturbances associated with the onset and maintenance of the voice problem. When the psychogenic causes are resolved, the voice disorder dissipates. Voice pathologists must develop and possess superior interview and counseling skills, as well as the skill to know when the emotional or psychosocial problem is in need of more intensive evaluation and therapy by other professionals.

Physiologic Voice Therapy

Physiologic voice therapy includes voice therapy programs that have been devised to directly alter or modify the physiology of the vocal mechanism. Normal voice production is dependent on a balance among airflow, supplied by the respiratory system; laryngeal muscle strength, balance, coordination, and stamina; and coordination among these and the supraglottic resonatory structures (pharynx, oral cavity, nasal cavity). Any disturbance in the physiologic balance of these vocal subsystems may lead to a voice disturbance.

Disturbances may be in respiratory volume, power, pressure, and flow. Disturbances may also manifest in vocal fold tone, mass, stiffness, flexibility, and approximation. Finally, the coupling of the supraglottic resonators and the placement of the laryngeal tone may cause or be perceived as a voice disorder. The overall causes may be mechanical, neurologic, or psychological. Whatever the cause, the management approach is direct modification of the inappropriate physiologic activity through exercise and manipulation.

Inherent in physiologic voice therapy is a holistic approach to the treatment of voice disorders. They are therapies that strive to balance the three subsystems of voice production at once, as opposed to working directly on single voice components, such as pitch or loudness. Examples of physiologic voice therapy include Vocal Function Exercises, Resonant Voice Therapy, and the Accent Method of Voice Therapy, all of which will be presented in this chapter.

Eclectic Voice Therapy

Eclectic voice therapy is the combination of any and all of the orientations of voice therapy. Successful voice therapy is dependent on the voice pathologist using all of the voice therapy techniques that seem appropriate for individual patients. Many patients may share the same diagnosis, but the etiologies and personalities, vocal needs, emotional reactions, and motivations to their voice problems may be different. Because of these differences, the same pathologies may require different management approaches. Therefore, the voice pathologist is advised not to adhere to any one philosophical orientation of voice therapy but to learn a broad range of management approaches. Utilizing a case study format, let us examine a composite patient with a voice disorder from the perspective of each voice therapy orientation.

Case Study 1

The patient was a 48-year-old woman who was diagnosed by the laryngologist as having moderate, bilateral Reinke's edema, with the left fold suggesting a more severe draping, polypoid degeneration. The patient was referred for a voice evaluation and a trial voice therapy program. If short-term therapy was not successful in improving her vocal fold condition and voice quality, then the patient would be scheduled for surgical intervention.

History of the Problem

The patient was referred to the otolaryngologist by her internist when, during a regular physical examination, she noticed that the patient's voice quality "sounded as deep as a man's." The patient stated that her voice had always been deep and that she really didn't think that there was much of a problem. When the otolaryngologist told her that she had vocal fold polyps, however, she became concerned enough to throw her cigarettes in the exam-room trash can and, by the time of the voice evaluation, had not smoked for 2 weeks. She reported that her voice quality was essentially the same throughout the day, though it tended to become "huskier" toward the end of a workday.

Medical History

The patient reported undergoing thyroid surgery 5 years ago during which her left thyroid lobe was excised. In addition, she underwent a tonsillectomy and an appendectomy as a teenager. She had also been hospitalized for chronic depression on two occasions. The last hospitalization lasted for 3 weeks and occurred 18 months ago. The patient continued to be treated for depression with medication and remained in bimonthly counseling.

Chronic medical conditions included asthma and frequent bronchitis; high blood pressure; elevated blood sugar; and rheumatoid arthritis. Daily medications were taken for depression, "nerves" (a sleep aid), thyroid, high blood pressure, and pain associated with the arthritis. Until 2 weeks prior, she had smoked 1½ to 2 packages of cigarettes per day for approximately 30 years. Her liquid intake was poor, consisting of approximately three cups of caffeinated coffee and four cans of caffeinated soda per day. Chronic throat clearing was noted throughout the evaluation. The patient indicated that on a day-to-day basis she felt "fair-to-poor" because of stress, fatigue, and arthritis pain.

Social History

The patient had been married for 29 years but had recently been separated from her husband for 3 months, causing much stress and tension. She had three grown children. The middle child, a 26-year-old son, had recently divorced and temporarily moved back into the house. Again, the patient pointed to the stress of this situation. The patient was not reticent to talk about her depression and indicated that an unhappy marriage and the feeling of an unfulfilled life were the causes.

A factory that made latex gloves for medical use had employed the patient for 6 years. She indicated that her specific job was in the "powder room" where the gloves were filled with powder and packaged. Apparently, the powder dust caused much coughing during the day. In addition, the packaging machines were noisy, requiring the workers to talk loudly to be heard. Most talking on the job was social among eight people who worked in a large, well-ventilated room.

Nonwork activities included walking her two dogs nightly, talking on the telephone with her daughter, and actively shopping at yard sales and flea markets with a close friend. All of these activities were curtailed when she didn't feel well physically and emotionally, however.

Oral-Peripheral Examination

The structure and function of the oral mechanism appeared to be well within normal limits for speech and voice production. The patient reported laryngeal sensations of dryness and occasional thickness. She demonstrated laryngeal area muscle tension and neck tension.

Voice Evaluation

The patient's voice quality was described as mild-to-moderately dysphonic, characterized by low pitch, increased loudness, and husky hoarseness.

Respiration: Patient demonstrated a thoracic, supportive breathing pattern. She tended to speak at the end of her respiratory volume, especially toward the end of phrases.

Phonation: A slight breathiness was noted during conversational voice. Occasional glottal fry was noted toward the end of phrases.

Resonance: Normal

Pitch: Patient demonstrated an unusually low pitch conversationally.

Loudness: Patient spoke unusually loud for the speaking situation.

Rate: Normal

Acoustic measures and aerodynamic analyses revealed the following:

- fundamental frequency = 136 Hz — (low for gender)
- frequency range = 106 to 320 Hz — (limited for gender)
- jitter percent /a/ = .56 — (normal < 1.04%)
- shimmer dB /a/ = .67 — (abnormally high > .35 dB)
- intensity (habitual) = 76 dB — (normal to loud)
- airflow volume = 2,300 mL — (WNL)
- airflow rate = 180 mL/s, all pitch levels — (WNL 75-200 ml/s)
- phonation time = 12.7 s — (low)
- subglottic air pressure = 8.6 cm/H_2O — (high 5-7 cm/H_2O)

Laryngeal videostroboscopic observation revealed a moderate bilateral vocal fold edema, worse left than right. Prominent blood vessels were noted bilaterally. Glottic closure was complete with mild ventricular fold compression. The amplitude of vibration was moderate-to-severely decreased left and moderately decreased right. The mucosal wave was severely decreased bilaterally. The open phase of the vibratory cycle was slightly dominant, while the symmetry of vibration was irregular by 50%. In short, the patient demonstrated an edematous, stiff, out-of-phase vocal fold vibratory pattern.

Impressions

The patient presented with a voice disorder secondary to many possible etiologic factors:

- long-term cigarette smoking
- laryngeal area muscle tension
- harsh employment environment in terms of dust and talking over noise
- poor hydration and large caffeine intake
- asthma and frequent bronchitis
- prescription medications causing mucosal drying
- frequent coughing and throat clearing
- emotional instability
- talking too loudly in general conversation
- using a low pitch

Recommendations

Hygienic Voice Therapy

General focus would be to identify the primary and secondary behavioral causes of the voice disorder and to modify or eliminate these causes. The primary causes would include:

- smoking
- laryngeal dehydration from poor hydration, caffeine intake, and prescription drugs
- voice abuse such as talking loudly over noise at work, coughing, and throat clearing
- inhalation of large quantities of powder.

Secondary causes that may be more the result of the problem as opposed to a cause would be:

- laryngeal area muscle tension caused by increased mass and stiffness
- low pitch caused by increased mass
- increased loudness caused by effort to force stiff, heavy folds to vibrate.

Therapy would focus on modification or elimination of the primary etiologic factors. The patient would be supported in her effort to stop smoking, encouraged to begin a hydration program and to reduce caffeine intake, given vocal hygiene counseling in an effort to reduce vocally abusive habits, and encouraged to wear a mask to filter her breathing at work. The secondary causes of tension, low pitch, and increased loudness would be expected to spontaneously improve as the primary causes were modified and the vocal fold condition improved.

Symptomatic Voice Therapy

General focus would use facilitating techniques to:

- raise pitch
- reduce loudness
- reduce laryngeal area tension and effort.

This direct symptom modification would follow an explanation of the problem and would run concurrently with modification of the vocally abusive behaviors including:

- smoking
- caffeine intake
- coughing and throat clearing.

Psychogenic Voice Therapy

General focus would explore the psychodynamics of voice disorder. This exploration would include:

- detailed patient interview to determine the cause and effects of stress, tension, and depression
- determination of the exact relationship of emotions on voice problems
- counsel the patient regarding the effects of the emotions on voice problems
- reduction of musculoskeletal tension caused by emotional upheaval
- support of ongoing psychological counseling.

Secondary focus would deal with modification or elimination of the abusive behaviors including:

- smoking
- caffeine intake
- coughing and throat clearing.

Inappropriate use of pitch and loudness would most likely be viewed as obvious symptoms of the voice problem. As the psychodynamics improve, the voice symptoms would be expected to improve.

Physiologic Voice Therapy

General focus would be to evaluate the present physiologic condition of the patient's voice production and develop direct physical exercises or manipulations to improve that condition. This patient demonstrated increased mass and stiffness of the vocal folds impairing the physical dynamics of vocal fold vibration. Indeed, she was required to build greater subglottic air pressure to initiate and maintain vibration that required a borderline high airflow rate. This increased pressure caused her to speak too loudly in conversation. She also attempted to overcome these problems by making physical adjustments, such as increasing supraglottic tension in an effort to maintain her voice. When added to the mucosal and muscular stiffness, vocal hyperfunction was the result. The management program would therefore include:

- Vocal Function Exercises designed to rebalance the three subsystems of voice production
- hydration program and decreasing caffeinated products to improve the mucous membrane of vocal folds
- discuss potential impact of her medications with the patient's physician
- elimination of habit coughing and throat clearing.

Eclectic Voice Therapy

It is obvious in the review of these orientations, that each management approach has certain strengths, as well as inherent weaknesses. It is also obvious that the orientations must overlap to be effective. You will be able to best treat your patients with the understanding and use of all of these orientations. Therefore, eclectic voice therapy is obviously the treatment of choice with any patient with a voice disorder. This particular patient would best be served when the management plan included:

■ elimination or modification of the vocal abuses and attention to the mucosal covering of the vocal folds
■ symptom modification
■ attention to the psychodynamics of the problem
■ direct physiologic exercise.

The remainder of this chapter presents specific treatment strategies categorized under the major therapy orientations including hygienic, symptomatic, psychogenic, and physiologic voice therapies. Also included are voice therapy strategies used with special cases of voice disorders.

Hygienic Voice Therapy

Treatment Strategies for Voice Abuse and Misuse

Hyperadduction of the vocal folds is vocally traumatic, especially when the trauma occurs frequently. Some common vocally traumatic behaviors that may be modified through voice therapy include shouting, loud talking, screaming, producing vocal noises, and habitual throat clearing. There are many opportunities for voice trauma among both adults and children. Home-makers may shout at their children for discipline, factory workers talk loudly over noise for extended periods of time, and teachers and lecturers may talk too loudly with inappropriate tone focus on a routine basis. Most children shout and make vocal noises. They shout during unsupervised play; they are encouraged to shout while participating in team sports; and they shout when they are angry. Even cultural styles and artistic voice use exhibit vocally "aggressive" productions in advertisements, character voices, music videos, and other media images. Both adults and children are also susceptible to the development of throat clearing either primarily as the result of frequent colds or allergies or secondary to the development of laryngeal pathologies. Let us examine some of the techniques used for modifying these vocally traumatic behaviors.

Vocal Hygiene Therapy Approaches

The most effective way of dealing with voice abuse and misuse is through **vocal hygiene counseling**. Once the abusive vocal behaviors have been identified, the first step of this approach is patient education. Patient education involves making the patient aware of the effects that trauma has on the laryngeal mechanism by utilizing graphic pictures and descriptions of the anatomy and physiology. Indeed, the most effective educational tool is the patient's own video of the stroboscopic evaluation. It is easier for patients to resolve their vocal problems when they truly understand the cause-and-effect relationships that may be displayed visually.

After the general abuses or misuses have been identified and explained in detail, it is important to determine exactly why the patient presents with these specific behaviors. If the abuse is shouting, for example, the voice pathologist will want to know when and why it occurs and whether the patient feels it is required. Once these factors are determined, the treatment plan will involve: (a) eliminating those abusive behaviors that may be eliminated (b) modifying those abusive behaviors which cannot be totally eliminated to reduce the traumatic impact on the vocal mechanism and (c) environmental manipulations to secure more favorable voicing conditions.

We may synthesize the vocal hygiene approach to a four-step outline:

1. Identify the trauma behavior
2. Describe the effects
3. Define specific occurrences
4. Modify the behavior

Let us examine several cases in the context of the vocal hygiene therapy approach.

Case Study 2: The Homemaker

A 35-year-old patient was referred with the diagnosis of bilateral vocal fold nodules. She had a several-year history of intermittent dysphonia that became persistent approximately 3 months before the voice evaluation. She reported that her voice was better in the morning than in the evening and that she had never experienced aphonia.

The patient's medical history was unremarkable except for a large intake of caffeine and little other liquid. She had never smoked and had always lived in a nonsmoking environment. Socially, she was a homemaker with three sons, ages 3, 8, and 12 years. She enjoyed crafts, decorating her newly purchased Victorian home, and, until recently, sang soprano in the church choir. Her voice problem precluded singing. Her two oldest sons played soccer, and her oldest son also played baseball and basketball. The patient's husband was a manufacturer's representative and was on the road three out of five working days. The patient admitted to frequent shouting when disciplining her children and cheering loudly during their many sporting events.

The patient's voice quality during the evaluation was moderately dysphonic, characterized by low pitch and a breathy hoarseness. Respiration was thoracic and supportive for conversational voice. She was able to sustain the /z/ for 7 seconds and the /s/ for 21 seconds. Phonation was characterized by voice breaks and the production of occasional glottal fry. A limited pitch range was demonstrated with the habitual pitch located near the bottom of the range. Limited inflection was noted conversationally. Resonance was normal and the loudness level was appropriate for the speaking situation. She was able to readily increase the loudness level to a shout. Rate was normal. The abusive behavior of throat clearing was noted throughout the evaluation. The patient complained that her voice quality worsened with use, suggesting laryngeal fatigue.

Instrumental measures yielded the following:

▨ fundamental frequency	168 Hz	(low < 180 Hz)
▨ frequency range	156 Hz–460 Hz	(very limited for soprano)
▨ jitter percent	.57%	(WNL < 1.04%)
▨ mean intensity	68 dB SPL	(WNL)
▨ shimmer dB	.47 dB	(high > .35 dB)
▨ airflow volume	3200 mL	(WNL)

▪ airflow rate   235 mL/s   (high > 200 mL/s)
▪ maximum phonation   13.6 s   (low)
  time
▪ subglottic air pressure 5.2 cm/H_2O (normal
                                                5-7 cm/H_2O)

Vocal traumas are common in many homemakers.[15] Homemakers often shout for disciplinary purposes and call their children home from long distances. Voice abuse behaviors in the home that may not be easily recognized include calling or reprimanding a pet, shouting from one room to another, calling someone to the telephone, talking to a spouse or relative who is hard of hearing, and talking loudly over the noise of the children, television, or CD player. By discussing the specific situations that relate to the patient, the voice pathologist and the patient may devise alternatives to the traumatic behaviors. The alternatives may be as simple as turning the volume down on electronic devices when speaking or as creative as blowing a whistle to call the children home for dinner. Some patients are advised not to answer when someone calls from another room but rather to make the caller seek them or to go to the caller before replying. Again, once the specific traumatic behaviors are identified, most motivated patients are able either to eliminate them or devise creative nontraumatic alternatives to aid in their own treatment processes.

The homemaker in Case Study 2 developed vocal nodules as a result of shouting and maintained inappropriate vocal health through habitual throat clearing, laryngeal dehydration, and laryngeal muscle strain. Following the four-step vocal hygiene plan, this problem was managed as follows:

1. Identify the abuse:
   ▪ shouting
   ▪ throat clearing
   ▪ caffeine intake
   ▪ laryngeal muscle strain
2. Describe the effect:
   ▪ accomplished with illustrations, as well as the patient's own stroboscopic evaluation
3. Define specific occurrences:
   ▪ shouting to discipline children and at sporting events

■ chronic habitual throat clearing
■ heavy caffeine intake
4. Modify the behavior:
  ■ attempt to discipline through discussion and behavioral consequences
  ■ substitute a mechanical noise maker for vocal enthusiasm at sporting events
  ■ eliminate habitual throat clearing through behavior modification program (discussed later this chapter)
  ■ introduce formal hydration program (6-8 eight ounce glasses of water or juices per day)
  ■ Vocal Function Exercise to balance the physiologic vocal system

Case Study 3: The Noisy Job Environment

Communication often is difficult and potentially vocally traumatic for people who work in noisy job environments. In these situations, the vocal abuse usually takes the form of loud talking or shouting over noise for extended periods of time. In defining specific occurrences, it is necessary to determine how much talking is job-related, that is, how much is necessary for the worker to carry out the duties of the job and how much is simply social discourse. Unnecessary communication may certainly be reduced, but this is not the total answer. The clinician will also want to know the type of noise, whether constant or intermittent, to determine if there are more appropriate times than others to talk.

Strategies for modifying this behavior may include moving as far away from the noise sources as possible, shielding the voice with the body by turning away from the noise source, and wearing ear protectors so background noise is masked and the speaker is better able to hear his or her own voice. Another beneficial principle to teach patients who must talk in noisy environments is to make the listener strain to hear them, not for them to strain their voices to be heard by the listeners. Describing the Lombard effect, in which the speaker will always talk slightly louder than the noise source, is often helpful for patients. Many patients do not realize how loudly they are talking in the noisy background because of the Lombard effect. Patients may also use electronic amplification of the voice. Personal amplifiers that fit in shirt pockets or attach to belts are available at reasonable prices. Direct voice therapy may also be used to teach the patient how to raise the voice in this environment without causing trauma. Finally, the most drastic step in working with a patient with a voice disorder caused by a noisy environment is to explore the possibility of removing the patient through job transfer to a less noisy environment.

For example, a 50-year-old male with a diagnosis of a postsurgical left unilateral vocal fold polyp was referred for voice evaluation and treatment. He worked as a foreman at a local automobile assembly plant. Being a nonsmoker, the polyp development was thought to be associated with his need to speak loudly in the work environment. The following vocal hygiene plan was developed during the diagnostic evaluation:

1. Identify the voice abuse:
   - talking loudly over noise on a daily basis
2. Describe the effect:
   - accomplished with video and discussion of physiology
3. Define specific occurrences:
   - discussing daily work duties with 22 workers
   - reporting daily activities to a supervisor
   - social discussions
4. Modify the behavior:
   - meet with workers, 2 to 4 at a time, in office away from noise source
   - make inspections on the line, then ask workers to come into the office as needed
   - decrease social conversations
   - make workers strain to hear
   - direct voice therapy concentrating on increasing loudness with improved abdominal breath support, appropriate pitch, and precise articulation

Case Study 4: The Public Speaker

Excessive loud talking with inappropriate tone focus and breath support by teachers, lecturers, politicians, preachers, actors, and other professional voice users may often be the cause of vocal difficulties. These inappropriate vocal behaviors or misuses may lead to vocal fatigue and, in some cases, to vocal fold mucosal changes, including edema and mass lesions. In the early stages of the problem, the public speaker often will describe to the voice pathologist, in a perfectly normal voice, extreme vocal difficulties that occurred during presentations or lectures. The history of the problem normally includes strong voice in the morning that weakens as the day progresses. Some of these patients report that by the end of the day that they are "lucky to have any voice at all." (A discussion of voice fatigue is found in Chapter 4.)

As the voice is tested during the diagnostic, there is a good chance that findings will be normal and that the abuse or misuse behaviors will not be evident. Clinicians should secure a taped sample of the public-speaking voice to determine the presence of vocal trauma during the presentation. This is easily accomplished by having the patient ask a lecture participant to audiotape or videotape record 10-minute samples at both the beginning and the end of a presentation.

If it is determined, after reviewing the tape, that excessive loudness, inappropriate pitch, and poor tone focus are causing strain of the vocal mechanism, then the need to define the specific situation is present. For example, how large is the room? Are the acoustics adequate? How many people are being addressed? Is amplification available? What is the seating arrangement in relation to the podium? How many hours of public speaking are done each day? When do breaks occur? What is the subject matter?

After defining the situations, the occurrences, and the specific environment of the speaker, the modifications are made. These may include moving the lecture site closer to the audience, using amplification, building vocal time-outs into daily lesson plans, or simply talking more softly while monitoring the back row of the audience to see if the speaker can still be heard.

If the patient continues to speak with the inappropriate voice components following these environmental controls, then direct modification of loudness, pitch, and focus may prove necessary. In the latter stages of therapy, large room presentations should actually be practiced using the improved voice components. (Modification of specific components is described under Symptomatic Voice Therapy.) Finally, direct Vocal Function Exercises for rebalancing airflow, muscle activity, and tone focus may be utilized.

For example, a 32-year-old female was referred for voice evaluation and treatment with the diagnosis of bilateral vocal fold nodules. The patient was a new college professor who taught courses in special education and remedial reading. The following vocal hygiene plan was developed during the diagnostic evaluation:

1. Identify the abuse/misuse:
   - excessive loudness during lectures
   - use of a high pitch
   - poor tone focus
2. Describe the effect:
   - accomplished with video and discussion of physiology
3. Define specific occurrences:
   - during 9 hours of lecture per week to an average class size of 25 students
   - during occasional (average once per month) guest lectures that involved half-day workshops
4. Modify the behavior:
   - ask the students to sit in the front of the room
   - build in more classroom discussion and less straight lecture
   - have more audience participation during workshops
   - use amplification when possible
   - direct modification of the voice components of loudness, pitch, and tone focus
   - Vocal Function Exercises

Case Study 5: Voice Abuse or Misuse in Children

By far the most common cause of voice disorders in children is vocal trauma including the potentially abusive behaviors of shouting, crying, loud talking, vocal noises, and throat clearing. Most children shout, and some shout more than others. Part of the natural childhood expression is through shouting. The problem, of course, arises when children who traumatize their voices develop laryngeal pathologies such as vocal fold nodules or chronic vocal fold edema.

When laryngeal pathologies occur, traditional management approaches have focused on ways of reducing or eliminating the abusive behaviors through behavior modification programs.[16]

These programs involve identifying the specific vocal abuses and then charting their occurrences on daily graphs prepared by the voice pathologist. Reduction in the occurrences of the abuses is recorded in some manner, and the child is given a physical reward. Although this approach has proved to be successful with many children, its limited scope proves less than adequate for many others. We suggest that other vocal hygiene questions must be considered when planning management strategies for vocally abusive children. These questions include:

- How does the child shout?
- Why does the child shout?
- Does the child make vocal noises?
- Does nonplay shouting occur?
- Has the laryngeal pathology created a physiologic imbalance of the vocal mechanism?
- Does habitual throat clearing occur?

Let us examine each question individually.

How Does the Child Shout?

Why, if most children shout, do some children develop laryngeal pathology and others do not? We might speculate that some children simply shout more than others do; or children are differentially susceptible to the development of laryngeal pathology; or maybe some vocal mechanisms are not as resilient as others are. Another reason that appears clinically significant is that different children shout in different ways. Some of the shouting behaviors may be more physiologically balanced and supported than others, and therefore not as traumatic to the vocal mechanism.

These speculations have led us to attempt a treatment strategy that has yielded successful results. That strategy is to teach the child how to shout. We believe that it is not practical or totally fair to ask a child to stop all shouting behaviors. Rather than trying to extinguish all shouting (especially during play), it is possible and effective to teach children to shout using a low-pitched voice with improved breath support and adequate forward focus. Using lower pitch reduces the natural stiffness and tension of the vocal folds inherent to higher pitch, thus reducing the glottal impact. This may be accomplished by teaching the child to use a "grown-up voice," "daddy's voice," or a "papa bear voice," depending on the child's age. With older children, we simply explore their lower pitch range and choose a pitch level in the lower midportion of the range. The patient practices speaking at that level in a comfortable conversational loudness level. They are then instructed in gradual steps to increase the loudness level until an appropriate "shout" is attained. At the same time, respiratory support, using abdominal breathing patterns, is established. As the pitch and loudness is modified, a forward focus tone placement is established to further reduce glottal impact and to enhance loudness (Forward Focus exercises are discussed later in this chapter). This is also a method that works well with cheerleaders who develop voice disorders.

Why Does the Child Shout?

This question explores the psychodynamics of the shouting behaviors. Andrews [10,17] explained the importance of modifying the psychosocial aspects of the child's shouting behavior for the more direct therapy interventions to be successful. The exploration and modification of these behaviors must involve cooperation of the parents. At times, major changes in family interactions must be developed. Reactions to the vocally abusive child often require major modifications in interpersonal strategies. In extreme cases, family counseling may be helpful in developing more appropriate family psychodynamics.

Does the Child Make Vocal Noises?

A traumatic vocal behavior that can be overlooked is the production of vocal noises. Most children make vocally traumatic noises during play, but, unless they are specifically asked about vocal noises during the evaluation, they will remain undetected. Some favorite noises include machine guns, cars, trucks, motorcycles, sirens, various character voices, and animal noises. Each year there appears to be a popular new set of noises that most often are influenced by popular toys, movies, television shows, or video games. Modification or elimination of these abusive noises is often desirable as a part of the treatment plan. Various mouth sounds and whistles that do not involve phonation may serve as acceptable substitutions. Extinguishing these phono-traumatic behaviors rarely proves to be difficult when play behavior and maturity levels change.

Does Nonplay Shouting Occur?

Another factor that needs to be identified and modified is nonplay shouting. Again, it is extremely helpful to have a parent involved in the entire management process. If such cooperation is available, parent education may help to modify occurrences of shouting in the home, such as shouting from room to room, calling people to the telephone, and arguing with brothers and sisters. Suggestions for the parent may include (a) not responding when the child calls from another room, forcing the child to physically seek the person being called; (b) not shouting for the child and expecting a response; and (c) attempting to control vocal sibling arguments. Without the parent's cooperation, nonplay shouting will probably continue, ideally with a modified low-pitched, abdominal-breath-supported, forward-focused shout.

Has the Laryngeal Pathology Created a Physiologic Imbalance?

Both children and adults with laryngeal pathologies are likely to develop an imbalance in the respiratory, laryngeal muscular, and resonatory aspects of voice production as the vocal mechanism adjusts itself to accommodate the presence of the pathology. When a physiologic imbalance is suspected, direct Vocal Function Exercises, the Accent Method of voice therapy, and Resonant Voice Therapy are holistic management approaches that have proven to be successful with this population. (These holistic therapies are described later in this chapter under Physiologic Voice Therapy.)

Does Habitual Throat Clearing Occur?

In a study by Stemple and Lehmann,[18] more than two thirds of the patients studied with vocal hyperfunction demonstrated a habitual throat-clearing behavior. As a primary etiology, throat clearing most commonly develops as a result of mucus drainage caused by colds, flu, and allergies or as a secondary symptom of esophageal reflux. Although drainage itself is not detrimental to the laryngeal mechanism, the throat clearing habit that results is extremely abusive because of the mechanical impact of the vocal folds and the grinding of the posterior laryngeal structures. In addition, acid burning caused by reflux in the posterior larynx creates a globus sensation, or "lump in the throat" feeling leading to habitual throat clearing. The behavior often continues even after the medical condition has resolved because of the inherent edema and irritation that leads to yet more throat clearing, simply as a result of habit. At times, this cycle continues until laryngeal pathology results.

Throat clearing may also develop secondary to laryngeal pathologies. This behavior occurs especially in the presence of mass lesions and vocal fold edema. Many patients report that they "feel" something in their throats that they try to clear. Some patients clear their throats to prepare the voice for phonation before they talk; others have no awareness of their throat-clearing habit.

The importance of eliminating this behavior cannot be overstated. We have seen clinical cases in which all etiologic factors except throat clearing were resolved, and the phonotraumatic nature of this behavior alone maintained the pathology. The techniques for significantly reducing throat clearing apply to both children and adults. The following example is a management approach that is appropriate for all ages; the language used will vary, of course, with the age of the patient.

> Throat clearing is one of the most traumatic things you can do to your vocal folds. When you clear your throat like this (demonstrate), you create an extreme amount of movement of your vocal folds, causing them to slam and rub together (demonstrate using your hands). You should understand that it is not unusual for you to have developed this habit. The vast majority of patients we see with your type of voice problem also have this habit. Sometimes people do not even know that they are doing it. But often they say that they feel something in their throat, like phlegm or mucus. The majority of the time, however, when you clear your throat, there is simply nothing there. The only thing you have accomplished is to create more vocal fold trauma.
>
> We have demonstrated to you with a tape recording of this evaluation that most of the time when you clear your throat, it occurs right before you begin to speak. Also, you are clearing many more

times than you realized. This is a sign that throat clearing is very much a habit. Like all habits, it is difficult to break. We are, therefore, going to try to make it easier by giving you a substitute habit that will (a) take the place of throat clearing, (b) accomplish the same thing as throat clearing, and (c) is not abusive. This substitute, nonabusive habit is a hard, forceful swallow. If you do, in fact, occasionally have an increased amount of mucus on your vocal folds, a hard swallow will accomplish the same thing as throat clearing, minus the vocal fold trauma. The only difference is that throat clearing feels good. It psychologically gives you more relief than the hard swallow, even though it physically accomplishes no more. It is your goal to overcome this psychological dependence. Understand that this habit is harmful and it must be broken.

To break this habit, you need to tell everyone in your family and any friends who are around you often (and whom you feel comfortable in telling) that you are not permitted to clear your throat anymore. When these "helpers" hear you clear your throat, and they will, they are to immediately point it out to you. Your task then is to "swallow hard." Obviously, it will not be necessary to swallow, because you just cleared your throat. Nonetheless, this is your first step in substituting the hard swallow for the throat clearing.

After your family and friends have pointed out your throat clearing to you several times, you will begin to catch yourself. You will clear your throat and almost immediately think "OOPS! I am not supposed to do that." Your response again should be to swallow hard. When you have caught yourself clearing your throat several times, you will begin to halt yourself just prior to clearing. Once again, you will substitute the hard swallow, but this time the throat clearing was stopped. By the time you have reached this point, you will be very close to breaking the habit totally. The final goal will be met when you realize that you are swallowing many fewer times than the number of times you used to clear your throat.

I want you to work very hard on this problem. I think you will be very surprised just how quickly you are able to break this habit. As a matter of fact, the majority of our patients have significantly reduced the habit within one to two weeks. Most patients, though, cannot do it alone. So please, find other people to help you by having them point out when this occurs.

Following this explanation, the patient will typically clear his or her throat more times than usual. The voice pathologist immediately points out each event, and the hard swallow substitution is initiated. Great gains in habit modification often are made during this initial session.

Zwitman and Calcaterra[19] made another suggestion for modifying throat clearing. These authors suggested a "silent cough" substitution for this behavior. The silent cough is accomplished by breathing deeply and forcing air strongly through abducted vocal folds. This technique also reduces the abuse of coughing. A modified Valsalva maneuver may also be used as a throat clearing substitution. The patient is instructed to lightly approximate the vocal folds as if lifting an object. The impounded subglottic air is then sharply released without vocalization.

As stated previously, several factors must be considered when planning therapy strategies for vocally abusive children. Charting and graphing may certainly serve as a positive behavior modification approach in modifying or eliminating traumatic vocal events; however, many more factors may be considered and other approaches utilized. A summary of a vocal hygiene plan for phonotraumatic children would include:

1. Identify the abuse/misuse:
   - shouting
   - loud talking
   - vocal noises
   - throat clearing
2. Describe the effect:
   - use pictures, diagrams, drawings, and video (Do not hesitate to give simple explanations of anatomy and physiology to children.)
3. Define specific occurrence:
   - These will be distinctly different with every individual child. No two children will follow the same management plan. Psychodynamics of the behavior must also be described.
4. Modify the behavior:
   - teach the child how to shout
   - modify or eliminate vocal noises
   - eliminate nonplay shouting
   - eliminate throat clearing
   - balance the physiology of voice production through direct therapy

Case Study 6: Can We Always Expect Success?

Voice abuse or misuse may occur in many settings under many different circumstances. These settings might include nightclubs, bars, bowling alleys, swimming pools, auction houses, sporting events, work environments, homes, schools, and churches. Wherever we communicate, the possibility of voice misuse is present. The lifestyles of patients often dictate the ease or difficulty they will have in attempting to make vocal modifications. Some patients are not willing to modify their lifestyles even for the health of the laryngeal mechanism. Voice pathologists must realize that their own concern for the patient's voice disorder does not always match that of the patient. For example, the patient who enjoys "getting rowdy" in bars may not respond well to the voice pathologist's greatest efforts for vocal reeducation. The patient who enjoys bowling in winter leagues may continue to bowl and abuse the voice by laughing, talking, and shouting above the noise level, as well as drinking dehydrating liquids and perhaps smoking. These are the patients who provide us with interesting challenges, but, we must remember that the ultimate responsibility for change rests with the patient. The following is an interesting example of the patient who failed to respond to a four-step vocal hygiene counseling program.

The patient was a 30-year-old female who was referred for evaluation and treatment with the diagnosis of chronic vocal fold edema. The patient reported experiencing intermittent dysphonia for several years, but the dysphonia became persistent about 6 months prior to the evaluation. The diagnostic evaluation yielded the following management plan:

1. Identify the phonotrauma:
   ■ shouting
   ■ straining the singing voice
2. Describe the effect:
   ■ accomplished with illustrations and review of stroboscopic examination
3. Define specific occurrences:
   ■ shouting to discipline her children
   ■ straining the voice during church singing on Sunday mornings and Wednesday evenings
4. Modify the behavior:
   ■ discussed various other strategies for disciplining children
   ■ patient agreed to discontinue singing until her voice improved
   ■ singing without strain would then be discussed

The patient's voice quality during the evaluation was moderately dysphonic, characterized by a low pitch, glottal fry phonation, pitch breaks, and breathiness. No significant change or improvement in voice quality was observed during a 3-week period of therapy sessions, which were held twice weekly. The patient denied shouting at her children and singing in church during this time.

Also during this period an interesting pattern of dysphonia was noted. The patient reported experiencing severe dysphonia and almost total aphonia every Sunday night and Thursday morning. When the patient was seen in therapy on Tuesdays and Fridays, the original moderate dysphonia was noted. Further questioning yielded the true cause of the patient's disorder.

As you may have guessed, she attended church services on Sunday mornings and Wednesday evenings. Although she refrained from singing, she joined the many people in the congregation who responded with vigorous vocal enthusiasm to the preacher's message. The need to add this behavior to those requiring modification was explained to the patient.

Although she made concentrated efforts to reduce her vocal enthusiasm during the church service, she had little success in doing so. Final attempts were made to counteract these periods of extreme vocal abuse through direct symptom modification. Because of the frequency of the abuse however, this, too, proved unsuccessful. The patient eventually was terminated from therapy with no improvement noted in her vocal condition. This patient made an informed decision that her vocal behaviors during the church service were more important to her than improving the quality of her voice.

Can we always expect success? Yes! Otherwise we may be guilty of a self-fulfilling prophecy. Will we succeed with all patients? The answer, unfortunately, is no. But only a concerted effort for a reasonable period of time will give us that answer.

Hydration

The vocal hygiene program not only considers elimination and modification of voice abuse behaviors, it must also attend to the health of the tissue lining of the true vocal folds and larynx.

Internal hydration is an important component of good vocal hygiene.[20] In our clinical experience, most of the patients who present with voice disorders are not well hydrated. It has been demonstrated that phonation threshold pressure is increased under experimentally induced laryngeal dehydration.[21] Increased phonation threshold pressure translates to increased effort by the patient to produce voice. Over an extended period of time this increased effort may lead to voice fatigue, laryngeal pathologies, or both.

We recommend that most of our patients begin a formal hydration program. This program involves consuming a minimum of 48 to 64 ounces of water per day. It is explained to the patient that what is swallowed does not touch the vocal folds. Rather the liquid and food is diverted around the vocal folds by the epiglottis and collects in the pyriform sinus cavity and then enters the esophagus. Should any of the swallowed substance mistakenly enter the larynx, a spontaneous protective cough would be initiated (as if it went down the wrong pipe). It is further explained that the vocal folds must be well lubricated for them to function normally. Secretory glands that lie in the ventricles provide this lubrication. The whole body must be well hydrated, otherwise the fluid secreted by the glands to the vocal folds will demonstrate increased viscosity. In other words, thick, sticky mucus will cover the vocal folds and interfere with vibration.

In this dehydrated state, patients often feel the sticky mucus and assume that sinus drainage is causing this problem. Often, the natural reaction is to take a dehydrating medication to reduce the mucus. Of course, this only exacerbates the problem. Another negative result may be the development of a throat-clearing habit.

When patients understand the importance of adequate hydration to maintaining a healthy vocal mechanism, they most often respond well by conforming to a hydration program. It is requested that the patient significantly reduce caffeine and alcohol intake, as these are both diuretics and contribute to dehydration. Patients are instructed to find a receptacle with a known liquid volume. They are instructed to drink liquid from that receptacle as many times as is needed during the day to guarantee the required liquid intake. Improved laryngeal hydration often leads directly to improved voice quality, as well as reduction in the physical sensations in the throat as reported by patients.

Confidential Voice

Initiation of a vocal hygiene program may require short-term vocal conservation especially when the vocal fold injury is recent, or the patient has just had surgery on the vocal folds. Colton and Casper[22] suggested the term "confidential voice" to describe an easy, quiet, breathy voice, as if speaking confidentially to someone at close range. When the voice is produced in this manner, the vocal folds have small amplitudes of vibration, and they do not strike each other forcefully. Confidential Voice Therapy does not involve a single procedural protocol from start to finish for all patients. Rather, the voice pathologist adapts CVT to fit the patient's particular need. The clinician will demonstrate to the patient how to produce quiet, easy, breathy voice. Whispered voice is not desirable. The main challenge to the patient is remembering to use the confidential voice in all speaking situations. The confidential voice is usually used in therapy for only a short period of time. After some recovery has been achieved, other therapy approaches are used to complete the voice recovery.

SYMPTOMATIC VOICE THERAPY

Chapter 3 describes the components of voice that include respiration, phonation, resonance, pitch, loudness, and rate. The inappropriate use of any one vocal component or combination of components may lead directly to the development of a voice disorder. Voice disorders may occur in patients who simply have faulty vocal habits and use, for example, a functionally breathy voice, soft voice, or voice that is too high or too low in pitch. Other patients may use the resonance system inefficiently or may focus the laryngeal tone inappropriately, whereas others talk either too fast or too slow. When inappropriate vocal components are used, direct symptomatic voice therapy may be in order.

It is important to understand, however, that inappropriate vocal components may also be the result of laryngeal pathologies and not their cause. A patient with Reinke's edema may have a voice quality that is breathy and low in pitch for example. Although the components of pitch and respiration are inappropriate, they are not the primary causes of the voice disturbance, just merely two of the symptoms. Modification of the primary etiology (such as smoking in the case of Reinke's edema) is the first line of treatment, with symptom modification following only when necessary. Let us examine symptom modification approaches for the primary components of voice production.

Therapy Approaches for Respiration

In reviewing the literature related to the role of respiration or breathing training in voice therapy, it becomes evident that a primary debate, which appeared in the early part of the 20th century, continues to this day. The debate questions whether respiratory control of voice production should be considered automatic and essentially ignored or should direct respiratory training be part of a voice therapy program. As we travel through the literature, some authors give direct respiratory exercises and breathing training and some do not. Some authors state that few voice patients have breathing patterns so faulty that they interfere with normal phonation. However, it is evident that some laryngeal pathologies certainly alter normal respiration.[2, 7, 11, 13, 14, 23-27]

The current conclusion that we have drawn from this debate is that respiratory training, whether direct or indirect, is a primary part of improving the disordered voice. The justification for this conclusion is that most therapy techniques modify air pressures and airflow in an attempt to bring about efficient voice production. Respiration is one of the three major subsystems responsible for the production of voice. Because physiologic balance of respiration, phonation, and resonance is the ultimate goal of voice therapy, the respiratory component cannot be ignored.

Symptomatic voice therapy techniques concentrate on direct modification of breathing for voice production. Breathing modifications are most often needed in individuals who talk with decreased breath support and professional speakers and singers who may require greater breath support during presentations than during normal conversational speech.

Limited Breath Support

Patients who continue to talk following the normal expiration of air are talking with limited breath support. Because this type of phonation requires increased laryngeal muscle tension, this behavior may strain the vocal mechanism and lead to the development of a voice problem. Suggestions for reducing this behavior include the following:

■ **Identification:** Identify the problem for the patient and describe its effect in detail, utilizing illustrations and descriptions of vocal fold anatomy and physiology.

■ **Ear training:** Monitor the patient's respiration strategy utilizing tape-recorded samples of the voice.

■ **Component modification:**
  - Practice breathing for voice by saying as many numbers as possible on one normal expiration. Stop before any force or strain is evident.
  - Mark a paragraph with phrase markers (see Appendix 7-1). Read the paragraph aloud with normal inhalations occurring at each phrase marker.
  - Tape-record an open discussion between the voice pathologist and the patient during the structured therapy period. Monitor the tape for inappropriate breathing patterns.
  - **Stabilization:** Ask the patient to monitor the voice daily during nontherapy conversational times. A good time to do this may be during dinner with the family.

Abdominal/Diaphragmatic Breathing Patterns

Some patients, especially those who use their voices for some type of public speaking, request strategies for learning "diaphragmatic breathing." Although the diaphragm is always active during respiration in normally healthy individuals, some use a greater amount of thoracic or chest breathing during respiration. Chest breathing patterns may be adequate for voice support, although a more efficient means of breathing for speech can be achieved when the abdominal/diaphragmatic movements predominate over other respiratory chest wall movements. A suggested approach for training this method follows.

■ By utilizing a box diagram (Figure 7-1), describe the various means of air exchange, including clavicular, thoracic,

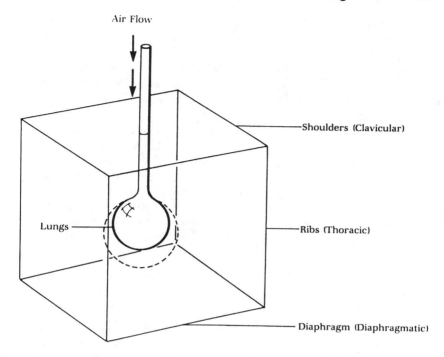

Air Flow

Shoulders (Clavicular)

Lungs

Ribs (Thoracic)

Diaphragm (Diaphragmatic)

Figure 7-1. Box diagram representing breathing patterns.

and diaphragmatic. The voice pathologist may say, "There are three ways in which air may be made to flow into the lungs. All three ways require some expansion of the thoracic cavity, where the lungs are located. The least efficient way to expand the cavity is to raise the top of the box or the shoulders. This allows for poor cavity expansion and would require much vocal effort and tension given the small amount of the air that enters the lungs. This type of breathing pattern is seldom used. The most common way of expanding the cavity is to raise the sides, or the rib cage. This larger expansion normally allows enough air to be inhaled to support voice during normal conversational speech. If you watch people breathe as they talk, you'll notice that most are using this method for inhalation."

"The most efficient method of air intake for the support of voice is through the downward contraction of the bottom of the box, or the diaphragm, and the outward expansion of the abdomen. The diaphragm is the dome-shaped elastic muscle that forms the bottom of the thoracic cavity. When it contracts downward, the abdomen is forced outward, and the cavity expands to its maximum extent. This expansion permits a greater flow of the air into the lungs. The air may then be used to better support your voice."

■ Following this explanation, the patient is requested to place one hand on the chest and the other hand on the upper abdominal wall. When inhaling, the abdominal wall will expand outward while the chest remains in a nearly fixed position with only minimal movement. Contraction of the diaphragm cannot be seen. The patient is asked to breathe in this manner without phonation while observing the proper hand movement on both inhalation and exhalation. Practice is then gradually expanded, utilizing vowels, words, phrases, paragraph reading, and conversational speech. The public speaking voice may also be practiced in the therapy session utilizing the new breathing method.

A variation of this method for training diaphragmatic breathing is to ask the patient lie down in a supine position. A book then may be placed on the abdomen while the patient is asked to observe the natural movement of the abdomen during breathing. As the patient inhales, the book will rise. The opposite movement will be observed during exhalation. As in the previous example, the patient is asked to breathe in this manner without phonation and then gradually introduce the voice component. This technique is simply used to introduce the patient to proper abdominal movement during respiration. The voice pathologist must understand that breathing in a supine position is different physiologically than breathing in an upright position.

Therapy Approaches for Phonation

Symptomatic voice therapy may be used to modify inappropriate components of phonation. Inappropriate phonation is demonstrated by the use of hard glottal attacks, glottal fry phonation, and breathy phonation. As usual, the first step in modifying these behaviors involves identifying their presence to the patient. This may be accomplished by evaluating tape-recorded samples of the voice. The impact of the vocal misuse should also be identified through illustrations and discussion of vocal fold anatomy and physiology. Finally, the specific misuse should be described in detail as follows:

Hard Glottal Attack

A hard glottal attack is made when subglottic air pressure, or air that you build up below your vocal folds, is increased to a very high pressure level just before you say a word that begins with a vowel sound. Then, when you say that word, the vocal folds literally blow apart (demonstrate a hard glottal attack) like this. This action is very harsh on the vocal folds. It causes them to squeeze together very hard to maintain the high air pressure. Then when the vowel sound is produced, they rub and bang together as the pressure is released.

Another way of describing this behavior is to use the example of a garden hose:

A typical garden hose is attached to a faucet at one end and has a spray nozzle at the other end. When the nozzle is closed and the water is turned on at the faucet, a tremendous amount of pressure builds up through the whole system, with the greatest amount of pressure at the nozzle. If the nozzle is suddenly opened and then closed, the water gushes out and slams against the nozzle valve. If the nozzle were slightly open and the water was controlled at the faucet, however, the entire system would remain relaxed and little pressure would be exerted on the valve. We can relate the pressure in the hose to your subglottic air pressure and a nozzle to your vocal folds. What you need to do is to learn how to produce words that begin with vowel sounds without building up that pressure.

The patient is then taught to produce a soft glottal attack or an easy onset by initiating phonation with the sound /h/, utilizing vowels, vowel-consonant combinations, and progressing through words, phrases, paragraph reading, and conversation. The /h/ is extinguished as soon as possible in the process. Negative practice is effective as a stabilization strategy.

Glottal Fry Phonation

Glottal fry is the lower register of voice produced at the bottom of the normal pitch range. It may be recognized as an aperiodic staccato sound and is produced on tightly approximated vocal folds though free edges are vibrating. Aerodynamic measures reveal that glottal fry is produced with very reduced airflow (10-20 mL/s). We often observe glottal fry phonation at the end of phrases, as patients drop breath support, and in the voices of patients who complain of voice fatigue. Extended use of glottal fry phonation appears to be abusive to the vocal folds and should be modified. Because it normally occurs in conjunction with the use of an inappropriately low pitch, modification is made by training a slight increase in pitch and loudness. The increase in pitch and loudness requires improved respiratory support, which explains why this technique eliminates the glottal fry.

Breathy Phonation

Some patients have the habit of speaking with an incomplete adduction of the vocal folds, yielding a weak, breathy voice. A weak breathy speaking voice may also be the result of disengaging the thyroarytenoid muscles and speaking in a falsetto voice. Although some actors cultivate this type of voice to project an image of sultriness or sexiness (Marilyn Monroe), it is a vocal misuse. Its prolonged use can lead to laryngeal pathology.

Again, therapy would begin with identification of the problem and education of the effects that breathy phonation may have on the vocal mechanism. When phonation is breathy, causing wastage of air during phonation, the vocal folds are forced to vibrate inefficiently. The inherent poor breath support impairs vocal quality by causing secondary abusive glottal or supraglottal tension.

The major symptomatic therapy approaches for modifying the breathy voice involve training the patient to produce a more firm or engaged vocal fold approximation. The specific approach used will depend on the severity of the breathiness.

  ■ Mild breathiness may be modified through patient education and often through the use of a more precise articulation, especially on the plosive sounds /p/, /t/, and /k/.
  ■ Training the speaker to increase vocal intensity may often modify a moderate amount of breathiness. A slightly louder voice will force the vocal folds to approximate more firmly, thus decreasing the wastage of air. Ear training, comparing the breathy voice to the louder voice on a tape recorder, and negative practice are excellent modification approaches.

■ A more than moderate amount of breathiness may require these approaches, as well as a more rigorous therapy approach. This may include actually teaching the patient to approximate the vocal folds utilizing the previously described "misuse" of hard glottal attacks. Hard glottal attacks will give the patient an awareness of vocal fold approximation and muscle engagement. The vowels produced in this manner will have clearer tones that can be compared to the patient's breathy tones. An even more rigorous approach would be the use of pushing exercises. These exercises combine the isometric pushing of the arms at the same moment of phonation. These simultaneous activities create firmer adduction of the vocal folds through overflow muscular tension, thus decreasing breathiness. Once the clearer tone is experienced and stabilized, the glottal attack and pushing strategy are quickly extinguished so as not to develop a vocal hyperfunction habit. (A complete description of glottal attack and pushing exercises are described under voice therapy for vocal fold paralysis later in this chapter.)

Therapy Approaches for Resonance

Functionally inappropriate resonance may be one of the more difficult properties of voice to modify. Thus far in our discussion, we have been concerned with functional voice behaviors. When considering therapy for resonance disturbances, it is important for voice pathologists to be certain that the disorder is, in fact, functional and not organic in origin. There are many organic causes for resonance disturbances including various palatal clefts, insufficient functioning of the velopharyngeal port, surgical trauma, and neurological diseases and disorders. These organic causes are determined through medical examination, cinefluoroscopy, and manometric measures. The major characteristic of functional resonance disorders is the lack of consistency in the resonance quality and positive stimulability for more normal resonance characteristics.

Typical speech resonance patterns vary greatly from one geographic location to another. For example, resonance judged appropriate in the eastern states may not be acceptable in the midwestern states. These qualities often change naturally as speech and voice patterns are assimilated into the local patterns, or they may need to be modified through therapy. Another common cause of functional resonance disturbances is structural oral-pharyngeal change following tonsillectomy and adenoidectomy.

Treatment of organic resonance problems is usually limited to surgical and orthodontic or prosthodontic procedures. These may include the closing of clefts, the creation of pharyngeal flaps for inadequate velar closure, or the molding and fitting of prosthetic obturators to provide posterior velar competence. An interdisciplinary group of professionals that comprise a Cleft Palate/ Craniofacial Anomaly Team most often provides evaluation and treatment of organic resonance disturbances. Team members may include a speech-language pathologist, audiologist, orthodontist, prosthodontist, otolaryngologist, and oral and plastic surgeons. Voice therapy often follows medical treatment to guarantee that the combined treatments achieve maximum gain.

The voice pathologist is most concerned with modifying both functional hypernasality and hyponasality, as well as dealing with the more common use of an inappropriate tone focus. Treatment of resonance and focus problems often proves difficult and requires all the creative skills available. No management approach can be generalized to any population with a resonance disturbance. Techniques that work to improve voice quality for one individual may not work for others with the same problem.

For functional hypernasality and denasality problems, the direction of voice therapy is to boldly manipulate articulation, mouth opening, vocal tract postures, and phonation boldly in as many combinations as proves necessary to locate the most efficient resonant quality. Use of imagery, modeling, imitation, and negative practice are all strategies that may assist patients in achieving consistently appropriate resonance quality.

Hypernasality

■ **Identification:** As usual, the first step in the modification of any vocal property is to identify the problem and describe it in detail to the patient. Illustrations demonstrating the relationships between the resonance cavities are helpful.

Tape-recorded samples of the patient's voice compared to the voices of other individuals of similar age are helpful for ear training.

■ **Articulation therapy:** Often, maximizing the strength and precision of articulatory movements and decreasing any articulation errors will increase the intelligibility of the speech and decrease the perception of hypernasality.[28,29] Increasing articulatory precision will involve activating all the articulators in a somewhat exaggerated manner, with special emphasis placed on a wider mouth opening, thus decreasing the contribution of the nasal cavity in the treatment of the glottal sound.[30]

■ **Pitch and loudness modification:** Boone[31] discussed the positive decrease in the amount of nasal resonance in some patients who were taught to speak with increased intensity at a lower pitch level. Activation of the glottal tone through increased loudness focuses more of the speech energy into the oral cavity decreasing the contribution of nasal resonance.

■ **Nonspeech phonation:** The patient plays with the voice, making various nonspeech vocal sounds, such as animal and engine noises. If any of the nonspeech sounds demonstrate reduced nasality, then work from this sound by comparing it to the hypernasal sounds, training similar sounds, and expanding into speech sounds.

■ **Utilize articulation deep test:** The deep test of articulation is used to determine if any sounds in any phonetic contexts are made with normal or near normal levels of nasal resonance. If so, these phoneme productions are expanded into similar sound clusters, then words, phrases, and conversational speech.

■ **Do the obvious:** The patient's ability to produce a voice "... as if you have a cold" is explored. Some patients with functional hypernasality can easily produce a denasal voice quality when speaking in this manner. They simply were not aware that a slight modification of the "cold" voice would yield the normal nasal resonance. It pays to explore this ability early in the therapy program.

■ **Negative practice:** Negative practice may also be an effective therapy tool used with resonance disorders. When the patient first produces new normal resonance, purposeful productions of the same sounds utilizing the "old" hypernasal voice may reinforce and strengthen the use of normal resonance. The patient's ability to use both voices upon dismissal from therapy shows a true mastery of the therapeutic goals.

- ▪ **Instrumental feedback:** Many of the explorations mentioned above may be aided by instrumental assessment and biofeedback. The Nasometer (Figure 7-2; Kay Elemetrics Corporation) is an instrument that measures and visually demonstrates the degree of nasalance on a computer screen. This instrument provides for excellent patient monitoring and feedback, as well as a useful resonance evaluation tool.

Denasality

Functional denasality may occasionally occur, especially following the removal of nasal obstructions. Wilson[30] suggested that the patient's auditory feedback system does not quickly adjust as he or she continues to attempt to maintain the status quo even though the nasal cavity is no longer obstructed. Once the disorder has been identified and described in detail, approaches used to modify the behavior include:

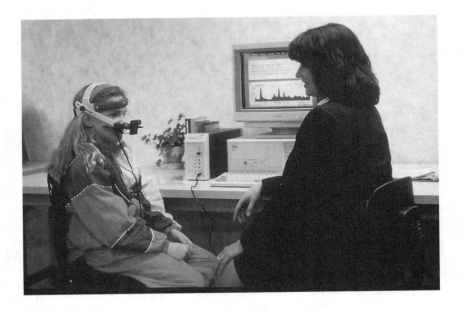

Figure 7-2. Nasometer (Kay Elemetrics Corporation).

Utilizing the normal nasal sounds: In this approach, the voice pathologist should determine the patient's ability to produce /m/, /n/, and /ŋ/ with normal resonance. If this is possible, /m/ and /n/ may be combined with vowel sounds and expanded through words, phrases, and so on. If the nasal sounds are also produced with the denasal quality, attempts may be made to train nasalization of /m/ using the singing voice. Humming, with the lips closed in the /m/ position, forces the production of more nasal resonance. These productions may be slowly modified by (a) opening the mouth while humming and saying /ma/, (b) expanding to other vowel sounds, (c) eliminating the hum, and (d) then expanding into other sounds, words, phrases, and so on.

Utilizing hypernasal resonance: Some patients who demonstrate a functional denasal voice are readily able to produce an exaggerated hypernasal voice quality. If this is so, then different gradients of velar closure may be demonstrated and stabilized, leading to normal velopharyngeal functioning.

Nonspeech phonation: (Explained under hypernasality) this approach may also be an effective means of initiating normal voice resonance.

Negative practice: (Explained under hypernasality.)

Tone Focus

Focus refers to the resonance of the voice in the supraglottic vocal tract. Constriction of the supraglottic airway at any point will alter the focus of voice production. When the vocal tract is relaxed and open without supraglottic constriction, the glottal sound source can resonate freely and maximally, creating what is called a "forward focus" or "placement" of tone. The ideal placement of this tone is forward, as this placement allows the voice to resonate fully throughout the pharyngeal, nasal, and oral cavities without effort or tension. Tension at any point in the vocal tract will alter both the free resonance of the tone and voice quality. In addition to changing the quality, less-than-ideal tone placement may result in voice that fatigues easily and lacks flexibility and vibrancy.

Poor tone focus may be observed in patients who functionally constrict the pharynx, retract the tongue, and elevate the larynx as the habitual manner in which voice is produced. Poor tone focus may also be the result of laryngeal pathologies which, when present, force the patient to constrict the upper airway to accommodate the presence of the pathology. This constriction often leads to what is commonly termed a back-focused tone. The voice qualities associated with several laryngeal pathologies commonly present with a backward tone focus. These pathologies include edema and mass lesions of the vocal folds which require the patient to constrict the glottic and supraglottic structures because of the presence of the increased mass; bowed vocal folds and other incomplete glottic closures caused by laryngeal myasthenia and laryngeal fatigue, paresis or paralysis; and adductor spasmodic dysphonia, which forces the patient to tense the vocal mechanism as a means of pushing the voice through the spasms. As the inappropriate focus becomes habituated, direct voice therapy approaches commonly must be utilized to reintroduce a more ideal and less tense placement of the tone.

Following is a therapy approach that we have found useful for improving tone focus using nasal sounds and sensory feedback to "tune the patient in" to the nebulous concept of focus:

- **Patient education:** We begin by teaching the patient about the concept of resonance by demonstrating how one sentence may be said with various resonance characteristics. Patients are made aware of how celebrity impersonators change the resonance of the voice to sound like other people. The concepts of frontal, back, and mid-focus are introduced by first demonstrating a tight, constricted, back-focused phrase that the patient is asked to imitate. Because this type of tone placement often is implicated as the problem, most patients, although somewhat embarrassed, are able to produce this voice. Second, a breathy, poorly focused tone is imitated followed by an exaggerated, almost nasal forward focus. It is explained to the patient that, although the ultimate goal was not to talk in a nasal quality, practicing this placement would help to approximate the desired focus. Practice of this exaggerated forward placement would be one step toward learning the desired placement.
- **Nasalized phrase production:** The clinician instructs the patient to slowly and softly chant the following phrases on a comfortable pitch level slightly above the fundamental frequency:

OH MY OH MY OH MY OH MY . . .

OH ME OH ME OH ME OH ME . . .

OH NO OH NO OH NO OH NO . . .

OH MY NO OH MY NO OH MY NO . . .

OH ME OH MY OH ME OH MY . . .

The forward resonance of each phrase is exaggerated to the extreme and the clinician instructs the patient to feel and sense the energy of the tone in the nose, on the lips, in the front of the face, and so on. Tape recordings of the phrases are made for both the clinician and the patient, and ear training is accomplished as needed.

Once the phrases are produced to the satisfaction of the voice pathologist, negative practice is used. The patient is asked to alternate between forward and back focuses to demonstrate the mastery of the focus technique on these simple phrases.

■ **Introduce intensity and rate variations:** Using the same phrases, the clinician asks the patient to repeat each phrase multiple times using the following routine:

Very slow and very soft

Faster and louder

Fast and loud

Slower and softer

Very slow and very soft

Changing the rate and loudness of the chanted phrases adds a new dimension to the exercise that forces the patient to concentrate on maintaining the forward placement even as the intensity and rate are increased. The pitch remains the same.

■ **Introduce inflected phrase and normal speech:** When the patient has succeeded in mastering the first three steps, the practice phrases may be modified from the single pitch chant to a more "sing-song" or over-inflected vocal presentation and then directly into a normally spoken phrase:

soft and slow

louder and faster

exaggerated inflection

normal speech

The proper focus of the tone is closely monitored during each one of the steps utilizing the phrases. Negative practice is judiciously used throughout each session. Some patients move quickly through each of these steps and master a forward focus with ease. Others require many therapy sessions to master the appropriate focus. The final step is to expand the ability to produce a forward focus from these phrases into expanded phrases and sentences, paragraph reading, and conversational speech.

Other clues suggested by Lee[32] to help make patients aware of forward focus include playing a comb wrapped with waxed paper with the lips. The lips are made to vibrate by phonation, and the comb resonates this vibration making patients more aware of the forward placement of the tone. Make a motorcycle noise by vibrating the lips together (this technique works well with children) and trilling the tongue on the top of the alveolar ridge while moving the lips to shape different sounds.

The above therapy techniques isolate the resonance component of voice production. Later in this chapter, resonance will be integrated with phonation and respiration in a holistic voice therapy program known as Resonant Voice Therapy.

Therapy Approaches for Pitch

Pitch levels that are either too high or too low are represented in many different types of laryngeal pathologies. The decision to modify pitch should be based on whether it is a primary etiologic factor (the actual cause of the voice disorder) or whether it is merely a symptom of the pathology. If an inappropriate pitch is present because of laryngeal pathology, it is likely to reach a normal level without direct component modification once the path-ology is resolved. Direct pitch modification can be somewhat difficult and has the potential of causing laryngeal harm if the new pitch level is trained artificially high or low. Let us examine some of the more common reasons for the use of inappropriate pitch levels and identify those that may benefit from direct symptom modification.

Increased vocal fold mass as a result of edema and mass lesions of the vocal folds may cause a lowering of the fundamental frequency. The primary etiology is whatever caused the pathology. If the cause proved to be the inappropriate use of pitch, therapy would focus on direct pitch modification.

An example of inappropriate pitch as a primary cause of laryngeal pathology would be the use of a pseudoauthoritative voice. Conscious efforts by both men and women to sound more authoritative or self-assured by using a forceful deep voice, especially in work settings, may lead to the development of a voice disorder. In this case, the therapy of choice would be a direct symptom modification approach, as well as a discussion of why the need to use this voice is perceived by the patient.

Another example of an intentional pitch modification occasionally seen in therapy is the patient who is trying to "save" the voice. These are patients who are experiencing some vocal difficulties. In an attempt to counteract these difficulties, they try to "save" the voice by habitually lowering the pitch and volume. The patients have the misconception that by talking in this manner, they are reducing the impact of whatever is causing the vocal difficulty. In reality, just the opposite is true. Habitual use of an inappropriately low-pitched voice is a vocal misuse and can lead to the development of pathology. Direct pitch modification is then in order.

Patients who develop a hormonal imbalance after surgery, because of malfunction of the endocrine system, or as a side effect to medications present an interesting problem. These factors often cause a permanent change in the vocal folds, causing a permanent pitch modification. In this etiologic scenario, laryngeal pathology is not likely to occur unless the patient's auditory feedback system attempts to modify the pitch level back to the original level. Counseling against direct pitch modification is often the treatment of choice here.

Emotional and physical disturbances often will lead to a voice of depression. The way a person feels physically and emotionally is directly reflected in the vocal quality. People who are depressed, agitated, upset, physically ill, mourning, or going through other emotional conflicts often have a low-pitched, poorly supported voice quality. The primary etiology is the emotional stress, but secondary use of the inappropriate vocal components may lead to a voice disorder.

Two other factors that lead to the inappropriate use of pitch are whole body and laryngeal fatigue. The person who is constantly fatigued is likely to use poor breath support and permit the pitch level to lower because of a lack of effort behind the speaking voice. Fatigue may also affect the components of respiration and loudness. Sensations of general and laryngeal fatigue often lead to an effort to talk. As a result, patients often drop the pitch and respiratory support, which actually exacerbates the problem. These patients are encouraged to "energize" the voice with increased loudness and breath support, which will increase the pitch to a more appropriate level.

Upward pitch changes may also cause voice problems. Recall that as vocal intensity increases so does the frequency level. This problem may be remediated through direct pitch modification. Finally, pitch change may actually be desirable as requested by a gender dysphoria patient. Let us now look at some therapy approaches for pitch modification.

Case Study 7: The Pseudo-authoritative Voice

A 25-year-old male with the diagnosis of bilateral contact ulcers without evidence of reflux was referred for evaluation and treatment. Voice quality during the evaluation was moderately dysphonic, characterized by low pitch, glottal fry phonation, inappropriate loudness, and breathiness. The patient reported experiencing vocal difficulties soon after beginning a new job as a bank manager trainee 5 months prior to the evaluation. Other than occasional shouting at sporting events, no other vocal abuses were identified. Results of the evaluation revealed that the patient's contact ulcers were the result of using a loud, low-pitched pseudo-authoritative voice in his work setting. Being in his first position of authority, the patient attempted to project a "strong" image. Inappropriate use of the low, loud voice involved rubbing and grinding of the arytenoid cartilages that lead to the development of the contact ulcers. The treatment plan involved three major steps:

The first step was to identify the causes and to explain to the patient in detail what contact ulcers are and what lead to their development. When dealing with a male patient, it generally is not wise to explain that the pitch must be raised. The mental impression he gains would be that of a major pitch modification when, in fact, a minor modification is needed. It is better to explain that he is talking at the bottom of his voice range and that therapy will be designed to return it to its normal level. Tape-recorded samples were then used to demonstrate the vocal symptoms in question. The voice pathologist also imitated examples of the voice components.

The second step was an attempt to identify a more appropriate pitch level. As previously stated, this is somewhat risky with the pathological voice. However, a higher pitch that is comfortable for the patient, and produced with little effort, will normally prove adequate. Cooper[26] suggested having the patients say, in a natural conversational voice, "um-hum" as if answering "yes" to a question. The "hum" part of the production is usually produced in a relaxed tone near the patient's present, most comfortable pitch level.

The third step was to match the appropriate pitch level to a musical note on a pitch pipe, which served as a reference note. The patient was then asked to match that level while repeating single-syllable words and short phrases. The phrases were gradually lengthened and inflectional patterns were introduced. Sentences, paragraph reading, and conversational speech marked his progress, which was monitored with immediate audio replays (Facilitator by Kay Elemetric Corporation) and by tape-recorded samples. Negative practice was also used. It is positive for a patient to have total control of the voice, and negative practice helps the patient meet this goal.

Case Study 8: The Voice Saver

The patient was a 31-year-old male who was referred for evaluation and treatment with the diagnosis of mild, bilateral vocal fold edema. The patient had only recently begun experiencing vocal difficulties. As a young assistant pastor of a large parish, he was required to hold meetings, counsel youth, visit the sick and elderly, teach a Bible studies class, and deliver a sermon one Sunday per month. He noticed 4 weeks prior to the evaluation that his voice routinely tired and became hoarse every day in the early afternoon. The patient denied any vocal abuse and did not feel that he gave enough group presentations to cause the vocal problem. His medical history was unremarkable, and the social history did not yield evidence of the typical forms of voice abuse except for throat clearing, which was noted throughout the evaluation.

The patient's voice quality during the evaluation was described as moderately dysphonic, characterized by low-pitch, low-intensity, glottal fry phonation, and an unusual amount of breathiness. The use of these inappropriate voice components could account for the patient's voice difficulties, but the severity of voice quality did not fit the observations made through the laryngeal videostroboscopy or the diagnosis of mild edema.

The patient was therefore asked if this voice was typical of his voice when it would fatigue. "Oh, no!" He replied, and to the voice pathologist's surprise, his reply was in a normal voice. "I'm talking down like that to save my voice."

Further questioning revealed that the patient had a chest cold for 2 weeks prior to the onset of his daily voice fatigue. Much coughing and throat clearing during the cold was reported. When the cold subsided, the throat clearing persisted, continuing the mild edema of the vocal folds and an imbalance of voice subsystems. Introduction of the "saving" voice only caused more vocal misuse. Successful therapy focused on vocal hygiene counseling, elimination of throat clearing, and balancing of the voice subsystems through Vocal Function Exercises. Attempts to save the voice were extinguished.

It is said that experience is the best teacher. After that experience, we have found several patients who were trying to "save" the voice in much the same manner. This especially seems to occur in people who do a great deal of talking or singing on a daily basis. They report that they begin to experience laryngeal fatigue and therefore let the voice drop lower in pitch, decreasing the phonatory effort and respiratory support. This, of course, is a misuse of the vocal components that leads to an imbalance in the three subsystems of voice production, thus accelerating sensations of laryngeal fatigue.

The most positive short-term approach to counteract fatigue is to train the patient to use more breath support for voice, slightly increase the loudness, and to maintain the higher, more appropriate pitch level. Even though this requires more perceived physical effort, the improved balance of the vocal components will often reduce the sensations of fatigue and, indeed, refresh the voice production.

Case Study 9: Emotional Voice Changes

The patient was a 23-year-old woman who was referred for evaluation and treatment, with a diagnosis of mild-to-moderate vocal fold edema. The patient's voice quality during the evaluation was a mild dysphonia, characterized by low pitch, low intensity, and breathiness. She reported that she began experiencing vocal difficulties just one month prior to the evaluation, and the usual diagnostic questions were posed, probing for the etiologic factors associated with the development of the disorder. No form of vocal abuse could be identified, and the medical history was unremarkable.

Questions regarding her social history, specifically "how long have you been married?" elicited an emotional and tearful response, however. This line of questioning was followed. The patient volunteered that just prior to the onset of her vocal difficulties she discovered that her husband of 11 months had been unfaithful. Rather than confront him with this information, she remained silent and was contemplating divorce.

The relationship of emotional tension and depression on the vocal components and the resulting voice quality were explained. Often, the patient's understanding of why the voice lowers, weakens, becomes breathy, and tires easily is enough to relieve the additional anxiety of the vocal problem. In all cases, the need for further counseling is determined, and the appropriate referrals are made. This particular patient was referred for family counseling to attempt to resolve the primary cause of her laryngeal pathology. Direct vocal component modification was not appropriate or necessary in this situation.

Therapy Approaches for Gender Dysphoria Voice Change

The voice pathologist may be called upon to aid in the feminization of the male-to-female transsexual voice and speech patterns. Individuals who desire gender reassignment therapy and surgery are often referred to gender dysphoria clinics. The programs these clinics offer include step-by-step procedures leading to the final surgical modifications necessary to accomplish the permanent gender reassignment. The procedures also include psychological counseling, electrolysis for the removal of body hair, and hormone treatments to enhance female characteristics. In addition, patients are required to live the part of the desired gender for 1-year prior to surgery.

The effects of hormones administered for the purpose of feminization are minimal as related to voice change. Therefore, the individual is required to make numerous changes to create a more feminine speech pattern. The patient must elevate the fundamental frequency, modify the resonance characteristics, and alter inflection and intonation patterns, precision of articulation, and even type of vocalized pauses.[33-35] It is desirable to modify these speech and voice characteristics even prior to the gender reassignment surgery.

Pitch modification is actually the first and easiest part of the feminization of the voice. We choose to test the entire frequency range of the patient and then attempt to place the new fundamental frequency as close to the comfortable mid-range as is possible. In the normal laryngeal mechanism, pitch modification is potentially harmful if muscle tension results. Tension is monitored throughout therapy to assure that voice misuse does not occur. The new pitch range is defined on a monitoring instrument (in our case, a Kay Elemetrics Visi-Pitch), and the patient practices producing words, phrases, sentences, paragraph readings, and conversations until the pitch level is habituated. At the same time, a slightly breathy phonation is taught and, when necessary, the patient is taught to retract the tongue slightly, which also tends to elevate the larynx in the neck. These slightly altered tongue and larynx positions tend to shorten the length of the vocal tract and reduce the available area for supraglottic resonance, which tends to feminize the voice.[35]

Along with the direct modification of the voice and vocal tract, patients must also learn to increase their rate of speech and lengthen their pauses, while at the same time increasing the precision of articulation.[36,37] Because female speakers use increased intonation, inflection patterns also must be increased through practice with the voice pathologist. Finally, vocalized pauses, coughing, and throat clearing must be modified. A harsh, low-pitched "uh" or throat-clearing sound would certainly destroy the effect of the new voice and speech production. Patients must be trained to produce these sounds within a new acceptable range.

Therapy Approaches for Loudness Modification

Functional misuse of the intensities of voice may lead to the development of laryngeal pathologies. The vocally abusive behaviors of shouting and loud talking have been previously discussed under Vocal Hygiene. Habitual misuses of conversational voice levels that are either too loud or too soft also may lead to voice disorders. The first step in dealing with patients with either of these behaviors is to refer them for a complete hearing evaluation. The voices of patients with sensorineural hearing loss often are produced with too much intensity, caused by the inability to monitor the voice adequately. Those with conductive hearing losses may talk too softly, caused by the ability to hear through bone conduction and their inability to monitor competing background noise. When an auditory disorder has been ruled out or treated, several intensity modification approaches may be followed:

- Make the patient aware of the problem by utilizing the diagnostic voice evaluation tape. Compare the patient's vocal intensity to that of the voice pathologist on the tape. Use illustrations and discussion to explain what effect the inappropriate use of loudness has had on the laryngeal mechanism.
- Raise the patient's awareness level regarding how people react to the voice. For example, if the patient talks too loudly, do people back away, look away, or cut the patient short? Does the patient perhaps project an overbearing image? People who talk too softly frequently may be asked to repeat themselves, may be ignored, or may project a bashful image.
- Practice direct manipulation of many different intensities. Record these using short phrases for ear training purposes.
- Utilize an electronic VU meter, a hand-held sound level meter or another commercial intensity monitor (such as a Visi-Pitch) to stabilize productions at a reasonable intensity level. Habituate this level through words, phrases, paragraph readings, and conversational speech.

Therapy Approaches for Rate Modification

Seldom is the rate of a patient's speech deviant enough to cause laryngeal pathology. If rate becomes inappropriate enough to create a voice disorder, it is typically because the rate is too fast. Speaking with too fast a rate may create vocal hyperfunction. A modification approach for reducing rate follows:

■ Make the patient aware of the problem by reviewing the voice on the diagnostic evaluation tape recording and comparing it to the rate of the voice pathologist on the same tape. Use illustrations of vocal fold anatomy and discussion of physiology to explain how a faster rate creates vocal hyperfunction.

■ Many patients who attempt to slow down the rate of speech attempt to accomplish this by pausing longer between words and phrases. Although this is helpful, it is more effective to have the patient exaggerate vowel prolongation in words within moderately long phrases. This exercise is totally opposite their normal habit.

■ From deliberate vowel prolongation in phrases, the patient may move into reading song lyrics and poetry. The inherent rhythms and inflectional patterns are ideal for indirectly teaching timing and melody, both of which are lacking.

■ When the patient has sufficiently mastered the reading of lyrics and poetry, begin paragraph readings of prose material. Monitor progress through tape recordings or the use of a Facilitator (Kay Elemetrics Corporation).

■ Begin negative practice. Listen to tape recordings of the same material read by the patient at an increased rate and at a normal rate.

■ Stabilize the new rate in structured conversational speech within the therapy setting. Use negative practice and expand the physical settings until the new rate is stabilized.

Treatment Approaches for Laryngeal Area Muscle Tension

Vocal hyperfunction may be characterized by intermittent periods of laryngeal area tension, as may occur when someone shouts or clears the throat. It may also be a persistent general laryngeal area muscle tension. The term muscle tension dysphonia (MTD) has been used as a descriptor for chronic laryngeal area muscle tension. This tension may either be the cause of a voice disorder or may be the result of compensations made for the presence of a disorder. Several techniques that may be used to reduce persistent laryngeal area muscle tension are progressive relaxation, chewing exercises, the yawn-sigh facilitating technique, and EMG biofeedback.

■ **Progressive relaxation:** Reduction of whole-body tension may serve as an indirect method of reducing laryngeal area tension. Progressive relaxation techniques presented by Jacobson[38] are designed to teach patients to recognize the differences between muscles that feel tense and muscles that feel relaxed. The most popular exercise involves alternately tensing and relaxing all the muscles from the scalp to the toes. This technique may prove especially helpful in reducing tension for patients who are diagnosed with MTD.

■ **Chewing exercises:** In 1952, Froeschel[39] described the chewing method for laryngeal tension reduction. This method is based on the theory that phonating during vegetative chewing will relax all the structures involved in articulation, resonance, and phonation. Wilson[30] described a detailed approach in utilizing the chewing method with children. Using this technique, patients are taught to imagine they are chewing food. They are encouraged to utilize a wide excursion of their jaws and tongues while simulating chewing food. When a relaxed chewing method has been achieved, vocalization of a neutral vowel is added to the chewing exercise. Complete relaxation of the laryngeal area is encouraged during phonation. When adequate progress has been made in relaxed phonation, short words and phrases are added to the chewing exercise. Finally, the chewing behavior itself is extinguished as more relaxed phonation is expanded into longer phrases, paragraph readings, and conversational speech.

■ **Yawn-sigh approach:** Another approach for reducing laryngeal area tension is the yawn-sigh facilitating technique as first described by Boone.[2] Patients are asked to initiate the first half of a yawn behavior. The yawn serves to expand the pharynx and to stretch and then relax the extrinsic laryngeal muscles, thus lowering the larynx in the neck to a more neutral position and permit a more forward placement of the tongue in the oral cavity. The subsequent sigh should then be more relaxed with less tension noted in the phonation of the tone. From the sigh phonation, the patient is taught to appreciate the sensation of laryngeal relaxation. The yawn-sigh technique is then paired with vowels and then gradually expanded into words, phrases, paragraph readings, and conversational speech.

- **Biofeedback training:** The basis of biofeedback is that self-control of physiological functions is possible with continuous, immediate information about the internal bodily state. Electromyographic biofeedback has been used successfully in the rehabilitation treatment of a wide range of neuromuscular disorders. EMG biofeedback training permits patients to monitor electrical activities of their muscles and to exert some control over these areas. This form of biofeedback training has permitted patients to view the tension of the extrinsic laryngeal muscles and to reduce or increase these tension levels utilizing auditory and visual feedback.[40, 41] Stemple et al[41] demonstrated the successful use of EMG biofeedback in reducing laryngeal area tension and improving the vocal folds and voice production with a group of patients with vocal fold nodules.

Case Study 10: Ventricular Phonation

Occasionally patients increase laryngeal area muscle tension to such an extreme that they begin phonating using the false vocal folds. This may be a functional disorder or it may result from the patient's attempt to compensate for gross laryngeal pathology.

The patient was a 55-year-old lawyer who was referred for evaluation and treatment with the diagnosis of ventricular phonation. The problem had begun 6 weeks prior to the evaluation at about the same time that he was told he was being considered for a county judgeship. Voice quality was moderately dysphonic, characterized by harshness; however, the patient had gained a fair level of control and consistency of the voice. The major complaint was that the voice tired easily. He was not unduly concerned by the quality, which was puzzling to the voice pathologist. Results of the evaluation yielded no probable etiologic factors other than the patient's anxiety associated with the pending appointment. Laryngeal videostroboscopic observation of the vocal folds confirmed the ventricular folds as the source of voice. After further discussion, the patient recognized that he had developed the voice disorder to satisfy a psychological need. He would use the voice difficulty as an excuse if he were not appointed judge. However, the voice had habituated and needed to be changed.

Indirect therapy methods were first attempted utilizing general progressive relaxation and EMG biofeedback. The patient was readily able to reduce laryngeal tension levels, but this did not modify or reduce ventricular phonation. Direct vocal manipulation was then employed. This followed the basic treatment approach presented by Boone.[31] This approach suggests that the voice pathologist use the following five steps:

1. Ask the patient to inhale and exhale in a prolonged manner with a wide-open mouth. He or she should not attempt to phonate at this time.
2. Repeat the same procedure with the patient phonating vowels during inhalation. This often is facilitated by the use of a higher pitch. Inhalation phonation can only be accomplished with the true vocal folds.
3. When true vocal fold inhalation phonation is achieved, ask the patient to match this sound on exhalation phonation in the same breathing cycle. It is extremely important that the voice pathologist be persistent during this step in therapy. It is critical that patients are required to persist until they achieve appropriate target exhalation phonation.
4. When exhalation phonation is achieved, begin modifying this to a normal pitch level. This may be accomplished by singing down a musical scale in two to three-note intervals on a vowel sound until the desired level is approximated.
5. Vary the vowel sounds and move on through syllables, words, phrases, and paragraphs. Stabilize the improved true vocal fold phonation during conversational speech.

It may also prove helpful to use digital manipulation of the thyroid cartilage. The position of the larynx during ventricular phonation is often high in the neck. Grasping the thyroid cartilage and holding or massaging it down during inhalation and exhalation phonation cycles may be effective.

Direct vocal manipulation proved effective in modifying this patient's voice, but only after he was appointed to the bench. Exercises to rebalance the subsystems of voice were used to return the voice to a healthy condition (see Vocal Function Exercises).

Psychogenic Voice Therapy

Patients who develop a disordered voice in the context of a structurally normal larynx are among the more interesting challenges in voice therapy. Several terms have been used to describe these disorders including functional dysphonia, functional aphonia, psychogenic voice disorders, and conversion voice disorders. Muscle tension dysphonia (MTD) has also found its way onto this list of functional voice disorders. Psychological or personality disorientation often is presumed with psychogenic voice pathologies. Nonetheless, such labels collectively reflect etiological presuppositions when clear thresholds or discrete boundaries separating these various diagnostic categories are lacking. It is more likely that these voice disorders comprise a complex blend of psychological, social, and physiologic factors.[42] Beyond the controversy and confusion surrounding these disorders, is the voice pathologist's exceptional role in treating these patients. That role includes sorting through all of these factors to determine the most appropriate method of improving the voice quality.

The major types of laryngeal pathologies that we will discuss under the category of psychogenic voice therapy include conversion aphonia, conversion dysphonia, the mutational falsetto, and juvenile voice. The management plans for all of these voice pathologies include four major stages.

■ Stage 1 is the medical evaluation. As with all voice disorders, it is essential that the presence of organic pathology be ruled out prior to the initiation of therapy. The report of normal laryngeal structures will also confirm the diagnosis of a functional disorder, in the presence of inappropriate and often unusual vocal symptoms.

■ Stage 2 is the diagnostic voice evaluation. During the evaluation, the voice pathologist will develop the history of the pathology and will learn how the patient functions socially and physically within the environment. An impression of the patient's personality will evolve. The diagnostic time is also used to prepare the patient for vocal change. This is accomplished by explaining to the patient how the vocal mechanism works and by describing what is happening physiologically within the larynx to create the present voice quality. Although no attempt is yet made to explain why this is occurring, the physiologic description provides the patient with a rationale for the vocal problems.

■ Stage 3 of vocal treatment is the direct manipulation of the voice. The type of manipulation will vary depending on the type of pathology. Vocal manipulation most often begins during the diagnostic evaluation. The expected result is a dramatic change in the voice toward normal phonation during the first treatment session.

■ Stage 4 involves probing to determine why the disorder developed. For example, in conversion voice disorders the voice quality change is felt to represent a symbolic somatization of psychodynamic conflict. It is the patient's subconscious effort to escape an unpleasant situation or the memory of the situation that promotes the reaction. Aronson[11] suggested that the most appropriate professional to deal with this type of disorder is the voice pathologist, whose complete understanding of the vocal processes and counseling background provide the basic skills and abilities to remediate these pathologies. Once normal voicing has been achieved, it is a natural transition to begin examining why the problem existed. By this time, the voice pathologist has gained the trust of and a rapport with the patient. With interview questions that are structured in a nonthreatening manner, the voice pathologist can usually determine the cause of the problem. Patients frequently volunteer the necessary information, which often opens a floodgate of emotion.

Once the cause or causes have been identified and discussed, the voice pathologist needs to determine if further professional counseling is advisable. If so, the appropriate referral should be discussed with the patient and should be made with the patient's consent. Let us now closely examine several types of functional dysphonias and the voice therapy techniques for treating them.

Conversion Aphonia

Conversion voice disorders, called hysteric, hysterical, nervous, functional, and psychosomatic aphonia, have been discussed in medical journals for scores of years. Many curious and unconventional treatments have been advocated in the literature.

Russell[4] suggested that hysteric aphonia was a mental or moral ailment that required moral treatment. The method of cure was "to rouse the will, and thus rid the body of its thousand morbid things."

Ward[5] advocated the application of an astringent to the vocal folds along with simultaneous electric shock. The pain of both procedures would influence the patient to talk. Goss,[3] Ingalls,[43] and Bach[44] also utilized painful "remedies" such as bitter tonics, iron, quinine, arsenic, and strichnia.

Winslow[45] and Howard[46] described two of the more imaginative remedies. According to Winslow.[45(pp1129-1130)]

> My method of treatment is as follows: the patient is seated before me and a careful history of the case is taken. Then with the laryngeal mirror I make a careful examination of the larynx, noting the movements of the vocal cords and the condition of the mucous membrane from the pharynx down as far as I can see. If I am satisfied that the case is one of functional aphonia, I remove the mirror. The patient is then asked to take 10 or 12 deep breaths. He is next told to raise the arms above the head 10 or 12 times. Now looking the patient directly in the eye, I say to him that there is a little piece of cartilage in his throat which is slightly out of position and as soon as I put my finger down his throat and fix it, he will be able to use his voice (this is to bring about the proper psychological attitude of the patient). Then standing to his right with my left arm under the his neck, the index finger of the left-hand pushing on the cheek, between the upper and lower jaw (done to keep the patient from biting), the index finger of the right-hand is shoved down the throat beyond the epiglottis and held there until the patient makes an attempt to get away. I continue to hold my finger there until it becomes quite uncomfortable. At this stage the patient will, as a rule, make a sound like a grunt and as soon as this happens I take my finger from the throat and begin to count fairly loud from 1 to 5, at the same time urging the patient to count with me. If this does not work I repeat the count, from 1 to 5, much louder than before. It may be necessary to yell while counting before the patient begins to use his voice. When the voice is restored, I keep working for some time so that the patient will become accustomed to it. The attitude of the operator should be firm but gentle, and he must, by his demeanor, inspire the patient with the idea that he will restore the voice.

Howard[46(p 104)] described his case as follows:

> Mrs. M.T., aged 51, whose nervous system had been below par since her husband had committed suicide a year-and-a-half ago, in January, 1922, contracted influenza. Prior to February 1, she enjoyed the full

use of her voice, but that morning she found that she could not talk above a whisper. A diagnosis was made of functional aphonia, also known as hysterical nervous aphonia. The patient was informed that there was no paralysis of the cords; that people affected in this way always recovered, and that the voice usually came back suddenly, just as it had left. The next day, she was told that we would put her to sleep and apply medicine to the parts, and that when she woke up she could talk. She was given ether, and, while she was under the anesthetic, the region was painted with one-percent silver nitrate as a local fillip to the parts. In coming out of the anesthetic, and while only partly conscious, she mumbled something above a whisper. She was encouraged to talk louder and asked to count out loud, and she did so. She has since then been talking normally.

Although these techniques are fun to review, the problem with all these so-called remedies is, of course, that their practitioners were not necessarily honest with the patients. Deceit is not necessary (nor ethical) in modifying the vocal condition of conversion aphonic patients. Patients with this pathology have an unconscious need for the voice disorder and deserve an honest professional management approach. By the time patients with conversion aphonia are referred to a voice pathologist, they are often truly seeking relief from the disorder and are subconsciously ready for change. Often, the event that precipitated the need for the conversion reaction has passed. Some patients may continue to receive secondary gains from the disorder and resist all therapeutic modifications, but the majority of patients will respond quickly to direct voice therapy. It is extremely important to understand that these patients are not malingering. They truly believe that they have lost their voices and are seeking your help with the hope of voice restoration. With this orientation in mind the following treatment strategies may be applied.

■ **Nonspeech Phonatory Tasks:** Following the interview period of the diagnostic evaluation, the voice pathologist will present a physiologic description of the vocal mechanism, using simple line drawings, pictures of the vocal folds, or the patient's own laryngeal videostroboscopic examination tape. These visual displays are used to demonstrate how the adductory muscles are not pulling the vocal folds together, causing the voice to be whispered. The clinician may give this type of explanation:

> For some reason, the muscles that pull the vocal folds together are simply not pulling the way that they should. Therefore,

the vocal folds are not closing all the way. When they don't close all the way, they can't vibrate and so all we can hear is a whisper. Our goal in therapy today is to manipulate the vocal muscle system in whatever way we need to encourage the vocal folds to come together.

With this approach, the voice pathologist has given the patient a nonthreatening, reasonable explanation as to why phonation is not occurring. No comment is yet made regarding the patient's inherent ability to phonate. In fact, the "blame" for lack of phonation has been removed from the patient and placed squarely on the faulty laryngeal mechanism.

Traditional therapy approaches then examine the patient's ability to phonate during nonspeech phonatory behaviors such as coughing, throat clearing, laughing, crying, sighing, and gargling. When phonation is identified on one of these behaviors, it is then shaped into vowel sounds, nonsense syllables, words, and short phrases. The voice pathologist must remain patient, supportive, and persistent throughout. Most patients have not phonated for several weeks. The possibility of proceeding too quickly and frightening the patient away from phonation is present. Once good, consistent phonation is established under practice conditions, the voice pathologist begins to gently insist that it be used during the therapy conversations. When voice is regained in this manner, it is seldom lost again, and patients do not substitute other conversion symptoms.[47]

■ **Manual Circumlaryngeal Therapy (Digital Massage):** Aronson[11] suggested that all patients with voice disorders, regardless of etiology should be assessed for excess laryngeal musculoskeletal tension, either as a primary or a secondary cause of the persisting dysphonia. If tension is an etiologic factor, then reducing it releases the capability of the larynx to produce normal voice. Roy, Bless, Heisey, and Ford[48] demonstrated the efficacy of manual circumlaryngeal therapy with functional dysphonia patients including those with aphonia. A seven-step program of digital massage for decreasing laryngeal tension was suggested by Aronson.[11(p200-201)]

1. Encircle the hyoid bone with the thumb and middle finger, working them posteriorly until the tips of the major horns are felt.

2. Exert light pressure with the fingers in a circular motion over the tips of the hyoid bone and ask if the patient feels pain, not just pressure. It is important to watch facial expression for signs of discomfort or pain.

3. Repeat this procedure with the fingers in the thyrohyoid space, beginning from the thyroid notch and working posteriorly.

4. Find the posterior borders of the thyroid cartilage just medial to the sternocleidomastoid muscles and repeat the procedure.

5. With the fingers over the superior borders of the thyroid cartilage, begin to work the larynx gently downward, also moving it laterally at times. Check for a lower laryngeal position by estimating the increased size of the thyrohyoid space.

6. Ask the patient to prolong vowels during these procedures, noting changes in quality and pitch. Clearer voice quality and lower pitch indicate relief of tension. Because these procedures are fatiguing, rest periods should be provided.

7. Once a voice change has taken place, the patient should be allowed to experiment with the voice, repeating vowels, words, and sentences.

Aronson further stated that the rate of improvement varies depending on the cause of the tension. With the conversion dysphonic patient, changing voice quality should be expected within the first session. Circumlaryngeal therapy may be used with other laryngeal tension disorders.

Falsetto Voice Technique: Another therapy technique used for reestablishing normal voice in the aphonic patient relies on first establishing a normal falsetto voice production. This approach is based on breaking the current inappropriate laryngeal muscle posturing by substituting the falsetto voice muscle posture and then gradually lowering the voice to the normal habitual pitch. The patient again is instructed in the physiology of the laryngeal mechanism and how it relates to the vocal difficulties. The clinician explains that he or she is going to manipulate the vocal mechanism in a manner that will force the muscles to pull the vocal folds together. The voice pathologist then produces a falsetto tone on the sound /aɪ/ and tells the patient in a matter-of-fact manner that everyone can produce this tone, even those who are having vocal difficulties. The clinician again demonstrates the falsetto, and instructs the patient to produce the same sound. Some patients initially resist the falsetto production, but in our experience, with a little coaching, the majority of patients will eventually produce the tone. The falsetto is then stabilized briefly on vowels.

It is explained to the patient that we are going to use the modified laryngeal muscle posture created by the falsetto to encourage the vocal folds to pull together normally. The patient is then given a list of two-syllable phrases and asked to read them in the falsetto voice (Appendix 7-1). During this exercise, the patient is constantly encouraged to read swiftly and loudly. After the voice stabilizes in a relatively strong falsetto, the patient is halted and asked to match the clinician singing down the scale about three to four notes from the original falsetto tone. The patient is then asked to continue reading the phrases at this new pitch level. The same procedure is repeated two or three more times until the patient is approximating a normal pitch level fairly closely. The patient is continually encouraged to produce these phrases louder and faster until eventually the voice "breaks" into normal phonation.

Occasionally the patient will approximate normal phonation but then hesitate as if somewhat reluctant to produce normal voice. When this occurs, the patient is instructed to "drop way down" and produce a guttural voice quality while reading the phrases. The guttural voice is simply another method of changing the inappropriate muscle posturing. After a few minutes, the patient is taken back to the falsetto voice with the break into normal phonation usually occurring soon after.

■ **Visual Biofeedback:** Providing the patient with a reasonable physiologic explanation as to why the voice is whispered is an important part of encouraging a return to normal phonation. Another technique that we have found useful is the use of direct visual feedback using laryngeal videoendoscopy. While the patient is being scoped, either with a rigid or flexible endoscope, an explanation is given related to the positioning of the vocal folds and how that positioning relates to the present vocal problem. The patient is able to monitor the video over the voice pathologist's shoulder. The patient is then instructed in various manipulations of the vocal folds such as deep breathing, light throat clearing, laughing, and attempts to produce tones of various loudness levels and pitches. We have had surprising success in the quick return of normal voicing using these procedures.

It is extremely important that the voice pathologist be patient when applying any of these therapy techniques. The normal time frame from aphonia to normal voice is approximately 30 to 45 minutes (quicker with visual feedback). The voice pathologist must not only be tolerant and persistent but must also present a matter-of-fact, confident manner. Voice pathologists are not cheerleaders. They are simply confidently presenting a technique that they know will work. Why do these techniques work?

■ The patient is ready for change.
■ The voice pathologist has given a reasonable explanation for why the voice is gone.
■ The voice pathologist has demonstrated confidence in the therapeutic techniques.

Following return of voice, it is necessary to explore the actual cause for the conversion reaction. It is desirable to do this in a direct manner. For example, the voice pathologist may say:

I'm very pleased that the muscles are all functioning well now and that your voice has returned to normal. It sounds very good. The thing that still puzzles me somewhat is why the muscles stopped closing the folds in the first place. I can tell you quite frankly that with many other patients that we have seen with the same problem, the cause is often related to an upsetting event or some form of emotional stress. Can you think of anything that has been going on lately that might have contributed to this kind of stress?

By this time the patient has developed strong confidence in the voice pathologist and may provide freely information related to the psychosocial problems that could be related to the development of the voice disorder. In discussing these problems, the voice pathologist attempts to accomplish two major objectives: (a) give the patient total and final control over the laryngeal mechanism; and (b) determine the patient's general emotional state to decide the need for further professional counseling. To this point, the voice pathologist has been manipulating the voice. The patient now must understand that despite the actual cause of the aphonia, he or she is in total control of voice and does not need to permit the problem to recur. If it does, the patient now knows how to regain control of the voice (using whatever manipulations were used). The patient is in control. Finally, just because the need for the conversion reaction may no longer be present, this does not mean that formal family, psychiatric, or psychological counseling would not be useful. If the voice pathologist feels that the psychosocial problem has not resolved and further counseling is in order, the suggestion should be discussed with the patient and appropriate referrals should be made.

Conversion Dysphonia

Aphonia is the most common conversion voice disorder, but many other vocal symptoms with varying degrees of dysphonia may occur as conversion voice disorders. The voice pathologist recognizes these vocal symptoms as a conversion disorder when a medical examination yields normal appearing vocal folds, when the history of the problem yields limited reason for the occurrence of the voice disorder, with the recognition of an atypical voice quality when compared to "normal" dysphonias, and when the patient retains the ability to produce normal phonation while producing nonspeech vocal behaviors such as a throat clear.

Treatment for conversion dysphonia follows the same approach and therapy techniques as those suggested for the aphonic patient. The major thrust of therapy continues to be (a) explanation of what the vocal folds are doing physiologically, (b) direct vocal manipulation, and (c) follow-up counseling as required. It is important to note that some very bizarre sounding dysphonias can occur. Seldom, however, can a conversion voice disorder patient create a vocalization that the voice pathologist cannot also produce. True hoarseness is difficult to imitate. A helpful aid in determining exactly how the patient is producing voice and for confirming the conversion disorder diagnosis is to imitate the vocal behavior.

Functional Falsetto

Functional falsetto is the production of the preadolescent voice in the postadolescent male. Variously termed mutational falsetto, persistent falsetto, and puberphonia, the high-pitched falsetto voice often draws unwanted attention to the postpubescent, physically mature patient. In fact, when not recognized and treated early, the unusual voice quality is often responsible for shaping the psychosocial character of the individual. Young males who present with this disorder have normally developed and normal appearing larynges and vocal fold systems. However, the falsetto voice register is produced instead of the normal modal register. To accomplish this register, the suprahyoid muscles elevate the larynx, and the cricothyroid muscles are active while the thyroarytenoid muscles disengage. To maintain this register, respiration is usually shallow, with minimal subglottic air pressure. In fact, one of the diagnostic signs of functional falsetto is that the patient is not able to build adequate subglottic air pressure to produce a shout.

It has been suggested that functional falsetto may be the result of psychogenic factors such as failure of an adolescent male to accept an adult male role, over-identification with the mother, or social immaturity.[11] We would agree with Colton and Casper[14] who suggested that this disorder may simply result from attempts to stabilize unstable pitch and quality characteristics present in the male pubescent voice. Whatever the reason for the development of this voicing behavior, most patients are ready and willing to modify the voice with direct therapy. It has been our experience that this diagnosis is often missed in the young postadolescent male because of the presence of a mild dysphonia, which often accompanies the falsetto production. The dysphonia may be caused from strain placed on the laryngeal mechanism as the patient attempts to produce a more appropriate sounding voice. Voice pathologists working with males in this age group should be cognizant of this problem.

Several therapy techniques may be used to modify mutational falsetto voices. As with all functional voice disorders, the first step is to guarantee the presence of a normal laryngeal mechanism through a laryngeal examination by an otolaryngologist. The second step is to offer the patient a reasonable explanation for the vocal difficulty. Consider, for example, an explanation similar to the following:

> Often, as we grow, our many muscles grow so fast that for a while we may experience a lack of coordination or even clumsiness. I'm sure that you've known people whose legs have grown so fast in one year

that it looks as if they are going to trip whenever they run. Well, our vocal folds are also made of muscles, and sometimes they grow so fast that we have to learn to use them correctly. That's why when voices begin to change, they crack and the voice breaks and sometimes it sounds funny.

In your case, all the muscles changed and grew physically just the way they were supposed to grow, but they are not yet functioning properly. They need just a little bit of training to get them to work correctly. Our goal for today is to encourage the vocal folds to vibrate differently than they have vibrated before. I want you to do things I ask you to do with your voice and do not be surprised by some of the changes that we're going to hear.

This simple, brief explanation prepares the patient to accept the therapy procedure by providing a reasonable rationale for the problem. The third step is to utilize direct vocal manipulation. The following procedures are recommended:

▪ Ask the patient to produce a hard glottal attack (HGA) on a vowel. Demonstrate how the vowel should be produced with effort closure. When the glottal attack is produced correctly, the pitch will break into the normal lower register as the falsetto positioning of the intrinsic and extrinsic laryngeal muscles for the HGA cannot support initiation of this form of effort closure. If the pitch does not break, grasp the larynx with your thumb and index finger and hold it in a lowered position in the neck as the vowel is produced. If, after several trials, this fails to elicit the desired sound, depress the tongue with a tongue depressor as the patient produces the glottal attack.

▪ When the lower pitch is produced, identify it immediately as the appropriate voice sound. Have the patient repeat it several times using the glottal attack. Then produce several different vowel sounds when attempting to reduce and then extinguish the effort of the glottal attack. Stabilize the normal voice on vowel prolongation.

▪ Immediately move from vowels into words and phrases while maintaining the lower voice register. Attempt to expand the phrases through paragraph readings and into conversational speech during the initial therapy session.

Using this approach, the voice change is expected to be sudden and the progress of therapy rapid. The best way of accomplishing this sudden improvement is for the voice pathologist to be aggressive with the therapy approach. It must be remembered that the voice is new to the patient. His auditory feedback system does not yet identify the new voice as belonging to him. Initially, the voice may want to shift back into the falsetto. Positive encouragement may be necessary.

Follow-up sessions may be needed to stabilize the new voice. We often give the patient Vocal Function Exercises to build the strength and balance of the laryngeal mechanism. In addition, in our effort to aid the patient in developing total control of the voice, we will often use negative practice by having the patient shift back and forth between the two voices. Interestingly, as the "new" voice is increasingly used, patients find it more difficult to produce the falsetto voice.

Most patients are somewhat excited by and proud of the new voice, but some are embarrassed by the sudden voice quality change. These patients may require a gradual desensitization program as a part of the stabilization process. A desensitization program involves establishing with the patient a personal hierarchy of communication experiences ranging from the least difficult to the most difficult speaking situations. A typical hierarchy may include:

1. talking to strangers in a fast-food restaurant or store
2. talking to family members
3. talking to selected friends
4. talking in the classroom.

One of our patients was a 17-year-old who developed normal voicing from falsetto over the Christmas holidays. The patient handled his drastic voice change in a humorous manner. He returned to school using the falsetto voice for half of the day in the classroom. During his afternoon math class, he began coughing and asked to be excused to get a drink of water. When he returned to class he exclaimed excitedly in his normal voice, "Mr. ＿＿＿, they must have put something in the water; listen to my voice!"

We have also had another experience that made the therapeutic intervention rather easy. The patient was easily able to produce the glottal attack. When it was explained to him that this was the desired voice, he replied in a normal modal voice register, "Okay, I can do that all day long if I have to." Indeed, this young man had experimented with the modal voice register. He was not aware, however, that this was supposed to be his voice. As with all of these patients, we make liberal use of taped samples of the falsetto voice and the "new" voice. When this patient realized the excellent quality of the modal voice, he simply began using it on a regular basis. From that experience, we have learned to first ask the patient before initiating any other therapy approaches, "Do you have any other voice?"

Other methods of initiating normal pitch levels include working from throat clearing and coughing and other non-speech phonations. Vegetative sounds such as these are usually spontaneously produced in the modal range and can be used as a point of departure for voice therapy. It should also be noted that a female falsetto voice production may also benefit from therapy. Our experience with these cases has been with older women who complain of a lack of power and strength in the voice. When examined stroboscopically, perceptually, and instrumentally, it becomes evident that they are producing voice in the falsetto register. In most cases, this form of voice production has been a lifelong habit and is more resistant to modification. In some cases, these patients appear to have modified pitch (upward) in response to normal pitch lowering associated with aging changes. The same therapy approaches utilized with the male are used with the female falsetto patient.[1]

The Juvenile Voice

The juvenile female voice is not often seen in voice therapy clinics because the problem is more one of aesthetics than one that is considered a pathological problem. An unusual high pitch characterizes the voice quality of juvenile voice with associated breathiness. In fact, the voice may or may not be produced in the falsetto register. What characterizes the juvenile voice is the "childlike" quality.

Our experience has been with women who complain of laryngeal fatigue and later-day hoarseness. The vast majority of these individuals have recently become involved in activities that require increased voice use. For example, one patient who had been a lifelong homemaker recently volunteered as a museum guide. She found that she could not project her voice well and that her voice fatigued very easily. When these patients seek treatment, they are not aware of the functional ineffectiveness of their vocal habits. It is the role of the voice pathologist to describe the inappropriate voice components and to seek production of an improved voice. As with a symptomatic voice therapy approach, various facilitating techniques may be utilized in this exploration. One technique the we have found useful with the juvenile voice population is as follows:

▓ Test the patient's entire singing pitch range. The juvenile voice patient's phonation for singing is often stronger and produced with improved respiratory support than is the speaking voice.

▓ Ask the patient to produce a strong high note on the vowel /o/.

▓ Gradually lower the note in 2-to-3 note steps. When the point has been reached where the voice is produced in the lower one third of the range, or chest voice, stabilize at this level by sustaining various vowel sounds. Use auditory feedback with the tape recorder or Facilitator or visual feedback using a pitch display device.

▓ Progress from sustained vowels to words, phrases, paragraph readings, and conversational speech.

▓ Introduce Vocal Function Exercises to balance the three subsystems of voice production. (Vocal Function Exercises are covered later in this chapter).

Unlike functional falsetto, modification of the juvenile voice is gradual and takes place over time. The desired voice quality demonstrates more mature vocal characteristics with a lower pitch, less breathiness, and overall improved timbre.

Paradoxical Vocal Fold Movement (PVFM)

As described in Chapter 4, paradoxical vocal fold movement is characterized by wheezing or inspiratory stridor caused by inappropriate closure of the true vocal folds throughout the respiratory cycle. PVFM is often mistaken for asthma and is treated with many pulmonary medications without relief of the symptoms.[49] During acute attacks, patients with PVFM often require emergency medical treatment and in severe cases have undergone tracheostomy. Treatment involves a combination of medical, psychological, and behavioral approaches.

Pharmacologic interventions including bronchodilators have been used in an attempt to relieve symptoms; however, success depends on the etiology of the disorder. Some centers use an inhalation therapy called "heliox," a mixture of helium (80%) and oxygen (20%) to relieve at least the acute symptoms and maintain symptom reduction even after cessation of the treatment.[49] Psychiatric or psychological intervention in the form of psychotherapy using methods of relaxation and supportive therapy has also been effective when emotional or psychological issues and family dynamics have been involved.[50]

Voice symptoms ranging from complete aphonia to mild hoarseness may be present in the PVFM patient, but the primary role of the voice pathologist is to aid in restoring the airway. As with most disorders, educating the patient regarding the disorder is the first step. Videolaryngoscopy is an excellent tool for this purpose. It should be remembered that these patients often have been treated for an asthmatic condition for many years. It may be quite disconcerting to suddenly be told that, in fact, they have a different disorder altogether. Patients are readily able to understand the disorder when observing inappropriate movements of the vocal folds during respiration. Our normal protocol examines the vocal folds during forced inspiration and expiration as well as during quiet breathing. We then encourage an increase in respiratory effort by having the patient walk briskly up and down steps or on a treadmill, which is in our office. This exercise often induces greater adductory movement of the vocal folds. (This is only done in a medical setting, with emergency protocol in place.) Finally, we ask the patient to simulate an attack while monitoring the larynx. This simulation is often very revealing. When videolaryngoscopy is not available, the patient may be educated with picture descriptions of inappropriate and appropriate vocal fold movements during respiration.

Because the patient now understands the disorder, direct treatment approaches may be applied. Martin, Blager, Gay, and Wood[51] described a nonthreatening treatment approach that facilitates laryngeal relaxation by maintaining continuous airflow through the glottis during abdominal breathing. By focusing on self-awareness, the patient is encouraged to become aware of sensations of heightened laryngeal and respiratory tension during an episode in comparison to laryngeal sensations when voluntary control is exercised. Therapy techniques include relaxation exercises to relax the oropharyngeal and upper body musculature, using abdominal breathing without laryngeal constriction or tension, and focusing on prolonged exhalation. Martin et al [51] further recommended inhaling through the nose with the lips closed, a relaxed tongue posture, and prolonged audible exhalation through pursed lips or while producing /s/.

Physiologic Voice Therapy

Whenever a voice disorder is present, we may assume that its presence has caused a change in the functioning of the physiology responsible for voice production. These changes may interrupt airflow causing inappropriate subglottic air pressure (as with a mass lesion of the vocal folds) or they may cause airflow to be unimpeded by the normal glottal resistance (as with a unilateral vocal fold paralysis). Physiologic changes may take the form of a general laryngeal muscle imbalance (as may occur in voice fatigue) or increased laryngeal area muscle tension (as in muscle tension dysphonia). Finally, supraglottic tension or an inappropriate coupling of the resonators may restrict the treatment of the glottal pulse. When any one or more of these voice subsystems is affected by pathology, the remaining subsystems must adjust to accommodate the change of the affected part. The hallmark of physiologic voice therapy is direct physical exercise and manipulations of the laryngeal, respiratory, and the resonance systems in an effort to improve voice quality. When all three systems are addressed in one exercise, then this is considered holistic voice therapy.

Case Study 10: Laryngeal Muscle Imbalance

The patient was a 35-year-old female who was referred for evaluation and treatment with a diagnosis of "voice disturbance."

Voice quality during the diagnostic evaluation was normal. The patient complained, however, of laryngeal fatigue when speaking and more recently when singing; she also described ineffective use of the lower range of her singing voice. Although she could maintain a "reasonably good" singing quality if she "forced" the voice, she was sure that the forcing contributed to the fatigue. In addition, she reported feeling a "shortness of breath" as if she were "running out of air" before the end of a musical phrase. An operatic contralto, she was currently engaged to sing her first solo as a professional. She indicated that this particular aria, which she had practiced many times a day, stretched her vocal range to its lower limit.

The evaluation yielded no significant etiologic factors or voice changes except for the symptoms described by the patient. Stroboscopic evaluation of vocal function revealed grossly normal appearing vocal folds bilaterally as the folds were free of any apparent edema or other visible pathology. The mucosal waves and amplitude of vibration were normal at comfort level. Glottic closure, however, demonstrated an unusual anterior glottal chink, which became larger as the pitch was lowered. The patient was able to sustain an upper range tone for 49 seconds and a lower tone for only 21 seconds. Her measured airflow rates were consistent, with a higher airflow rate measured at low pitch.

We speculated that this voice quality reflected imbalance between predominant cricothyroid muscle function and predominant thyroarytenoid muscle function was greater than normal, especially considering the expected increased stiffness of the folds at higher pitches. It was our impression, therefore, that this laryngeal muscle imbalance, most likely caused by voice strain, contributed to the fatigue in her speaking voice and the ineffectiveness of her lower singing range. The therapy focused on strengthening and balancing the voice subsystems and was successful in remediating her symptoms. Stroboscopic observation of the vocal folds following voice therapy demonstrated the anterior chink to be gone as glottic closure was complete at all pitch levels. We speculated that this patient had spent so much time pushing her voice "to its lower limit" while practicing her aria that she altered the coordination within the laryngeal musculature.

Stemple, Stanley, and Lee[52] studied voice and vocal fold changes following prolonged voice use in a vocally normal group of subjects. Results of their investigation were consistent with the example described above in that a significant number of subjects demonstrated the unusual anterior glottal chink following the voicing task. In addition, subjects experienced much difficulty in matching the lower limits of their pretest voices. These authors speculated that laryngeal muscle strain may have contributed to these results.

This 35-year-old singer demonstrated that at least two parts of her vocal mechanism had been negatively affected by laryngeal muscle imbalance. When the muscular system became strained and imbalanced, the respiratory system was forced to adjust and, through increased air pressure and airflow, could maintain a "reasonable" singing voice for a short period of time. For this the elite vocal performer, "reasonable" was not good enough. Indeed, we would speculate that had she continued to force the voice, that she would have developed a back-focused tone with a combination of all the faulty subsystems leading to more serious pathology.

Case Study 11: The Postsurgical Patient

The patient, a 55-year-old insurance sales representative, was referred for evaluation and treatment following two surgeries for removal of bilateral vocal fold polyps. Voice quality during the evaluation was moderately dysphonic, characterized by low pitch, loudness, and breathiness. He could not readily increase loudness to a shout. The patient was disturbed by the results of surgery, because it was his impression that his voice quality would be "normal" following the surgery. The voice evaluation indicated that the patient originally had a voice disorder caused by several etiologic factors. These included (a) excessive loud talking (b) the use of a low-pitched telephone voice (c) smoking 1½ packages of cigarettes per day and (d) habitual throat clearing. Presurgical voice therapy had modified all factors except those for smoking, which was reduced but not eliminated.

The presurgical vocal mechanism had adjusted the voice subsystems to accommodate the presence of the bilateral polyps. Once the polyps were removed, the subsystems were essentially in disarray and had not automatically rebalanced to provide the expected improved voice quality. Indeed, the patient had maintained the back-focused, strained voice production that had been required to produce voice prior to his surgeries. He continued with a vocal hyperfunction. Direct, physiologic voice therapy was used to accomplish the task of improving the voice.

Case Study 12: The Geriatric Voice

The patient was a 74-year-old male who was referred by the otolaryngologist with the diagnosis of bowed vocal folds. He was looking forward to the voice evaluation because of the restrictions that his voice was placing on his life. Two years prior to the evaluation, the patient was widowed, and he lived alone. He was a social individual who enjoyed going to weekly lunches with his friends, attending a variety of sporting events, and, until recently, singing in the church choir. He presented with a moderate dysphonia, characterized by dry breathy hoarseness. He found it difficult to compete vocally with background noise and noticed that his voice fatigued easily with use. Recently, the patient had begun declining social invitations because it was difficult to carry on conversations with his friends. The problems with his weak voice were exacerbated by the fact that several of his close friends were hard of hearing.

The geriatric population often complains of voice weakness, fatigue, and chronic hoarseness. As described in Chapter 2, several physiologic changes occur in the aging larynx, which may account for voice quality changes. The aging larynx suffers a decrease in muscle fiber, a stiffening of the vocal fold cover, and continued calcification of the laryngeal cartilages. Many geriatric patients present to otolaryngologists and voice pathologists complaining of these various vocal symptoms. Often, they are told that this is part of the aging process and that they would have to "live" with the problem.

Many geriatric people are widowed and live alone, often with little opportunity to talk for extended periods of time. Combine the natural physiologic changes in the larynx with the lack of voice use and these individuals develop voice problems that interfere with their communication ability when they do have the need and desire to speak. In our clinic, geriatric patients have found great success using a systematic vocal exercise program as a means of strengthening voice production by improving the relationships of the three subsystems of voice production: respiration, phonation, and resonance.

As previously stated, a voice pathologist must develop a large armamentarium of voice therapy treatment techniques. With experience, each clinician will choose techniques that feel comfortable, that make sense and can be easily explained to the patient, and that work well for that clinician. Physiologic voice therapy programs integrate all of the voice subsystems into the rehabilitative effort. The following are examples of comprehensive physiologic voice therapy programs that may be applied to many patients with various pathologies of varying etiologic origins. The strength of each of these approaches is their comprehensive holistic nature. Each approach attends to all three subsystems of voice production. They are hygienic treatments, symptomatic treatments, and physiologic treatments that address respiration, phonation, and supraglottic placement of the glottal tone all at once. As seen from the previous case discussions, their applications are many including both hyperfunctional and hypofunctional disorders.

Vocal Function Exercises (VFE)

The Vocal Function Exercise program is based on an assumption that has not been determined empirically. Nonetheless, this assumption and the clinical logic that follows has been supported through many years of clinical experience and observation using this exercise program. For our purposes, it is useful to consider that the laryngeal mechanism is similar to other muscle systems and may become strained and imbalanced through many etiologic factors. Indeed, the analogy that we often draw with patients is a comparison of the rehabilitation of the knee to rehabilitation of the voice. Both the knee and the larynx are comprised of muscle, cartilage, and connective tissue. When the knee is injured, rehabilitation includes a short period of immobilization for the purpose of reducing the effects of the acute injury. The immobilization is followed by assisted ambulation and then the primary rehabilitation begins in the form of systematic exercise. This exercise is designed to strengthen and balance all of the supportive knee muscles for the purpose of returning the knee to as close to its normal functioning as possible.

Rehabilitation of voice may also involve a short period of voice rest following acute injury or after surgery to permit healing of the mucosa to occur. The patient may then begin conservative voice use and follow through with all of the management approaches that seem necessary. Full voice use is then resumed quickly and the therapy program often is successful in returning the patient to normal voice production. We would suggest, however, that on many occasions patients are not fully rehabilitated because one of the important rehabilitation steps was neglected. That step is the systematic exercise program that is often necessary to regain the balance among airflow, to this laryngeal muscle activity, to the supraglottic placement of the tone.

Vocal Function Exercises first described by Barnes[53] and modified by Stemple[27] strive to balance the subsystems of voice production. The exercise program has proven successful in improving and enhancing the vocal function of speakers with normal voices.[54] In addition Sabol, Lee, and Stemple[55] demonstrated the effectiveness of Vocal Function Exercises in the exercise regimen of singers.

The program is simple to teach and, when presented appropriately, seems reasonable to patients. Indeed, many patients are enthusiastic to have a concrete program, similar in concept to physical therapy, during which they may plot the progress of their return to vocal efficiency. The program begins by describing the problem to the patient, using illustrations as needed or the patient's own stroboscopic evaluation video. The patient is then taught a series of four exercises to be done at home, two times each, twice per day, preferably morning and evening. These exercises include:

1. Sustain the /i/ vowel for as long as possible on the musical note (F) above middle (C) for females and boys, (F) below middle (C) for males. (Notes may be modified up or down to fit the needs of the patient. Seldom are they modified by more than 2 notes in either direction.)

   Goal: based on airflow volume. In our clinic the goal is based on reaching 80 to 100 mL/s of airflow. So, if the flow volume is equal to 4000 ml, then the goal is 40 to 45 seconds. When airflow measures are not available, the goal is equal to the longest /s/ that the patient is able to sustain. Placement of the tone should be in an extreme forward focus, almost, but not quite, nasal. All exercises are produced as softly as possible, but not breathy. The voice must be "engaged." This is considered a warm-up exercise.

2. Glide from your lowest note to your highest note on the word "Knoll."

   Goal: No voice breaks. The glide requires the use of all laryngeal muscles. It stretches the vocal folds and encourages a systematic, slow engagement of the cricothyroid muscles. The word "Knoll" encourages a forward placement of the tone as well as an expanded open pharynx. The patient's lips are to be rounded and a sympathetic vibration should be felt on the lips. (May also use a lip trill, tongue trill, or the word "whoop.") Voice breaks will typically occur in the transitions between low and high registers. When breaks occur, the patient is encouraged to continue the glide without hesitation. When the voice breaks at the top of the current range and the patient typically has more range, the glide may be continued without voice as the folds will continue to stretch. Glides improve muscular control and flexibility. This is considered a stretching exercise.

3. Glide from your highest note to your lowest note on the word "Knoll."

   Goal: No voice breaks. The patient is instructed to feel a half-yawn in the throat throughout this exercise. By keeping the pharynx open and focusing the sympathetic vibration at the lips, the downward glide encourages a slow, systematic engagement of the thyroarytenoid muscles without the presence of a back-focused growl. In fact, no growl is permitted. (May also use a lip trill, tongue trill, or the word "boom.") This is considered a contracting exercise.

4. Sustain the musical notes (C-D-E-F-G) for as long as possible on the word "Knoll" minus the "Kn." (Middle C for females and boys, octave below middle C for males.

Goal: Remains the same as for exercise No.1. The "oll" is once again produced with an open pharynx and constricted, sympathetically vibrating lips. The shape of the pharynx to the lips is likened to an inverted megaphone. The fourth exercise may be tailored to the patient's present vocal ability. Although the basic range of middle C, an octave lower for males, is appropriate for most voices, the exercises may be customized up or down to fit the current vocal condition or a particular voice type. Seldom, however, are the exercises shifted more than two notes in either direction. This is considered a low-impact adductory power exercise.

Quality of the tone is also monitored for voice breaks, wavering, and breathiness. Quality improves as times increase and pathologies begin to resolve.

All exercises are done as softly as possible. It is much more difficult to produce soft tones; therefore, the vocal subsystems will receive a better workout than if louder tones were produced. Extreme care is taken to teach the production of a forward tone that lacks tension. In addition, attention is paid to the glottal onset of the tone. The patient is asked to breathe in deeply with attention paid to training abdominal breathing, posture the vowel momentarily, and then initiating the exercise gesture without a forceful glottal attack or an aspirate breathy attack. It is explained to the patient that maximum phonation times increase as the efficiency of the vocal fold vibration improves. Times do not increase with improved "lung capacity." Indeed, even aerobic exercise does not improve lung capacity, but rather the efficiency of oxygen exchange with the circulatory system, thus, giving the sense of more air.

The musical notes are matched to the notes produced by an inexpensive pitch pipe that the patient purchases for use at home or a tape recording of live voice doing the exercises may be given to the patient for home use. Many patients find the tape-recorded voice easier to match than the pitch pipe. We have found that patients who complain of "tone deafness" can often be taught to approximate the correct notes well with practice and guidance from the voice pathologist.

Finally, patients are given a graph on which to mark their sustained times which is a means of plotting progress. Progress is monitored over time and, because of normal daily variability, patients are encouraged not to compare today to tomorrow and so on. Rather, weekly comparisons are encouraged. Estimated time of completion for the program is 6 to 8 weeks. Some patients experience minor laryngeal aching for the first day or two of the program similar to muscle aching that might occur with any new muscular exercise. As this discomfort will soon subside, they are encouraged to continue the program through the discomfort should it occur.

When the patient has reached the predetermined therapy goal, and the voice quality and other vocal symptoms have improved, then a tapering maintenance program is recommended. Although some of the professional voice users choose to remain in peak vocal condition, many of our patients desire to taper the VFE program. The following systematic taper is recommended:

- Full program 2 times each, 2 times per day
- Full program 2 times each, 1 time per day (morning)
- Full program 1 time each, 1 time per day (morning)
- Exercise #4, 2 times each, 1 time per day (morning)
- Exercise #4, 1 time each, 1 time per day (morning)
- Exercise #4, 1 time each, 3 times per week (morning)
- Exercise #4, 1 time each, 1 time per week (morning)

Each taper should last 1 week. Patients should maintain 85% of their peak time, otherwise they should move up one step in the taper until the 85% criterion is met.

In short, Vocal Function Exercises provide a holistic voice treatment program that attends to the three major subsystems of voice production. The program appears to benefit patients with a wide range of voice disorders because it is reasonable in regard to time and effort. It is similar to other recognizable exercise programs: the concept of "physical therapy" for the vocal folds is understandable; progress may be easily plotted, which is inherently motivating; and it appears to balance airflow, laryngeal activity, and supraglottic placement.

Resonant Voice Therapy (RVT)

Resonant Voice Therapy is another holistic voice therapy program. The program was developed by Katherine Verdolini[56] and is based on the work of Arthur Lessac.[57] Resonant voice is defined as voice production involving oral vibratory sensations, usually on the anterior alveolar ridge or higher in the face in the context of easy phonation. Resonant voice is a continuum of oral sensations and easy phonation building from basic speech gestures through conversational speech. The therapy goal is to achieve the strongest, "cleanest" possible voice with the least effort and impact between the vocal folds to minimize the likelihood of injury and maximize the likelihood of vocal health.

As with Vocal Function Exercises, the training methodologies are experiential, focusing on the processing of sensory information. The patient is constantly asked to monitor the "feel" and to concentrate on the auditory feedback. The training model assumes similar approaches for voice restoration for voice disorders and enhancing the normal voice (excellence training). The following fundamental characteristics guide RVT:

- The fundamental perceptual target is focused oral vibratory sensations in the context of easy phonation.
- The training methodology is experiential, involving an emphasis on the processing of sensory information (what the patient feels and hears).
- The singular training focus (resonance) is expected to affect multiple levels of physiology (breathing and laryngeal).
- Large numbers of repetitions are used, in varying speech/ singing and environmental contexts relevant to the learner.
- Both neuromuscular ("hardware") and cognitive ("software") shifts in voice production are expected.

■ Training is strongly goal (results) driven, involving a dogged insistence upon the greatest possible precision in the achievement of the perceptual tasks.

Each RVT session begins with a series of stretching and breathing maneuvers. These maneuvers may include the following:

■ **Stretches** (3-10 seconds per stretch)
  1. Shoulders
   • Touch elbows in back
   • Stretch arms in front
  2. Neck
   • Drop head down slowly in fractions
   • Rotate head up until right on top of the neck, feel neck muscles
   • "Turn off" when the crown and ball of head are balanced
   • Lift head away from the neck
   • Cross fiber stretch toward shoulders with fingers
   • Tilt ear to shoulder and stretch out opposite arm
  3. Jaws
   • Massage the masseters, pull down and forward
   • Push thumbs into masseters with slightly open mouth
  4. Floor of Mouth
   • Press thumb into floor of mouth
   • First make no sound, then produce a vowel with no tongue stiffness
  5. Lips
   • Lip trill
   • No voice
   • Continuous voice
   • Alternating off/on
  6. Tongue
   • Tongue trill
   • No voice
   • Continuous voice
   • Alternating off/on
   • Protrude tongue out and down, hands behind back
   • Voiceless breathing
   • Voiced
  7. Pharynx
   • Yawn

- Yawn-sigh with voice
- Stretch the pharynx with these maneuvers

8. Breathing
- Breathe out all air on /f/; do not breathe in until necessary;
- When necessary, simply release the abdomen, it will breathe for you
- Breathe-release-breathe-release-breathe-release with and without voice

Following the stretching and breathing maneuvers the patient is taught a basic training gesture. The training gesture is essentially a special type of humming that gradually builds into functional phrases and ultimately conversational voice. The following is a 7-step RVT program based on the work of Verdolini and developed within our own clinical voice practice.

■ **Basic Training Gesture**: The patient is asked to either stand or sit with good posture; to take a comfortable breath and to vocally sigh from a high to low pitch repeating the /m/. The pharynx is to be wide open and the energy of the /m/ is to be focused in the facial bones. Attempt to develop a connection between the abdominal respiratory support muscles and the face and lips.
- h-m-m-m-m . . . As a sigh
- Extreme forward focus is required with appropriate breath support
- Make the connection from the abdominal muscles to the lips
- Patient should feel very relaxed at the end of this gesture

■ **RVT Hierarchy Step 1 (All Voiced):** Begin to add nonlinguistic speech contexts on repetitions of /mamamama/. You will note that all exercises in this step use voiced sounds that do not require laryngeal articulation. Other vowels may be added as desired to vary the training contexts.
1. mamamama. . . (sustained pitch) on _____. (Choose comfortable conversational tone.)
   - Vary the rate only
   - Discover the vibrations; experiment with broad and narrow vibrations
   - Eventually focus on the narrow vibration; "like a narrow beam of light"
   - Increase the ease of production by reducing the effort by $\frac{1}{2}$ and $\frac{1}{2}$ again

- Increase "lift" (as if pitch were increasing)
2. mamamama . . .
   - Slow-fast-slow
   - Soft-loud-soft on _____ (comfortable conversational tone)
   - Vary the intensity and the rate of the sustained mama-mama . . .
3. mamamama . . . as speech (Make up nonlinguistic phrases using only the mamamama)
   - Use nonlinguistic phrases; vary the rate, pitch, and loudness; make the connection from the abdominal muscles to the lips
4. Chant the following voiced phrases on the musical note _____ ; totally exaggerate articulation and forward resonance (comfortable conversational tone)
   - Mary made me mad
   - My mother made marmalade
   - My merry mom made marmalade
   - My mom may marry Marv
   - My merry mom may marry Marv
   - Marv made my mother merry
5. Over-inflect these same phrases as speech. Be diligent about making the connection from the abdominal breath support to the front of the face.

◼ **RVT Hierarchy Step 2 (Voiced-Voiceless):** You will note that the exercise difficulty has been increased with the addition of the voiceless consonant. This requires rapid laryngeal articulation, which more closely approximates the requirements of conversational voice production.

1. mamapapa . . . vary the rate on _____ (comfortable conversational tone)
2. mamapapa . . . slow-fast-slow
   soft-loud-soft on _____ (comfortable conversational tone)
3. mamapapa . . . as speech
   - use nonlinguistic phrases; vary the rate, pitch, and loudness; make the connection from the abdominal muscles to the lips
4. Chant the following voiced/voiceless phrases on the musical note _____; (comfortable conversational tone) Totally exaggerate articulation and forward resonance
   - Mom may put Paul on the moon
   - Mom told Tom to copy my manner

- My manner made Pete and Paul mad
- Mom may move Polly's movie to ten
- My movie made Tim and Tom sad

5. Over-inflect these same phrases as speech

■ **RVT Hierarchy Step 3 (Any Phrase):** The task is now made more difficult by introducing other phrases. The chanted phrase should be said in an extreme forward focus with exaggerated articulation. The over-inflected phrase, and the more natural production must both maintain the same forward connection and ease of phonation.

1. Chant five to seven syllable phrases on the note _____. (Comfortable conversational tone; use phrases in Appendix 1)
2. Overinflect the same phrases with an extreme forward focus
3. Repeat the same phrases in a more natural forward speech/voice production

■ **RVT Hierarchy Step 4 (Paragraph Reading):** This step begins combining strings of phrases which expands the difficulty of the task once more. Maintain the exaggerated focus only as long as is necessary to confirm that the task has been mastered.

1. Read a paragraph with phrase markers; separate each phrase only by the natural inhalation of air
2. Exaggerate focus and then repeat with a more normal speech/voice production
3. Repeat the above with paragraphs without phrase markers (Appendix 7-1, Paragraphs)

■ **RVT Hierarchy Step 5 (Controlled Conversation):** It is now time to begin carryover to conversation of the new "forward-focus" voicing behavior. Any topic of interest is fair game for discussion from job and family to vacations and hobbies. The patient may want to establish practice times at home, such as at the dinner table, because it is difficult to concentrate on how one is talking while talking. If the foundation has been successfully established in the previous steps, however, then this challenge will be lessened.

- Practice forward speech placement in conversation
- Do not permit glottal attacks, glottal fry, etc

■ **RVT Hierarchy Step 6 (Environmental Manipulations):** Quiet conversation, as in Step 5, is an easier task than actually placing the patient in everyday situations where there is background noise and other commotion. This step encourages the patient to continue to use the new vocal habits despite ambient distractions.

- Simulate actual speaking environments consistent with patient's needs (actual/simulated)
- Use tapes of background noise
- Go to noisy setting such as a cafeteria
- Practice in a lecture environment

■ **RVT Hierarchy Step 7 (Emotional Manipulations):** Challenge the use of resonant voice by animating the discussion with topics that elicit laughter, loud talking, anger, indignation, and other emotions. Use materials and topics that increasingly engage and challenge the patient based on personality, interests, work experience, passions.

■ **RVT Hierarchy Home Exercises:** Home exercise is an essential part of RVT. In this day and age of managed care, therapy is often limited to a few actual sessions. In therapy, the patient is given the skills and tasks that must be mastered during home practice. It is evident when a patient has neglected to follow the practice recommendations.

- The critical portion of each exercise for each week is tape recorded as a home exercise example. The home program involves 15 to 20 minute sessions, two times per day with "minis" as needed
- Stretches
- Basic RV gesture
- Selected level of hierarchy

Several studies now indicate that easy, resonant voice tends to be produced with vocal folds that are barely touching or barely separated.[58,59] This posture appears to produce the strongest, clearest voice output for the least amount of vocal fold impact stress. This posture also requires the least amount of lung pressure to vibrate the vocal folds. Therefore, resonant voice is a relatively strong, clear voice, which appears to provide some protection from injury and is physically easy to produce.[56] Preliminary evidence indicates that the Resonant Voice Therapy program provides for efficient vibration of the vocal folds and a balance among the three subsystems of voice production. We have found the Resonant Voice Therapy program extremely useful as a means of training a forward focus voice production.

Resonant Voice Therapy and Vocal Function Exercises are extremely complementary in a therapy program used for a wide variety of voice disorders including both hyperfunctional and hypofunctional disorders.

Accent Method

Another holistic treatment approach is the Accent Method developed by Dr. Svend Smith of Denmark and described in detail by Kotby.[60] This voice therapy approach is designed to:

- increase pulmonary output
- reduce glottic waste
- reduce excessive muscular tension
- normalize the vibratory pattern during phonation.

The technique is based on the principles of the myoelastic-aerodynamic theory of phonation. The originators state that because voice production is created by subglottal air pressure and transglottal airflow, stronger air pressures below the vocal folds result in an increased amplitude of vibration and a more stable closed phase of the vibratory cycle. The stronger closed phase improves the filtering process of the vocal tract as a result of a longer duration of the vocal fold contact within one period and a higher airflow through the glottis in the opening phase of the vibratory cycle. Together they counteract the damping effect of the resonances in the vocal tract. The expected acoustic effects of treatment are:

- increased energy of the fundamental frequency
- increased energy in the second and third formant frequencies
- reduced irregular pitch perturbations
- optimal fundamental frequency
- increased frequency range
- increased dynamic range.[60]

A summary of the Accent Method procedures follows:

- **Facilitates abdominal breathing:** Ideally, the patient is placed in a recumbent position and normal abdominal breathing is elicited. The patient is instructed to place one hand on the stomach to monitor the abdominal movements while the clinician demonstrates abdominal breathing and upper body relaxation. A brief description of the lowering action of the diaphragm is given to demonstrate the appropriate increase in chest cavity size as air is inspired. The patient is asked to gain a consciousness over the abdominal movements for both inhalation and exhalation. Abdominal muscle control is important for achieving changes in pitch and loudness.

The patient is then instructed to watch the clinician as fricativelike sounds are demonstrated. The sounds are first sustained individually and then with a two-beat rhythm. The two-beat rhythm is accented, with the first sound being weak and the second sound produced with more force. A sample of this sequenced breathing exercise would be:

Inhale /s/----------Inhale /sh/----------Inhale /f/----------

The two-beat accented rhythm would be:

s-S----------

sh-SH----------

f-F----------

(The second sound is accented and sustained)

Throughout the accented practice, changes in body position (sitting, standing, walking, swinging the arms) are used to encourage regulation and adaptation of the breathing patterns.

■ **Utilize rhythmic vocal play:** When the correct breathing pattern has been established, phonation is begun. Voice is initially introduced with a soft, breathy onset of the tone. Again, the clinician demonstrates the rhythm and the patient imitates the accented pattern. Each stressed sound (the second accented sound) is accompanied by a smooth abdominal contraction. Eventually, the exercises are carried out at three different speeds: largo, andante, and allegro (slow, moderate, and fast) tempos (Figure 7-3). In implementing the Accent Method, the clinician can utilize arm

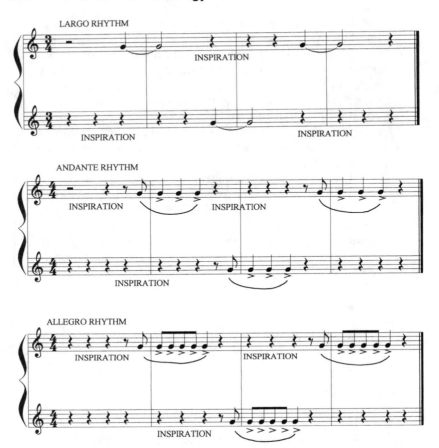

Figure 7-3. Largo, andante, and allegro rhythms.

movements, tapping, or even beating on a drum to help establish the rhythm. Many vowel and consonant combinations may be used.

The largo tempo consists of one or two main stresses in a three-beat rhythm in which breathy phonation and consonant resistances are used at the lips and the tongue. A sample largo sequence includes:

zh-ZH

zz-ZZ-ZZ

yoi-YOI

yoi-YOI-YOI

In the andante tempo, phrases are increased in size to three main beats in a four-beat rhythm and the breathiness of the voice is eliminated. This step introduces variability in pitch, intensity, timbre, vowel shape, and time. A sample andante sequence includes:

woo-WOO-WOO-WOO

yea-YEA-YEA-YEA

yee-YEE-YEE-YEE

In the allegro tempo, the voice exercises consist of an unstressed vowel followed by five stressed vowels. This speed is doubled as the main beats are divided into two faster beats. Phrase length, intensity, and a rich variety of sounds are incorporated into the practice as well as the other tempo patterns. This step encourages more variety to the voice and approaches the natural prosody used in conversation. A sample sequence of the allegro tempo would be:

yea-YEA-YEA-YEA-YEA-YEA

da-YA-YA-YA-YA-YA

ba-BA-BA-BA-BA-BA

no-NO-NO-NO-NO-NO

- **Transfer rhythms to articulated speech:** The final stage of the Accent therapy involves transferring the rhythms to real speech. The transfer process includes (1) repetitions following the clinician's model, (2) reading aloud using passages marked for phrasing and stresses, (3) monologue, and (4) conversation.

The Accent Method can be used for many different types of voice disorders. It is a therapy method that is widely used outside of the United States. There are many reasons why the method is effective in treating voice disorders. First, it is a programmed approach that follows a logical order of progression.

Second, it trains new motor patterns of voice production assisted by the emphasis on steady, rhythmic body movements. Third, the Accent Method, like Vocal Function Exercises and Resonant Voice Therapy, at once works to improve the balance among the three subsystems of voice production: respiration, phonation, and resonance.

Lee Silverman Voice Treatment (LSVT)

The Lee Silverman Voice Therapy program has been the most studied of all types of voice therapy programs. Developed by Lorraine Ramig PhD, and her colleagues at the University of Colorado, the LSVT has been proven to significantly improve the voice quality of patients with Parkinson disease.[61,62] LSVT is a very specific, intensive treatment program that emphasizes "loud" speech. The loud voice generates improved respiratory support, articulation, and even facial expression and animation.

Five basic concepts are followed in the LSVT program. These concepts include (1) think loud; think shout; (2) speech effort must be high; (3) treatment must be intensive; (4) patients must recalibrate their loudness level; (5) improvements are quantified over time.

Using visual feedback from a sound level meter, patients are taught the effort that is necessary to increase their loudness level. They are told to "think loud, think shout." Because most Parkinson patients use poor breath support and talk softly, they must learn that the effort to produce adequate loudness must be high. The most efficacious way of accomplishing this task is through intensive treatment. During the treatment, patients are taught to recalibrate their loudness level because the loudness that they think is normal is actually too soft. Finally, LSVT requires excellent record keeping so that the efficacy of the treatment may be demonstrated.

Efficacy studies have demonstrated that the program is most effective if therapy sessions are held daily, 4 days per week, for 4 consecutive weeks. Patients are also asked to practice therapy exercises daily at home. It is suggested that voice pathologists who claim to use LSVT receive special training in this method. An LSVT training manual is available from the National Center for Voice and Speech, and a certification course is required to use this therapy program with Parkinson patients.[63-65]

Team Management of Specific Laryngeal Pathologies

Voice problems arise under many conditions and, as described in Chapter 3, numerous etiological factors may play a role. In general, however, three overriding categories prevail: voice use patterns and voice demands, medical or organic factors, and psychosocial or emotional contributors.[66-68] Of course, there is considerable overlap between these three groupings. Inappropriate voice behaviors or excessive vocal demands may result in organic manifestations (eg, polyps or nodules); psychological trauma or excessive emotional stress may trigger the onset of focal dystonia. In this chapter, we have discussed the treatments that are specific to voice disorders associated with voice use patterns and voice demands and psychosocial and emotional contributors. In the remainder of this chapter, we will discuss treatment alternatives for medical or organic voice disorders that often require a team approach.

With medically related voice disorders, the voice pathologist plays a supportive role by assisting in the correct diagnosis and prognosis for change based on the assessment of laryngeal anatomy, vocal fold vibratory pattern, vocal function measurement, and rehabilitative options for voice treatment. Collaboration between otolaryngologists and voice pathologists continues to expand through joint examination of the laryngeal image and vocal function; efficacious cotreatment alternatives that include medications, phonosurgery, and voice rehabilitation; and clinical delivery models that encourage a team approach to voice disordered patients. More than ever, it is critical that the voice pathologist be aware of the medical pathologies in an otolaryngology patient population that affect voice production. Several of the medical pathologies of voice that require team treatment include vocal fold cover lesions, gastroesophageal reflux disease (GERD), vocal fold paralysis, and spasmodic dysphonia.

Vocal Fold Cover Lesions

Many benign vocal fold pathologies are the result of acute or chronic traumatic hyperfunctional voice use and respond readily to voice rehabilitation as previously described in this chapter. When standard voice therapy fails to improve voice quality, however, the otolaryngologist or voice pathologist may recommend surgery. The term phonosurgery refers to laryngeal surgeries that seek to improve voice quality as their primary goal. This definition is distinct from traditional concepts of laryngeal surgery, which seek to remove disease, with voice outcome as a secondary consideration. Recent advances in surgical instruments, bio implant materials, and development of alternative surgical techniques have created a new awareness of phonosurgical options that are available to enhance voice quality in patients with laryngeal pathology.[69] In cases of nonmalignant mucosal lesions of the vocal folds, phonosurgery will be used to excise the lesion with a simultaneous goal of preserving the vocal fold mucosa and restoring the vocal fold edge.

In our voice clinic, the voice pathologist plays a major role in treating patients who must undergo phonosurgery. First, a laryngeal videostroboscopic examination will be conducted to evaluate vocal function and determine the extent of disruption in the vibratory pattern caused by the lesion. The surgeon will study the stroboscopic image, which will help plan the surgical approach. Prior to surgery, the patient will undergo preoperative counseling with the voice pathologist. This counseling will involve vocal hygiene issues including hydration, elimination of abusive vocal behaviors, and sometimes initiation of conservative voice use. In cases where surgery cannot be performed for several weeks, the patient will start direct voice therapy including Vocal Function Exercises. The patient is also given strict instructions for immediate postsurgical voice use. Our surgeons choose to place patients on absolute voice rest for one week following surgery. In addition, they are encouraged to increase hydration and are placed on precautionary reflux precautions, including medications. (Reflux precautions will be described below.)

Seven to 10 days after surgery, the patient returns for a postsurgical laryngeal videostroboscopic examination. When sufficient healing is evident, postsurgical voice rehabilitation is begun. We believe that the postsurgical treatment has been significantly enhanced by the preoperative counseling and strict postoperative regimen.

Gastroesophageal Reflux Disease (GERD)

As described in Chapter 4, GERD is the reflux of gastric acid including bile, pepsin, and trypins from the stomach back into the esophagus and possibly into the pharynx. It is thought that reflux occurs normally in all individuals at some time. Reflux may cause irritation of the mucosal lining of the esophagus, pharynx, and larynx as it is released from the stomach. Gastroesophageal reflux becomes gastroesophageal reflux disease once histological changes take place within the esophagus. Symptoms of GERD may include dysphagia, odynophagia (or painful swallow), chest pain, a globus or lump in the throat sensation, onset of asthma during middle age, bloating, belching, and hiccups.[70] Long-term chronic gastroesophageal reflux may have detrimental effects on the esophagus. These include damage to the epithelial layer of the mucosal lining; the basal layer of the mucosal lining becomes thickened with extension of the papillae and loss of service cells in early inflammatory stages; stasis of the lumen, which is created with advanced inflammation; muscular atrophy; and severe gastroesophageal reflux has been implicated in gastrointestinal bleeding, Barrett's esophagus, and cancer. Individuals with GERD tend to be obese and are nocturnal refluxers. They tend to have lower esophageal dysfunction and complain of chronic heartburn.

Patients most often seen in a voice clinic by the otolaryngologist and voice pathologist experience laryngeal-pharyngeal reflux (LPR). Most of these individuals are upright refluxers and experience upper esophageal dysfunction. Most suffer from hoarseness; globus sensation; a sense of increased mucus; and chronic throat clearing, coughing, or both. Only 18% of these patients complain of heartburn.[71] Consistent reflux into the larynx can negatively influence voice production. Beyond the obvious hoarseness, patients often complain of voice fatigue. Koufman[71] suggested that

LPR might be responsible for edema, ulceration, granulation, polypoid degeneration, vocal nodules, laryngospasm, arytenoid fixation, laryngeal stenosis, and carcinoma of the larynx.

Treatment of GERD and LPR incorporates three treatment levels. Level 1 involves conservative measures including dietary and lifestyle changes along with over-the-counter medications, such as antacids and H2 blockers. Dietary precautions include decreasing the intake of fatty foods, spicy foods, tomato-based products, citrus fruits and fruit drinks, caffeine, carbonated beverages, alcohol, peppermint and spearmint, menthol, and onions. Lifestyle changes include decrease or elimination of smoking, losing excess weight, wearing loose clothing that does not bind the midriff, elevating the head of the bed at night, not exercising or singing too soon after eating, and waiting 3 to 4 hours before lying down after eating.

Level 2 involves all of the dietary and lifestyle precautions mentioned in Level 1. In addition, prescription H2 blockers such as cimetidin, rantidin, and famotidine are used to control mild to moderate GERD and LPR. H2 blockers control the acid, but the pepsin remains active. When H2 blockers prove not to be effective then a hydrogen pump inhibitor, omerprazole, is the medication of choice. Most laryngeal manifestations of LPR can be controlled through medication and conservative measures.

Level 3 treatment is for severe reflux. Severe reflux requires the use of omeprazole, dietary and lifestyle changes, and often surgery. The most common type of surgery is a fundoplication, which essentially tightens the sphincter between the stomach and the esophagus, decreasing the regurgitation of the stomach contents into the esophagus.

LPR is a common disease in the voice clinic. The voice pathologist is responsible for supporting the antireflux regimen, as well as providing the most appropriate direction for voice therapy. In the acute stages of voice change, therapy may involve decreasing or eliminating throat clearing and coughing, encouraging conservative voice use, and initiating new functional voicing behaviors. We have found it useful to encourage the placement of voice into an extreme forward focus, thereby decreasing the medial impact on the arytenoid cartilages and vocal folds. Resonant Voice Therapy is often our treatment of choice with LPR patients.

Unilateral Vocal Fold Paralysis

Patients with unilateral vocal fold paralysis present with varied vocal symptoms, ranging from mild to severe dysphonias depending on the resting position of the paralyzed fold. When the paralyzed fold is located near the midline, voice quality is less impaired. The impairment increases when the paralyzed fold is located further from the midline. Typically, voice is characterized by breathiness, low intensity, and diplophonia. Often, the patient will produce voice in a falsetto register because it becomes too much effort to maintain engagement of the thyroarytenoid muscle. Recall from Chapter 4 that this loss of vocal power and quality is due to inadequate closure of the vocal folds at midline, because the paralyzed vocal fold remains lateral to the midline and cannot meet its contralateral pair. Also, the loss of vocal fold body and tonicity result in bowing, flaccidity and weakness of the paralyzed fold. Both factors contribute to the asymmetric, aperiodic, and incomplete vibratory closure during phonation seen in patients with unilateral vocal fold paralysis.

Treatment choices for unilateral vocal fold paralysis include voice therapy, phonosurgical management, or a combination of the two. The selection of treatment is dependent on several factors. These factors include whether the cause for the paralysis is known or unknown, presence or absence of aspiration, the immediate voice needs of the patient, distance from the time of onset of the paralysis, and the resting position of the paralyzed fold to the midline and the presence or absence of vocal fold bowing.

When the cause for the vocal fold paralysis is known and it is determined that damage is permanent and there is no chance for return of function, then any form of management may begin immediately. When the cause for the paralysis is idiopathic or there is some question as to the return of function, most surgeons will routinely observe patients for 6 to 12 months before permanent surgical intervention.[72] When aspiration is a problem, some surgeons choose to inject Gelfoam into the paralyzed vocal fold as a means of temporarily improving glottic closure. Gelfoam is reabsorbed in a 2- to 3-month period of time, giving the paralyzed fold more time to recover.

Recently, clinical laryngeal electromyography (LEMG) has become a valuable diagnostic and prognostic test for patients with vocal fold paralysis. LEMG is effective in localizing the neural site of lesions, which aids in determining the cause and the prognosis of the paralysis. With LEMG, the nature and stage of the neuropathy, as well as the prognosis for recovery, may be determined. The presence of spontaneous neural activity, for example, indicates ongoing degeneration, and the finding of severely decreased recruitment indicates a poor prognosis for complete recovery.[73] The use of this diagnostic test might preclude much of the waiting that is inherent in the treatment of unilateral vocal fold paralysis.

The phonosurgical management alternatives for unilateral paralysis address both the midline glottic incompetence and the loss of vocal fold body. The traditional surgical treatment has been injection of a synthetic alloplastic, Teflon paste, into the lateral margin of the paralyzed fold. The paste forms a solid mass, which displaces the paralyzed edge medially to improve midline competence. This technique has been used routinely for more than 50 years with good success. Occasional complications have been reported, because of migration of the Teflon material into other sites of the body. Granulation of tissue around the Teflon has also been reported. When injected too superiorly or medially, the Teflon may impair the vibratory properties of the free edge of the paralyzed fold.[74] In most surgical voice centers, Teflon injection is no longer the treatment of choice.

New bioimplants have been explored as injectable alternatives to Teflon. A cross-linked bovine collagen has been developed for vocal fold injections.[75-77] The bioimplant is injected superficially into the lamina propria of the vocal fold where it incorporates into the cellular structure of the fold and reportedly enhances the vibratory properties in both paralyzed and scarred vocal folds. Unfortunately, this bovine collagen bioimplant is no longer readily available, although new human autologous collagen is being developed for vocal fold injection.

A third injectable alternative for the management of paralyzed vocal folds is autogenous fat. This technique has received variable reviews because of its rapid rate of resorption, which limits its long-term success. The success of this technique may be improved by an initial overinjection of fat to compensate for expected partial resorption.[78] The autogenous fat technique has the obvious advantage of being a natural, soft, flexible material, which vibrates well and does not pose any risk for antibody or foreign body response.

Another surgical approach to medialization of the paralyzed vocal fold is laryngeal framework surgery. Laryngeal framework surgery is manipulation of the cartilagenous framework that houses the vocal folds. The procedure offers certain advantages over injection methods for the treatment of unilateral paralysis. First, it is completely noninvasive of the vocal fold body and mucosa; second, it is potentially reversible, barring excessive scarring of the surgical site. The Type 1 Thyroplasty utilizes a surgical implant (silastic block) that is inserted and locked into a small window of the lamina of the thyroid cartilage. The silastic implant will actively "push" the paralyzed fold toward the glottal midline to improve glottic closure. The exact size and placement of the implant is critical; if positioned too high or low, a vertical level mismatch will result, and voice quality will be suboptimal. In our practice, the voice pathologist is involved in monitoring the position of the vocal folds and the quality of the voice during surgery. The patient is under a local anesthesia during the surgery. The voice pathologist places a flexible laryngeal videoendoscope and monitors the relative position of the vocal folds as the paralyzed fold is medialized. The patient's voice quality is also monitored perceptually. The combination of visual and auditory perceptual monitoring often leads to excellent postsurgical voice quality.

Isshiki and his colleagues introduced the concept of laryngeal framework surgery in 1974.[79] He and other otolaryngologists have continued to develop new types of framework surgery that manipulate the cartilage to alter the vocal fold configuration and restore voice in patients with unilateral paralysis, vocal fold bowing, and pitch disorders.[80-83] Laryngeal framework surgery is being explored now for use in managing pediatric laryngeal disorders.[84]

Along with a fold medialization, surgeons often enhance the adduction of the paralyzed vocal fold through a procedure known as arytenoid adduction. In this procedure, the vocal process of the arytenoid is manually adducted toward the midline of the glottis. Once positioned appropriately, it is sutured in place, thus improving the posterior closure of the vocal folds.

Injection techniques and laryngeal framework surgery address the deficit of midline closure in their approaches to management of unilateral vocal fold paralysis. To address the loss of vocal fold body and tonicity posed by atrophy and weakness of the denervated vocal fold, reinnervation techniques have been developed. These techniques include nerve muscle pedicle[83] and nerve anastomosis (synkinesis).[85] The principles behind neuromuscular reinnervation techniques include transplanting muscle blocks that can provide innervation to the paralyzed muscle, and the contraction characteristics of the donor muscle or nerve will be imparted to the paralyzed muscle. Thus, selection of an appropriate donor nerve or muscle (ie, one that is compatible with the contraction properties of the original) is important. Neuromuscular pedicle reinnervation is limited to a single muscle, usually the lateral cricoarytenoid (LCA) or thyroarytenoid (TA), which are the main vocal fold adductors.

An alternative to the nerve-to-muscle reinnervation is nerve-to-nerve reinnervation. Recurrent laryngeal nerve (RLN) to RLN reinnervation is not consistently successful and does not always provide functional return of adductor and abductor activity. Furthermore, RLN-to-RLN anastomosis may result in dysphonia because of jerky movements and excessive synkinesis of adductor and abductor muscles simultaneously. Crumley[85] has developed a nerve anastomosis procedure using the ansa cervicalis as a donor to the recurrent laryngeal nerve. Because the ansa nerve delivers a slower firing rate, no jerky movements or paradoxical vocal fold bulging result. Instead, a quiet tonicity of the vocal fold body is achieved (synkinesis), providing a better vibratory source for voice production.

Although reinnervation techniques increase the likelihood of vocal fold tonicity, they do not restore vocal fold mobility, and subsequent medialization procedures may still be necessary for an optimal result. Both surgical treatments can be used in combination with laryngeal framework surgery, and some otolaryngologists have advocated this combination approach to decrease the glottal gap and improve the tonicity of the vocal fold body.[83]

Voice therapy for unilateral vocal fold paralysis often can be very effective. The goal of therapy is to improve glottic closure without causing supraglottic hyperfunction. Historically, descriptions of voice therapy for this population have discussed the process of strengthening the nonparalyzed vocal fold for the purpose of crossing the glottal midline for better approximation of the folds. There is question as to whether a strengthening process actually occurs. Nonetheless, by whatever process is operational, improvement in voice quality will occur when glottic closure is improved.

In an attempt to compensate for a lack of glottic closure, some patients with unilateral vocal fold paralysis develop a vocal and laryngeal hyperfunction. This hyperfunction actually decreases the efficiency of vocal function and usually impairs voice quality to a greater level than what might be expected from the paralysis alone. The task of voice therapy with these cases is to decrease this hyperfunctional behavior.

Several therapy techniques have been suggested for use with unilateral vocal fold paralysis patients. They include:

- hard glottal attack exercises
- pushing exercises
- lateral digital pressure
- head tilt method
- half-swallow boom technique
- Vocal Function Exercises.

We have been known to try all of these techniques with an individual patient in an attempt to find a strategy that works.

Because of the potential for developing vocal hyperfunction, the hard glottal attack and pushing exercises have fallen out of favor with some voice pathologists. These exercises continue to be useful with vocal fold paralysis patients who also use the falsetto register for voice production, however. Because of the effort to produce voice caused by the lack of glottic closure, some patients default to the high-pitch, breathy voice of the falsetto. When this is the case we attempt to engage the thyroarytenoid muscle of the nonparalyzed fold using the hard glottal attack. The technique used is similar to that described for the adolescent male with functional falsetto. To produce a hard glottal attack the patient is instructed to:

- breathe in
- build air pressure without letting your air out; posture the vowel at the same time
- release the vowel.

In the first week, the patient is given the list of vowels and vowel-consonant combinations to practice twice per day for 1 week:

- Say each vowel two times using a hard glottal attack:
  a, e, i, o, oo
- Say each word two times using a hard glottal attack:
  eat, it, ate, etch, at, ooze, oats, ought, out, up, I'm

When the patient returns 1 week later, the glottal attack exercise is reviewed. If progress has been adequate, the exercise is made more challenging by asking the patient to again produce the glottal attack with the addition of stretching the vowel while gliding down to a lower pitch. Gliding down in pitch encourages contraction of the thyroarytenoid muscle, whereas sustaining the tone for a longer period of time encourages low impact adduction. The patient is instructed to practice this modified hard glottal attack exercise, using the above vowels and words, two times each, two times per day for 1 week.

When the patient returns for the third therapy session, the glottal attack exercise with the stretched vowel and the glide to lower pitch is reviewed. If progress has been adequate, the same exercise is made more challenging by asking the patient to incorporate an isometric push. The isometric push may be accomplished by pressing the hands together in front of the body or pulling up on the arms of a chair at exactly the same time that the air pressure is being built and the vowel is being postured. The isometric push is then released when the vowel is released.

It has been our experience that, if patients are able to extinguish use of the falsetto voice, improvement will most likely occur within a 3-week period of time. Continuing with glottal attack and isometric pushing exercises beyond this time frame may risk increased vocal hyperfunction. Remember that the purpose of introducing this exercise program is to develop use of the modal register for patients who are using the falsetto register as compensation for the unilateral vocal fold paralysis. It is important to monitor patient performance to ensure against inadvertent supraglottic hyperfunction during this therapy.

Lateral digital pressure, sometimes known as manual compression of the thyroid cartilage, has proven to be beneficial for improving the voice quality of some patients with unilateral vocal fold paralysis.[86] While the patient is sitting in an upright position, looking straight forward, and producing a vowel sound, the therapist uses his or her thumb and forefinger to apply pressure to one side of the thyroid cartilage. Different amounts of pressure are applied while the therapist explores any change that may occur in voice quality. Both sides of the thyroid cartilage receive pressure during the exploration. When improved voice quality is identified, the exercise will progress through words and phrases. The patient is taught to use his or her own digital pressure for practice at home. The ultimate goal of this approach is to improve voice quality while extinguishing the digital pressure.

The head-turn approach uses the natural repositioning of the vocal folds by simply turning the head to one side or the other. Again, the patient is instructed to sit in an upright position. While turning the head slowly to one side, he or she is asked to phonate. The therapist will monitor any change in voice quality while the head is being turned. When a head-turn position is found that improves voice quality, the exercise will progress through words and phrases. The position of the head is stabilized in therapy so that the patient may be able to practice using this same position at home. The ultimate goal of this approach is to improve voice quality while extinguishing the turning of the head.[86]

McFarlane et al[86] also suggested the use of what they termed the half-swallow boom technique. This technique is another means of repositioning the vocal folds for the purpose of exploring improved voice quality in the unilateral vocal fold paralysis patient. The patient is asked to take a breath and go through the motions of initiating the first part of a swallow. Apparently, the pharyngeal and laryngeal muscle movements that occur during the half-swallow improve glottic closure. At the peak of the half-swallow, the patient is asked to forcefully say "boom." When this technique is successful, the boom will demonstrate a louder and clearer voice quality. The muscle manipulations created by the half-swallow are stabilized on the boom and then expanded to other words and phrases.

The effect of these exercises is variable and often depends on the degree of vocal fold gap. To a certain extent, the prognosis for success of rehabilitative therapy can be predicted following the results of the videostroboscopic image. When light "touch" closure is achieved in glottic waveform, despite the position of the paralyzed fold, the likelihood of discrete benefits from behavioral therapy is greater than for vibratory patterns that display no touch closure whatsoever. When touch closure is present, we have found that low impact Vocal Function Exercises are extremely effective in improving the vocal function and voice quality of patients with unilateral vocal fold paralysis.

It is important to note that many patients with idiopathic etiologies for unilateral vocal fold paralysis have spontaneous return of function within 1 year of onset. For this reason, timing of surgical management is typically delayed at least 6 months to 1 year post onset. Voice therapy may facilitate recovery of serviceable voice during the waiting. Rehabilitation can also prevent the patient from adopting maladaptive compensatory strategies. Finally, the effects of vocal fold paralysis may have a strong emotional impact on patients, and therapy may serve as a time to monitor progress and support the patient's need to adjust communicative demands at home, work, and in social settings to accommodate the disorder. Occasionally, referral to mental health professionals for additional support may be appropriate.

Case Study 13: Unilateral Vocal Fold Paralysis

The patient was a 65-year-old, recently retired high school teacher. One month prior to the voice evaluation, he underwent an anterior approach to a cervical fusion. Upon recovering from the anesthesia, he noticed a severe hoarseness. He was not alarmed at that time, because it was his impression that the hoarseness was a temporary condition caused by intubation. When the hoarseness persisted for 2 weeks following the surgery, however, he sought the opinion of an otolaryngologist.

Results of the laryngeal examination confirmed the presence of a right true vocal fold paralysis. The patient was then referred for evaluation treatment to the voice center.

The patient presented with a moderate-to-severe dysphonia characterized by a weak, high, breathy pitch. Results of the laryngeal videostroboscopic evaluation demonstrated the posterior aspect of the paralyzed fold to be near the midline but, because of a significant bowing of the right fold, a large glottal gap was present, accounting for his poor voice quality.

Therapy was immediately employed, involving hard glottal attack exercises for the purpose of establishing use of his modal register. No improvement was made in voice production over a 3-week period of time. Other therapy methods, such as digital pressure, head tilt, and the half-swallow boom, were attempted without success. It was determined that the size of the glottal gap caused by the vocal fold bowing precluded improvement through behavioral therapy.

Because of the potential for spontaneous recovery of the right recurrent laryngeal nerve, permanent surgical intervention was not yet possible. This patient was extremely debilitated as a result of his poor voice quality, however. The weak voice interfered with many of his family and social activities. It was suggested in consultation with the otolaryngologist that this patient might benefit from a temporary Gelfoam injection of the paralyzed fold. Accomplished as an outpatient procedure, the gelfoam was injected into the lateral aspect of the right true vocal fold. Stroboscopic observation of the larynx following injection demonstrated significantly improved glottic closure. The patient's voice quality was also improved to a mild-to-moderate dysphonia characterized by a breathy hoarseness. In addition, his modal register was now being used.

The patient was extremely pleased with the improvement of voice quality. Gelfoam, however, provides only a temporary improvement because of absorption, which occurs within 2 to 3 months. The improvement resulting from this procedure gave the voice pathologist the opportunity to try other therapy approaches that might have provided a more permanent vocal change; Vocal Function Exercises were immediately employed. The patient practiced the exercise program for 9 weeks, making steady improvement in his maximum phonation times. His voice quality also steadily improved, so much so that there was speculation that the function of the right true vocal fold had returned. Subsequent stroboscopic evaluation, however, demonstrated that the vocal fold remained paralyzed. Even though the gelfoam had reabsorbed, glottic closure remained improved and the voice quality was adequate for the patient's daily voicing activities.

This was a case where the team approach was successful. Voice therapy was not effective as long as the large glottal gap was present. A more permanent medialization procedure was not possible. The combination of a temporary improvement in glottic closure and direct voice therapy lead to a significantly improved voice quality. As it turned out, this patient's right true vocal fold paralysis was permanent. He has not yet chosen to undergo a more permanent surgical procedure. Apparently, if he continues the maintenance program of the Vocal Function Exercises, his voice quality remains acceptable to him.

Spasmodic Dysphonia

Spasmodic dysphonia (SD) is a term that describes a family of strained, strangled voices. As described in Chapter 4, (SD) is a focal dystonia of the central motor system. As with other focal dystonias, SD is characterized by abnormal involuntary movements that are action induced and task specific. Perceptually, the voice symptoms are classified in two primary groups: adductor and abductor spasmodic dysphonia. Adductor spasmodic dysphonia, which appears to be the most common, is characterized by strained, strangled phonation with occasional intermittent stoppages of voice. The severity may range from very mild, intermittent symptoms to a very severe, persistent struggle to produce phonation. The abductor type is characterized by abductor vocal fold spasms causing sudden, intermittent explosions or escapes of air. Abductor spasms appear to occur most frequently on voiceless consonants.

The incidence of spasmodic dysphonia is low. The onset of the disorder is usually middle age (though we have treated patients as young as 9 years old) and tends to occur equally in men and women. Some patients experience a rapid onset of symptoms, whereas others experience a gradual onset over many years. Because of media publicity regarding the unusual treatment for spasmodic dysphonia, the diagnosis of this disorder has become more efficient in recent years. Nonetheless, we still see patients who have sought treatments from many laryngologists, speech pathologists, psychologists and psychiatrists, and chiropractors. They have been prescribed various drugs and holistic remedies and have gone through relaxation training, EMG and thermal biofeedback, hypnosis, acupuncture, acupressure, and faith healing.

Herbert Dedo[87] a San Francisco otolaryngologist, innovated the use of unilateral recurrent laryngeal nerve section for the treatment of adductor spasmodic dysphonia. Creation of the unilateral vocal fold paralysis decreased the opportunity for the vocal folds to spasm at the midline. This treatment enjoyed early favorable results.[88] However, long-term success has been debated due to relapse of symptoms within a few years of treatment.[66,89]

Botulinum toxin (BOTOX) injections for the treatment of spasmodic dysphonia have become a primary management option when symptoms persist and progress and are unresponsive to other behavioral treatment techniques.[90-92] For adductor spasmodic dysphonia, a small amount of BOTOX is injected into the vocalis muscle, resulting in decreased spasm activity for a period of 3 to 6 months. Individual responses vary, but the overall success of this treatment method in the management of adductor spasmodic dysphonia has been positive.

When used as a therapy for abductor spasmodic dysphonia, the BOTOX is injected into the posterior cricoarytenoid muscle on one side of the larynx. This injection decreases the ability of the vocal folds to spasm in the abducted position. Bilateral injections of the posterior cricoarytenoid muscles are avoided due to the potential compromise of the airway. Botox injections for abductor spasmodic dysphonia yield less predictable success.

Physicians use two techniques to inject BOTOX in the vocal folds for adductor spasmodic dysphonia. An intraoral technique using a long curved syringe[93] permits the otolaryngologist to visualize the vocal folds during the injection. Topical anesthesia is used to decrease the gag reflex. While the patient holds his or her tongue, the otolaryngologist visualizes the vocal folds with a laryngeal mirror in one hand and injects the folds with the syringe in the other hand. This procedure has the advantage of visual inspection of the injection site, ensuring correct placement of the toxin in the vocalis muscle. It does require excellent patient compliance to tolerate the curved syringe placement (Figures 7-4 and 7-5).

The most common method of injection, which can be used for both adductor and abductor spasmodic dysphonia uses percutaneous electromyography to discern correct locations in the intrinsic muscles (vocalis for ADSD and posterior cricoarytenoid for ABSD). After palpating the laryngeal cartilage landmarks, the otolaryngologist inserts the needles and injects the toxin. This method usually requires the collaboration of the otolaryngologist with a neurologist. The neurologist assists in the setup and interpretation of the electromyographic feedback (Figure 7-6). Placement of the EMG electrode in the correct muscle is verified using speech tasks designed to discriminate intrinsic laryngeal muscle activity. Both the timing and the quality of the sound of muscle activity recording indicate when the needle edge is located in the appropriate muscle body.

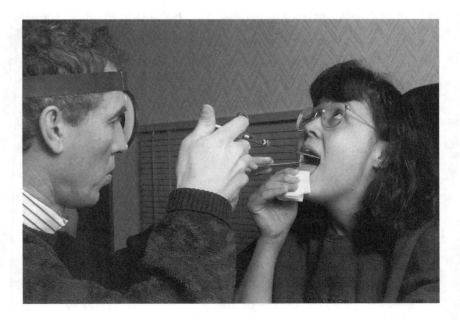

Figure 7-4. Botox injection using the curved syringe in an intraoral approach.

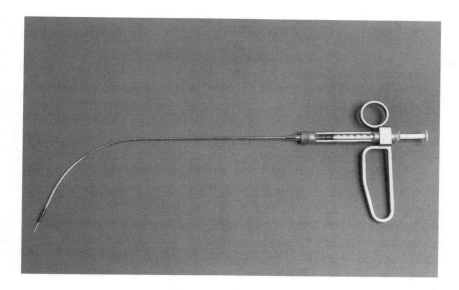

Figure 7-5. The curved syringe designed to inject the vocal folds through an intraoral approach.

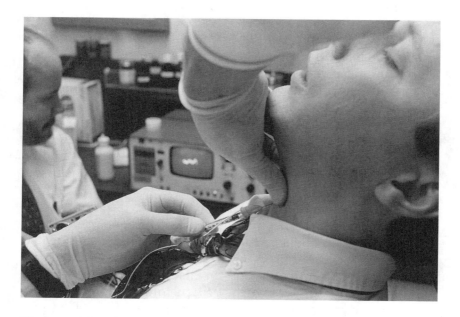

Figure 7-6. BOTOX injection using a percutaneous technique with EMG guidance.

The efficacy of rehabilitative voice therapy with spasmodic dysphonia is controversial, but many voice pathologists have reported good success with patients who are experiencing early or mild symptoms of SD or who used therapy in conjunction with BOTOX. Cooper[94] reported a long history of success in treating SD with behavioral therapy only. Beginning with a neutral "umhum" and expanding sequentially into vowels, syllables, words, and phrases, Cooper claimed to change the focus of the patients voice production and "cure" the spasmodic dysphonia. Others have not replicated his success rates, however. Other techniques for treatment of adductor spasmodic dysphonia include the use of increased pitch, increased breathy quality, use of /h/ onset in phonation, and relaxation training.

Most patients with adductor spasmodic dysphonia demonstrate a decrease in the frequency and severity of spasms when using a slightly elevated pitch. Using an increased breathy quality decreases the force of glottal impact thus decreasing the potential for spasm. The same logic is used to justify the use of the consonant /h/ at the onset of phonation. Because many spasmodic dysphonia patients develop an extreme hyperfunctional posture in an attempt to "push" the voice through the spasms, relaxation training often helps overcome this habit. Murry and Woodson[95] demonstrated that patients who follow up BOTOX injections with voice therapy often extend the effectiveness of the injections for a longer period of time than patients who do not have voice therapy.

In addition to the direct therapies mentioned above, the voice pathologist is responsible for educating the spasmodic dysphonia patient about the disorder. SD is an insidious disorder that often causes emotional upheaval. It can lead to depression, reclusive behavior, and, at the extreme, thoughts of suicide. The disorder has been known to ruin careers, friendships, and marriages. We believe that patients must be well educated regarding their disorder. Knowledge is power. Knowledge permits the patient to put a face on the disorder and to better plan ways of coping with it. Much written information regarding spasmodic dysphonia is shared with the patient. They are introduced to the National Spasmodic Dysphonia Association, which publishes information pamphlets, sponsors support groups, supports research, and holds a national convention for patients with spasmodic dysphonia. In addition, much supportive information regarding this disorder may be found on the World Wide Web.

Successful Voice Therapy

This chapter has provided the reader with a discussion of several orientations of voice therapy. One of the joys in providing therapy for patients with voice disorders is that many, if not most, improve. It is important to understand that the clinician and the patient share equally in the success or failure of voice therapy. The voice pathologist must be well grounded in anatomy, physiology, etiologic correlates, laryngeal pathology, and the psychodynamics of voice production. He or she must also possess outstanding skills in human interaction. These human interaction skills include the ability to talk to people, to skillfully and systematically divine the important aspects of the voice disorder and then to counsel appropriately.

The clinician must also understand all aspects of voice disorders, including the less obvious nuances of various pathologic conditions. By understanding voice disorders, realistic expectations of therapy will result and can be shared with the patient. The successful voice pathologist also will apply the management techniques appropriately. Every patient is an individual with different problems and individual needs. Patients with similar voice disorders will not necessarily respond to the same management approaches. Successful voice therapy is dependent on the clinician's awareness and use of all management techniques that seem appropriate. Misapplied techniques often result in failure.

Successful voice therapy can also be enhanced through patient education. For patients to be motivated to change vocal behaviors, they must understand why the change is required. Without a full understanding of the problem, the total management burden remains on the clinician. The clinician must use education to shift the burden for improvement to the patient. The patient must become any equal partner in the process of voice improvement.

Finally, the criteria for termination of therapy must be understood and agreed upon by both the voice pathologist and the patient. Documentation of the baseline voice production is essential to this process. Throughout the therapy program, it is necessary to subjectively and objectively plot progress for the purpose of accountability and to support the decision to continue or terminate therapy. It must be remembered that the patient lives with his or her voice on a daily basis. The patient may not appreciate the gradual, sometimes subtle changes that occur over time. Documentation of progress throughout the therapy program may demonstrate to the patient changes that they would not otherwise appreciate. These demonstrations are inherently motivating.

Assuming adequate preparation of the voice pathologist, the success of voice therapy may also be related to the patient. Successful voice therapy is dependent on the patient agreeing that a problem exists and having the motivation necessary to follow through and comply with the management suggestions. Patients also must be willing to share information. Information gathered during the patient interview is only valuable if it is complete and accurate. Even the most skilled clinician has experienced situations in which, after several sessions of therapy, the patient finally shares information critical to management decisions. Successful voice therapy is dependent on an open and honest relationship between patient and clinician. Ultimately, the patient has final control over the information he or she is willing to share.

Vocal image has a strong psychological influence on many people. Patients often find it difficult to modify even moderate-to-severe vocal disturbances because of the effect this change may have on their image. Voice therapy is comprised of a series of choices that both the clinician and the patient make. One choice that must be made by the patient is to shed the vocal image by following the management suggestions of the clinician. Successful voice therapy is dependent on the patient recognizing negative vocal behaviors and choosing the need to modify these behaviors.

Successful voice therapy, therefore, is a negotiation. The clinician's goal should always be the development of the best voice possible. This goal must be made clear to the patient. The patient's goal, however, may be beyond reasonable expectations or may be somewhat less than the best voice possible. It is the responsibility of the voice pathologist to negotiate the definition of each patient's successful voice therapy.

Some people are totally dependent on their voices for their livelihood. In one respect, these individuals are often a joy to work with in therapy because of their inherent motivation for improvement. On the other hand, their special needs and concerns require additional knowledge and understanding. Chapter 8 will introduce you to these individuals and provide you with a framework for successfully treating their voice disorders.

Appendix 7-1

Phrases And Sentences Graduated In Length

Two Syllable Sentences and Phrases

I am.	I will.	You can.	all right	Get up.
You are.	Oh no.	I'm fine.	King me.	black eye
He is.	Do it.	Look out.	Call me.	Cast off.
We are.	Don't go.	They're gone.	lost time	down here
You are.	What time?	Try it.	My my.	eat out
They are.	I'll try.	Why not?	No good.	free up
Come in.	Stop it.	no time	Oh my.	gee whiz
Get out.	Catch up.	too bad	part time	hot time
Keep out.	Watch out.	Get lost.	Guess what?	I'm fine.
Get up.	Thank you.	tee time	right now	last night
So long.	Go home.	Buy now.	Start up.	My mom.
Stand up.	Strike out.	Come back.	too much	next time
Sit down.	Turn right.	Don't go	used up	on top
Jump up.	first base	end run	Vote now.	post card
How much?	home plate	fast food	Where to?	rest stop
Push it.	Wake up.	great big	uptown	run down
Why not?	You bet.	grown up	Yes sir.	Step down.
Help me.	Good night.	Have some.	Yes ma'am	Sew up.
Prove it.	Goodbye.	I was.	Act now.	Where to?
Tell me.	too much	just so	Be good.	May I?

Three Syllable Sentences and Phrases

Pick it up.	Is that so?	Put that back.	See you soon.
Put it down.	Bake a pie.	Make salad.	Catch the ball.

Bring it here.	Ride the horse.	Fly away.	I said no.
I don't know.	Close the door.	Wear a tie.	more or less
Why not go?	Sweep the floor.	Go downtown.	Clean the tub.
Come over.	Start the game.	Race the car.	Wash dishes.
Go away.	Set the clock.	down the road	Fly the kite.
Here we are.	That's all right.	back by five	Build a house.
Good morning.	Go downtown.	I found it.	Light the lamp.
Can you go?	not so fast	Run it down.	Wind your watch.
Do it now.	Hit the ball.	Hurry up.	Don't touch it.
How are you?	Sleep all night.	Come back soon.	There she is.
Help me please.	Ring the bell.	It's snowing.	I'm sorry.
Is a time?	Don't do it.	like old times	Don't buy that.
I'm on time.	That's not true.	pretty eyes	Write a book.
Am I late?	Come back here.	far away	buy and sell
I told you.	Start a fire.	Go to sleep.	Look around.
over there	Mop the floor.	Call me soon.	Share the toy.
What about?	Go to school.	You look good.	Push and pull.
Should we go?	Write a check.	I feel fine.	a red light

Four Syllable Sentences and Phrases

It's very hot.	What could I do?	Give it to me.
Fry the bacon.	Will you be there?	Please say something.
Am I on time?	You should say so.	Is that enough?
Are you ready?	Am I early?	Write a letter.
I didn't know	Where do you sit?	Answer the phone.
Pick the apples.	I told you so.	When do we go?
a baby boy	That's not my fault.	Was I correct?
Feed the kitten.	How do you feel?	Do it again.
Don't wait for me.	Show it to me.	They all have jobs.
Can we go now?	Let's wait for them.	Open your eyes.

I don't know why.

How are you now?

Bring some money.

over the top

I like ice cream.

Open the door.

Bake apple pie.

I don't like that.

Should we go now?

Is that your car?

What time is it?

What have you done?

They are so slow.

Where do you live?

Turn to the left.

Fill the bird bath.

Turn on the light.

Walk down the hall.

Let's go swimming.

Play volleyball.

We must go now.

Did you know that?

How do you do?

Tell me the truth.

Did you hear me?

Keep on trying.

Put it away.

It stopped snowing.

Type the letter.

Let's go downtown.

Five Syllable Sentences

Give it to me now.

You are a good dog.

Come back when you can.

He has a nice car.

How much do you want?

There's not enough room.

The wind blew all day.

Do it before noon.

Do you want to go?

Go to the bookstore.

I want some pizza.

Do you have a dime?

The rain was welcome.

We designed our house.

She burst the balloon.

Speak clearly to them.

He is very shy.

There's not enough time.

They've sold their horses.

The crowd was pushed back.

He planted sweet corn.

The weather was cold.

Who pulled the alarm?

Bring a stronger rope.

I wouldn't do that.

Did he say maybe?

Stop, look, and listen.

Bring a keg of beer.

Answer the question.

I'm moving forward.

Use a safety pin.

Are you running now?

How did the race go?

The light bulb burned out.

Why don't you like it?

You made a mistake.

I'll come back today.

The dogs were barking.

Where did you grow up?

Have you talked to them?

We picked the berries.

Can you believe it?

Don't give it to me.

Let's watch some TV.

Open the window.

It's not all my fault.

We rode the rapids.

Keep on working hard.

I don't want to talk.

That's a better one.

I missed the last class.

They are very nice.

Is she your sister?

Let's play basketball.

You shouldn't do that.

We went to the bank.

The room was noisy.

They played in the sand.

Please open the door.

I was so nervous.

Six Syllable Sentences

Mike was cutting the grass.

What's not right must be wrong.

The player broke his arm.

Go to the store with me.

All the girls were laughing.

The fields were very dry.

Get there before they close.

Did you find your notebook?

Did you hear what she said?

Let's go skiing today.

Come in and close the door.

Do you like your new job?

Are you going tonight?

Promise that you won't tell.

Put everything away.

May I borrow that too?

Come whenever you can.

How are you this morning?

We heard that yesterday.

Beth was washing her clothes.

The player broke his leg.

The flags blew in the wind.

The children went swimming.

He slept under the tree.

It's time to go to class.

We don't want it to rain.

Please open window.

He couldn't start the fire.

Hit the ball to shortstop.

Do you think he's happy?

Don't wait till it's too late.

When should we come around?

Meet me at the courthouse.

Let's go to a movie.

Feed the dog his supper.

What's on TV tonight?

How much rent do you pay?

Who's on the telephone?

Seven and Eight Syllable Sentences

What movie would you like to see?

There's plenty of room in my house.

Sometimes I think you're very wrong.

Would you come by about seven?

May I have another piece?

I was raised in the Midwest.

Were you able to hear him speak?

The fisherman caught a large fish.

We grew roses on the back fence.

Show me how it should be done.

Yesterday he bought a new car.

I have too much to do today.

What do you want on your pie?

We ran a match race yesterday.

Come over this afternoon.

Please make sure your hands are clean.

The snow was a welcome sight.

All the fences were jumped with ease.

What's your favorite music?

I need to go to the bank.

Let's not take too much time here.

Why are there only seven?

The clock stopped at four thirty-nine.

Put it back where you found it.

The boy found it by the cooler.

We went skiing on the lake.

I eat breakfast every day.

Do you think we should start that now?

The trip was exciting.

Make sure you turn off your printer.

Nine and Ten Syllable Sentences

We need to go to the grocery store.

I scored one hundred percent on the test.

Let's go scuba diving this summer.

She had an interview this afternoon.

She has five brothers and four sisters.

Two of the brothers are in college.

That was the best time I ever ran.

Let's go to the ballgame on Saturday.

I couldn't believe how many were there.

She went to Florida during spring break.

Would you hold the door open for me?

I'm very happy that you could come.

He ordered a hamburger for lunch.

The snow melted before we could ride sleds.

We went fishing on Lake Superior.

I'm tired of cafeteria food.

What good movies have you seen lately?

I studied all night long for this test.

The marching band practiced before the game.

I'm going home for the holidays.

Do you have to work after class today?

There wasn't one parking space to be found.

Sometimes it's hard to keep up with the news.

You look absolutely marvelous.

What time do you think we should leave today?

The party was over by one-thirty.

I should be finished in time to leave then.

Why don't you take a fifteen-minute break?

Who was it that called on the telephone?

It's your turn to wash the dishes tonight.

Eleven to Fifteen Syllable Sentences

The instructor was rigid in his opinion.

There were eight hundred people in the psychology class.

With any luck, this course shouldn't be too difficult.

My pen ran out of ink in the middle of the test.

American history is my favorite class.

I would have helped you with that problem if you had only asked.

I want to jog for an hour before I begin to study.

My parents are coming to visit for the weekend.

How many more tests do you have this semester?

It's important that you listen closely in his class.

I wrote for so long that my hand began to cramp.

What was in the package you received this afternoon?

Most people wouldn't even consider doing that.

We stood in line for two hours to buy the tickets.

I just can't seem to get this program to run.

Most of this information can be found in the library.

Were you able to finish your project on time?

I was happy when classes were canceled because of the snow.

Everyone was shocked when he announced the surprise test.

The professor wouldn't start before she had had her coffee.

Two students from Taiwan were in my physics class.

We are going on a picnic if it doesn't rain.

My tape recorder could not pick up his voice.

What time do you want to leave the basketball game?

Our dormitory had a false alarm last night.

I can't wait until the Christmas holidays.

I swam ten laps this morning before eight o'clock.

Someone left his coat in the biology lab.

Make sure that you have all the facts and then proceed.

The library was so quiet, you could hear your heartbeat.

Sixteen to Twenty Syllable Sentences

The proposal was opposed by everyone who was eligible to vote.

How many times must we listen to the same thing over and over again?

I had steak, fried potatoes, and a tossed salad for dinner last night.

We knew as soon as we entered the room that someone had been there before us.

He posed the most important question that we would have to consider.

If I can raise the money, I'm going to fly to California.

Though we had been there only for a week, it seemed more like a month.

Let me know if there's anything I can do to help you get ready.

Since the building did not have air conditioning, the class was unbearable.

Nobody noticed when we entered the room a half-hour late.

Did you hear the plans to renovate the stadium for next year?

How many people do you think it will take to permit us to break even?

The runner developed the blister on his foot halfway through the race.

Students were caught painting victory signs on the railroad overpass.

How many months do you think it will take for us to finish this project?

We should be able to afford it if six of us rent the apartment.

He commuted to the university every day for five years.

She had already learned many of the skills in her co-op job.

I had eighteen more hours to complete for graduation.

The referee had obviously made a serious error in judgment.

The smoke was so thick in the lab that the sprinkler suddenly came on.

We carefully placed the project on the table for the instructor's inspection.

Someone threw an aerosol can in the fire, causing a loud explosion.

Would you rather take a written or an oral examination?

If you wait too long then you're going to miss a great opportunity.

I've been invited to go on vacation with my best friend's family.

It's impossible to measure the knowledge gained from this seminar.

Most people would not have the imagination to create such a thing.

Stop at the store on your way home and pick up a gallon milk.

We can't decide whether or not to participate in formal graduation.

Paragraph Readings

Passage 1

For the most wild yet the most homely narrative which I am about to pen,/ I neither expect nor solicit belief./ Mad indeed would I be to expect it,/ in a case where my very senses reject their own evidence./ Yet, mad am I not—/and very surely do I not dream./ But tomorrow I die, and today I would unburden my soul./ My immediate purpose is to place before the world,/ plainly, succinctly, and without comment,/ a series of mere household events./ In their consequences, these events have terrified—/ have tortured—have destroyed me./ Yet I will not attempt to expound them./ To me, they have presented little but horror—/to many they will seem less terrible than baroque./ Hereafter, perhaps, some intellect may be found which will reduce my phantasm to the commonplace—/ some intellect more calm, more logical, and far less excitable than my own,/ which will perceive, in the circumstances I detail with awe,/ nothing more than an ordinary succession of very natural causes and effects.

Edgar Allen Poe
from *The Black Cat*

Passage 2

Mr. President and Gentlemen of the Convention:/ If we could first know where we are, and whither we are tending,/ we could better judge what to do, and how to do it./ We are now far into the fifth year since a policy was initiated/ with the avowed object, and confident promise, of putting an end to slavery agitation./ Under the operation of that policy, that agitation not only has not ceased,/ but has constantly augmented./ In my opinion,/ it will not cease until a crisis shall have been reached and passed./ "A house divided against itself cannot stand."/ I believe this government cannot endure permanently, half slave and half free./ I do not expect the Union to be dissolved;/ I do not expect the house to fall;/ But I do expect that it will cease to be divided./ It will become all one thing or all the other./

Either the opponents of slavery will arrest the further spread of it,/ and place it where the public mind shall rest in the belief that it is in the course of ultimate extinction;/ or its advocates will push it forward till it shall become alike lawful in all the States,/ old as well as new,/ North as well as South. . . .

Abraham Lincoln

Passage 3

The wrath of God is like great waters that are dammed for the present;/ they increase more and more, and rise higher and higher, till an outlet is given;/ and the longer the stream is stopped, the more rapid and mighty is its course,/ when once it is let loose./ 'Tis true, that judgement against your evil work has not been executed hitherto;/ the floods of God's vengeance have been withheld;/ but your guilt in the meantime is constantly increasing,/ and you are every day treasuring up more wrath;/ the waters are continually rising, and waxing more and more mighty;/ and there is nothing but the mere pleasure of God that holds the waters back,/ that are unwilling to be stopped, and press hard to go forward./

If God should only withdraw his hand from the floodgate, it would immediately fly open,/ and the fiery floods and the fierceness and the wrath of God would rush forth with inconceivable fury/ and would come upon you with omnipotent power;/ and if your strength were ten thousand times greater than it is,/ yea, ten thousand times greater than the strength of the stoutest, sturdiest devil in hell,/ it would be nothing to withstand or endure it./

The bow of God's wrath is bent, and the arrow made ready on the string,/ and justice bends the arrow at your heart, and strains the bow,/ and it is nothing but the mere pleasure of God,/ and that of an angry God, without any promise or obligation at all,/ that keeps the arrow one moment from being made drunk by your blood.

Jonathan Edwards

Passage 4

In the long history of the world,/ only a few generations have
been granted the role in defending freedom in its hour of maximum danger./ I do not shrink from this responsibility;/ I welcome it./ I do not believe that any of us would exchange places
with any other people or any other generation./ The energy, the
faith, the devotion which we bring to this endeavor/ will light
our country and all that serve it,/ and the glow from that fire can
truly light the world./

And so, my fellow Americans,/ ask not what your country
can do for you;/ ask what you can do for your country./

My fellow citizens of the world,/ ask not what America will
do for you,/ but what together we can do for the freedom of man.

Finally, whether you are citizens of America or citizens of
the world,/ ask of us here the same high standards of strength
and sacrifice which we ask of you./ With a good conscience our
only sure reward,/ with history the final judge of our deeds,/ let
us go forth to lead the land we love,/ asking His blessing and
His help,/ but knowing that here on earth God's work must
truly be our own.

John F. Kennedy

Passage 5

While I was in San Francisco, I enjoyed my first earthquake. It
was one which was long called the "great" earthquake, and is
doubtless so distinguished till this day. It was just afternoon, on
a bright October day. I was coming down Third Street. The only
objects in motion anywhere in sight in the thickly built and pop-
ulous quarter, were a man in a buggy behind me, and a streetcar
wending slowly up a cross street. Otherwise, all was solitude
and a Sabbath stillness. As I turned the corner, around a frame
house, there was a great rattle and jar, and it occurred to me that
here was an item! —no doubt fight in that house. Before I could
turn and seek the door, there came a really terrific shock; the
ground seemed to roll under me in waves, interrupted by violent
joggling up-and-down, and there was a heavy grinding noise as
of brick houses rubbing together. I fell up against the frame
house and hurt my elbow. I knew what it was, now, and from

mere reportorial instinct, nothing else, took out my watch and noted the time of day; at that moment a third and still severer shock came, and as I reeled about on the pavement trying to keep my footing, I saw a sight! The entire front of a tall four-story brick building in Third Street sprung outward like a door and fell sprawling across the street, raising a dust like a great volume of smoke! And here came the buggy—overboard went the man, and in less time than I can tell it the vehicle was distrib-uted in small fragments along three hundred yards of the street. One could have fancied that someone had fired a charge of chair-rounds and rags down the thoroughfare. The streetcar had stopped, the horses were rearing and plunging, the passengers were pouring out of both ends, and one fat man had crashed halfway through a glass window on one side of the car, got wedged fast and was squirming and screaming like an impaled madman. Every door or of every house, as far as the eye could reach, was vomiting a stream of human beings; and almost before one could execute a wink and begin another, there was a massed multitude of people stretching in endless procession down every street my position commanded. Never was solemn solitude turned into teeming life quicker.

Mark Twain
from *The San Francisco Earthquake*

Passage 6

They tell us, sir, that we are weak; unable to cope with so for-midable an adversary. But when shall we be stronger? Will it be the next week, or the next year? Will it be when we are totally dis-armed, and when a British guard shall be stationed in every house? Shall we gather strength by irresolution and inaction? Shall we acquire the means of effectual resistance, by lying supinely on our backs, and hugging the delusive phantom of hope, until our enemies should have bound us hand and foot? Sir we are not weak, if we make proper use of the means which the God of nature hath placed in our power. Three millions of people, armed in the holy cause of liberty, and in such a country as that which we possess, are invincible by any force which our enemy can send against us. Besides, sir, we shall not fight our battles alone. There is a just God who presides over the destinies of nations; and who will raise up friends to fight our battles for us. The battle, sir, is not to the strong alone; it is to the vigilant, the active, the brave. Besides, sire, we have no election. If we were base enough to desire it, it is now too late to retire from the contest. There is no retreat, but in submission and slavery! Our chains are forged! Their clanking may be heard on the plains of Boston! The war is inevitable and let it come! I repeat it, sir, let it come!

It is in vain, sir, to extenuate the matter. Gentlemen may cry peace, peace but there is no peace. The war is actually begun! The next gale that sweeps from the north will bring to our ears the clash of resounding arms! Our brethren are already in the field! Why stand we here idle? What is it that gentlemen wish? What would they have? Is life so dear, or peace so sweet, as to be purchased at the price of chains and slavery? Forbid it, Almighty God! I know not what course others may take; but as for me, give me liberty, or give me death!

Patrick Henry

Passage 7

Friends and fellow-citizens: I stand before you tonight under the indictment for the alleged crime of having voted at the last Presidential election, without having the lawful right to vote. It shall be my work this evening to prove to you that in thus voting, I not only committed no crime, but, instead, simply citizen's rights, guaranteed to me and all United States citizens by Constitution, beyond the power of any State to deny.

The preamble of the Federal Constitution says:

"We, the people of the United States, in order to form a more perfect union, establish justice, insure domestic tranquility, provide for the common defense, promote the general welfare, and secure the blessings of liberty to ourselves and our posterity, do ordain and establish this Constitution for the United States of America."

It was we, the people; not we, the white male citizens; nor yet we, the male citizens; but we, the whole people, who formed the Union. And we formed it, not to give the blessings of liberty, but to secure them; not to the half of ourselves and the half of our posterity, but to the whole people women as well as men. And it is a downright mockery to talk to women of their enjoyment of the blessings of liberty while they are denied the use of their only means of securing them provided by this democratic-republican government the ballot.

For any State to make a sex qualification that must ever result in the disfranchisement of one entire half of the people is to pass a bill of attainder, or an ex post facto law, and is therefore a violation of the supreme law of the land. By it the blessings of liberty are forever withheld from women and their female posterity. To them this government has no just powers derived from the consent of the governed. To them this government is not a democracy. It is not a republic. It is an odious aristocracy; a hateful oligarchy of sex; the most hateful aristocracy ever established on the face of the globe; an oligarchy of wealth, where the rich govern the poor. An oligarchy of learning, where the educated govern the ignorant, or even an oligarchy of race, where the Saxon rules the African, might be endured; but this oligarchy of sex, which makes fathers, brothers, husbands, sons, the oligarchs over the mothers and sisters, the wives and daughters of every household which ordains all men sovereigns, all women subjects, carries dissension, discord and rebellion into every home of the nation.

Webster, Worcester and Bouvier all define a citizen to be a person in the United States, entitled to vote and hold office.

The only question to be settled now is: Are women persons? And I hardly believe any of our opponents will have the hardihood to say they are not. Being persons, then, women are citizens; and no State has a right to make any law, or to enforce any old law, that shall abridge their privileges or immunities. Hence, every discrimination against women in the constitutions and laws of the several States is today null and void, precisely as is every one against Negroes.

Susan B. Anthony

Passage 8

It chanced on Sunday, when Mr. Utterson was on his usual walk with Mr. Enfield, that their way lay once again through the by-street; and that when they came in front of the door, both stopped to gaze on it.

"Well," said Enfield, "that story's at an end at least. We shall never see more of Mr. Hyde."

"I hope not," said Utterson, "Did I ever tell you that I once saw him, and shared your feeling of repulsion?"

"It was impossible to do the one without the other," returned Enfield. "And by the way, what an ass you must have thought me, not to know that this was a back way to Dr. Jekyll! It was partly your own fault that I found it out, even when I did."

"So you found it out, did you?" said Utterson. "But if that be so, we may step into the court and take a look at the windows. To tell you the truth, I am uneasy, about poor Jekyll; and even outside, I feel as if the presence of a friend might do him good."

The court was very cool and a little damp, and full of premature twilight, although the sky, high up overhead, was still bright with sunset. The middle one of the three windows was half-way open, and sitting close beside it, taking the air with an infinite sadness of mind, like some deconsolate prisoner, Utterson saw Dr. Jekyll.

"What! Jekyll!" he cried. "I trust you are better."

"I am very low, Utterson," replied the doctor drearily, "very low. It will not last long, thank God."

"You stay too much indoors," said the lawyer. "You should be out, whipping up the circulation like Mr. Enfield and me. (This is my cousin - Mr. Enfield - Dr. Jekyll.) Come now; get your hat and take a quick turn with us."

"You are very good," sighed the other. "I should like to very much; but no, no, no, it is quite impossible; I dare not. But indeed, Utterson, I am very glad to see you; this is really a great pleasure; I would ask you and Mr. Enfield up, but the place is really not fit."

"Why then," said the lawyer, good-naturedly, "the best thing we can do is to stay down here and speak with you from where we are."

"That is just what I was about to venture to propose," returned the doctor with a smile. But the words were hardly uttered, before the smile was struck out of his face and succeeded by an expression of such abject terror and froze the very blood of the two gentlemen below. They saw it but for a glimpse for the window was instantly thrust down and they turned and left the court without word. In silence, too, they traversed the bystreet; and it was not until they had come into a neighboring thoroughfare, where even upon a Sunday there were still some stirrings of life, that Mr. Utterson at last turned and looked at his companion. They were both pale; and there was an answering horror in their eyes.

"God forgive us, God forgive us," said Mr. Utterson.

But Mr. Enfield only nodded his head very seriously, and walked on once more in silence.

Robert Louis Stevenson
from *Dr. Jekyll and Mr. Hyde*

Poetry Readings

Passage 1

Annabel Lee

It was many and many a year ago,
In a kingdom by the sea,
That a maiden there lived whom you may know
By the name of Annabel Lee;
And this maiden she lived with no other thought
Than to love and be loved by me.

She was a child and I was a child,
In this kingdom by the sea,
But we loved with a love that was more than love
I and my Annabel Lee
With a love that the winged seraphs of Heaven
Coveted her and me.

And this was the reason that, long ago,
In this kingdom by the sea,
A wind blew out of a cloud, by night
Chilling my Annabel Lee;
So that her highborn kinsmen came
And bore her away from me,
To shut her up in a sepulchre
In this kingdom by the sea.

The angels, not half so happy in Heaven,
Went envying her and me;
Yes! that was the reason (as all men know,
In this kingdom by the sea)
That the wind came out of the cloud,
chilling and killing my Annabel Lee.

But our love it was stronger by far than the love
Of those who were older than we
Of many far wiser than we
And neither the angels in Heaven above
Nor the demons down under the sea,
Can ever dissever my soul from the soul
Of the beautiful Annabel Lee;

For the moon never beams without bringing me dreams
Of the beautiful Annabel Lee;
And the stars never rise but I see the bright eyes
Of the beautiful Annabel Lee;
And so, all the night-tide, I lie down by the side
Of my darling, my darling, my life and my bride,
In her sepulchre there by the sea
In her tomb by the sounding sea.

Edgar Allen Poe

Passage 2

Bonny Barbara Allan

In Scarlet town, where I was born,
There was a fair maid dwelling,
Made every youth cry Well-a-away!
Her name was Barbara Allan.

All in the merry month of May,
When green buds they were swelling,
Young Jemmy Grove on his death-bed lay,
For love of Barbara Allan.

O slowly, slowly rose she up,
To the place where he was lying,
And when she drew the curtain by,
"Young man, I think you're dying."

O 'tis I'm sick, and very, very, very sick,
And 'tis a' for Barbara Allan";
"O the better for me ye's never be,
Tho your heart's blood were spilling,

"O dinna ye mind, young man," said she,
"When ye was in the tavern drinking,
That ye made the healths go round and round,
And slighted Barbara Allan?"

He turned his face unto the wall,
And death was with him dealing:
"Adieu, Adieu, my dear friends all,
And be kind to Barbara Allan."

And slowly, slowly rose she up,
And slowly, slowly left him,
And sighing said she could not stay,
Since death of life had left him.

She had not gane a mile but twa,
When she heard the dead-bell knelling,
And every jow that the dead-bell gave
Cried, "Woe to Barbara Allan!"

"O mother, mother, make my bed!
O make it soft and narrow!
Since my love died for me today,
I'll die for him tomorrow."

Unknown

Passage 3

The Old Cloak

This winter's weather it waxeth cold,
And frost it freezeth on every hill,
And Boreas blows his blast so bold
That all our cattle are like to spill.
Bell, my wife, she loves no strife;
She said unto me quietly,
"Rise up, and save cow Crumbock's life!"
Man, put thine old cloak about thee!"

HE

O Bell my wife, why dost thou flyte?
Thou kens my cloak is very thin.
It is so bare and over wom,

A cricket cannot creep therein.
Then I'll no longer borrow nor lend;
For once I'll new apparell'd be;
To-morow I'll to town and spend;
For I'll have a new cloak about me.

SHE

Cow Crumbock is a very good cow:
She has been always true to the pail;
She has help'd us to butter and cheese, I trow
And other things she will not fail.
I would be loth to see her pine.
Good husband, counsel take of me:
It is not for us to go so fine
Man, take thine old cloak about thee!

HE

My cloak it was a very good cloak,
It hath been always true to the wear;
But now it is not worth a groat:
I have had it four and forty year.
sometime it was of cloth in grain:
'Tis now but a sieve, as you may see:
It will neither hold out wind nor rain;
And I'll have a new cloak about me.

SHE

It is four and forty years ago
Since the one of us the other did ken;
And we have had, betwixt us two,
Of children either nine or ten:
We have brought them up to women and men:
In the fear of God I trow they be
And why wilt thou thyself misken?
Man, take thine old cloak about thee!

HE

O Bell my wife, why dost thou flyte?
Now is now, and then was then:
Seek now all the world throughout,
Thou kens not clowns from gentlemen:

They are clad in black, green, yellow and blue,
So far above their own degree.
Once in my fife I'll take a view;
For I'll have a new cloak about me.

SHE

King Stephen was a worthy peer;
His breeches cost him but a crown;
He held them sixpence all too dear,
Therefore he called the tailor 'lown.'
He was a king and wore the crown,
And thou'se but of a low degree:
It's pride that puts this country down:
Man, take thine old cloak about thee!

HE

Bell my wife, she loves not strife,
Yet she will lead me, if she can:
And to maintain an easy life
I oft must yield, though I'm good-man.
It's not for a man with a woman to threap,
Unless he first give o'er the plea:
As we began, so will we keep,
And I'll take my old cloak about me.

Passage 4

By-low, My Babe

By-low, my babe, lie still and sleep;
It grieves me sore to see thee weep.
If thou wert quiet I'd be glad;
Thou mourning makes my sorrow sad.
By-low, my boy, thy mother's joy,
Thy father breeds me great annoy
By-low, lie low.

When he began to court my love,
And me with sugared words to move,
His feignings false and flattering cheer
To me that time did not appear.

But now I see most cruelly
He cares not for my babe nor me
By-low, lie low.

Lie still, my darling, sleep awhile,
And when thou wak'st thou'llt sweetly smile;
But smile not as thy father did,
To cozen maids—nay, God forbid!
But yet I fear thou wilt grow near
Thy father's heart and face to bear
By-low, lie low.

I cannot choose, but ever will
Be loving to thy father still;
Where'er he stay, where'er he ride
My love with him doth still abide.
In weal or woe, where'er he go,
My heart shall not forsake him; so
By-low, lie low.

Unknown

REFERENCES

1. Stemple J. *Voice Therapy: Clinical Studies.* St Louis, Mo : Mosby Year Book; 1993.
2. Boone D. *The Voice and Voice Therapy.* Englewood Cliffs, NJ: Prentice-Hall; 1971.
3. Goss F. Hysterical aphonia. *Boston Med Surg J.* 1878;99:215-222.
4. Russell J. A case of hysterical aphonia. *Brit Med J.* 1864;8:619-621.
5. Ward W. Hysterical aphonia. *Chicago Med J Examiner.* 1877;34:495-505.
6. West R, Kennedy L, Carr A. *The Rehabilitation of Speech.* New York, NY: Harper and Brothers; 1937.
7. Van Riper C. *Speech Correction Principles and Methods.* Englewood Cliffs, NJ: Prentice-Hall; 1939.
8. Murphy A. *Functional Voice Disorders.* Englewood Cliffs, NJ: Prentice-Hall; 1964.
9. Brodnitz F. *Vocal Rehabilitation.* 4th ed. Rochester, NY: American Academy of Ophthalmology and Otolaryngology; 1971.
10. Andrews M. *Voice Therapy for Children.* San Diego, CA: Singular Publishing Group; 1991.
11. Aronson A. *Clinical Voice Disorders: An Interdisciplinary Approach.* New York, NY: Brian C Decker; 1980.
12. Aronson A. *Clinical Voice Disorders: An Interdisciplinary Approach.* 3rd ed. New York, NY: Brian C. Decker; 1990.

13. Case J. *Clinical Management of Voice Disorders.* 3rd ed. Austin, Tex: Pro-Ed; 1996.
14. Colton R, Casper J. *Understanding Voice Problems: A Physiological Perspective for Diagnosis and Treatment.* 2nd ed. Baltimore, Md: Williams and Wilkins; 1996.
15. Herrington-Hall B, Lee L, Stemple J, Niemi K, McHone M. Description of laryngeal pathologies by age, sex, and occupation in a treatment seeking sample. *J Speech Hear Disord.* 1988;53:57-65.
16. Wilson D. *Voice Problems of Children.* 3rd ed. Baltimore, Md: Williams and Wilkins; 1987.
17. Andrews M. Psychosocial aspects of children's behavior. In: Stemple J, ed. *Voice Therapy: Clinical Studies.* St Louis. Mo: Mosby Year Book; 1993:26-32.
18. Stemple J. Lehmann D. *Throat clearing:* the unconscious habit of vocal hyperfunction. Paper presented at: American Speech-Language-Hearing Association National Convention; November 1980; Detroit, Mich.
19. Zwitman D, Calcaterra T. The "silent cough" method for vocal hyperfunction. *J Speech Hear Disord.* 1973;38:119-125.
20. Verdolini K, Titze I, Fennell A. Dependence of phonatory effort on hydration level. *J Speech Hear Res.* 1994;37:1001-1007.
21. Jiang J, Ng J, Verdolini K, Hanson D. The effects of dehydration on phonation in excised canine larynges. *Ann Otol Rhinol and Laryngol.* In revision.
22. Colton R, Casper J. *Understanding Voice Problems: A Physiological Perspective for Diagnosis and Treatment.* Baltimore, Md: Williams and Wilkins; 1990.
23. Travis G. *Speech Pathology.* New York, NY: D Appleton and Company; 1931.
24. Fairbanks G. *Voice and Articulation Drill Book.* 2nd ed. New York, NY: Harper and Brothers; 1960.
25. Ainsworth S. *Speech Correction Methods: A Manual of Speech Therapy and Public School Procedures.* New York, NY: Prentice-Hall; 1948.
26. Cooper M. *Modern Techniques of Vocal Rehabilitation.* Springfield, Ill. Charles C Thomas; 1973.
27. Stemple J. *Clinical Voice Pathology: Theory and Management.* Columbus, Ohio: Charles E. Merrill; 1984.
28. Arnold G. Physiology and pathology of speech and language. In: Luchsinger R, Arnold G, eds. *Clinical Communicology: Its Physiology and Pathology.* Belmont, Calif: Wadsworth Publishing; 1965:337-510.
29. McWilliams B. Some factors in the intelligibility of cleft palate speech. *J Speech Hear Disord.* 1954;19:524-527.
30. Wilson D. *Voice Problems of Children.* 2nd ed. Baltimore, Md: Williams and Wilkins; 1979.
31. Boone D. *The Voice and Voice Therapy.* 2nd ed. Englewood Cliffs, NJ: Prentice-Hall; 1977.
32. Lee L. Refocusing laryngeal tone. In: Stemple J, ed. *Voice Therapy: Clinical Studies.* St. Louis, Mo: Mosby Year Book; 1993:49-53.
33. Coleman R. A comparison of the contributions of two voice quality characteristics to the perception of maleness and femaleness in the voice. *J Speech Hear Res.* 1976;19:168-180.
34. Nittrouer S, McGowan R, Milenkovic P, Beehler D. Acoustic measurement of men's and women's voices: a study of context effects and covariations. *J Speech Hear Res.* 1976;33:761-775.

35. Spencer L. Speech characteristics of male-to-female transsexuals: a perceptual and acoustic study. *Folia Phoniatrica.* 1988;40:31-42.

36. Terrango I. Pitch and duration characteristics of the oral reading of males on a masculinity-femininity dimension. *J Speech Hear Res.* 1966;9:590-595.

37. Wolfe V, Ratusnik D, Smith H, Northrup G. Intonation and fundamental frequency in male to female transsexuals. *J Speech Hearing Disord.* 1990;55:43-50.

38. Jacobson E. *Progressive Relaxation.* 2nd ed. Chicago, Ill: University of Chicago Press; 1938.

39. Froeschel E. Chewing method as therapy. *Arch Otolaryngol.* 1952;56:427-434.

40. Prosek R, Montgomery A, Walden B, Schwartz D. EMG biofeedback in the treatment of hyperfunctional voice disorders. *J Speech Hearing Disord.* 1978;43:282-294.

41. Stemple J, Weiler E, Whitehead W, Komray R. Electromyographic biofeedback training with patients exhibiting a hyperfunctional voice disorder. *Laryngoscope.* 1980;90:471-475.

42. Rammage L, Nichol H, Morrison M. The psychopathology of voice disorders. *Hum Comm Can.* 1987;11:21-25.

43. Ingalls E. Hysterical aphonia, or paralysis of the lateral cricoarytenoid muscles. *JAMA.* 1890;15:92-95.

44. Bach J. Hysterical aphonia. *Med News Philadelphia.* 1890;57:263-264.

45. Winslow P. Functional aphonia. *N Y Med J.* 1919;109:1129-1130.

46. Howard C. Report of a case of functional aphonia cured under general anesthetic. *JAMA.* 1923;80:104.

47. Stevens H. Conversion hysteria: A neurologic emergency. *Mayo Clin Proc.* 1968;43:54-64.

48. Roy N, Bless D, Heisey D, Ford C. Manual circumlaryngeal therapy for functional dysphonia: An evaluation of short- and long-term treatment outcomes. *J Voice.* 1997;3:321-331.

49. Christopher K, Wood R, Eckert R, Blager F, Raney R, Souhrada J. Vocal cord dysfunction presenting as asthma. *New Engl J Med.* 1983;308:1566-1570.

50. Selner J, Staudenmayer H, Koepke J. Vocal cord dysfunction: the importance of psychologic factors and provocation challenge testing. *J Allergy Clin Immunol.* 1987;79:726-733.

51. Martin R, Blager F, Gay M, Wood R. Paradoxic vocal cord motion in presumed asthmatics. *Semin Respir Med.* 1987;8:332-337.

52. Stemple J, Stanley J, Lee L. Objective measures of voice production in normal subjects following prolonged voice use. *J Voice.* 1995;9:127-133.

53. Barnes J. Voice therapy. Paper presented at: the Meeting of the Southwestern Ohio Speech and Hearing Association;1977; Cincinnati, Ohio.

54. Stemple J, Lee L, D'Amico B, Pickup B. Efficacy of vocal function exercises as a method of improving voice production. *J Voice.* 1994;8:271-278.

55. Sabol J, Lee L, Stemple J. The value of vocal function exercises in the practice regimen of singers. *J Voice.* 1995;9:27-36.

56. Verdolini K. Resonant voice therapy. In: Verdolini K, ed. *National Center for Voice and Speech's Guide to Vocology.* Iowa City, Iowa: National Center for Voice and Speech; 1998:34-35.

57. Lessac A. *The Use and Training of the Human Voice: A Biodynamic Approach to Vocal Life.* Mountain View, Calif: Mayfield Publishing Company; 1997.

58. Berry D, Verdolini K, Chan R, Titze I. Indications of an optimum glottal width in vocal production. *J Speech Hear Res.* In review.

59. Verdolini K, Drucker D, Palmer P, Samawi H. Laryngeal adduction in resonant voice. *J Voice.* 1998;12:315-327.

60. Kotby N. *The Accent Method of Voice Therapy.* San Diego, Calif: Singular Publishing Group; 1995.

61. Ramig L, Bonitati C, Lemke J, Horii Y. Voice treatment for patients with Parkinson disease: development of an approach and preliminary efficacy data. *J Medical Speech-Lang Pathol.* 1994;2:191-209.

62. Ramig L, Mead C, Scherer R, Horii Y, Larson K, Kohler D. Voice therapy and Parkinson's disease: a longitudinal study of efficacy. Paper presented at: The Clinical Dysarthria Conference; 1988; San Diego, Calif.

63. Ramig L, Pawlas A, Countryman S. *The Lee Silverman Voice Treatment: A Practical Guide for Treating the Voice and Speech Disorders in Parkinson Disease.* Iowa City, Iowa: National Center for Voice and Speech; 1995.

64. Ramig L, Countryman S, Thompson L, Horii Y. A comparison of two forms of intensive speech treatment for Parkinson disease. *J Speech Hear Res.* 1995;39:1232-1251.

65. Countryman S, Hicks J, Ramig L, Smith M. Supraglottal hyperadduction in an individual with Parkinson disease: a clinical treatment note. *Am J Speech Lang Pathol.* 1997;6:74-84.

66. Aronson A. *Clinical Voice Disorders: An Interdisciplinary Approach.* 2nd ed. New York, NY: Brian C. Decker; 1985.

67. Damste P. Diagnostic behavior patterns with communicative abilities. In: Bless D, Abbs J eds. *Vocal Fold Physiology.* San Diego, CA: College-Hill Press; 1987:435-444.

68. Rubin W. Allergic, dietary, chemical, stress, and hormonal influences in voice abnormalities. *J Voice.* 1987;1:378-385.

69. Ford C, Bless D. Introduction. In: Ford C, Bless D, eds. *Phonosurgery.* New York, NY: Raven Press; 1991:1-3.

70. Redmond E, Wetscher G. Introduction. In: Hinder R, ed. *Medical Intelligence Unit: Gastroesophageal Reflux Disease.* Austin, Tex: RG Landes Company; 1993:1-6.

71. Koufman J. Gastroesophageal reflux and voice disorders. In: Rubin J, Ed. *Diagnosis and Treatment of Voice Disorders.* New York, NY: Igaku-Shoin; 1995:161-175.

72. Kendall K. Evaluation and management of unilateral vocal fold paralysis: a survey, part II. *Phonoscope.* 1998;1:141-147.

73. Koufman J, Walker F. Laryngeal electromyography in clinical practice: indications, techniques, and interpretation. *Phonoscope.* 1998;1:57-70.

74. Ford C. Laryngeal injection techniques. In: Ford C, Bless D, eds. *Phonosurgery.* New York: Raven Press; 1991:123-141.

75. Ford C. A multipurpose laryngeal injector device. *Otolaryngol Head Neck Surg.* 1990;103:135-137.

76. Ford C, Bless D. Collagen injected into the scarred vocal fold. *J Voice.* 1992;1:116-119.

77. Ford C, Bless D, Loftus J. Role of injectable collagen in the treatment of glottic insufficiency: a study of 119 patients. *Ann Otol Rhinol Laryngol.* 1992;101:237-247.
78. Brandenberg J, Kirkham W, Koschkee D. Vocal cord augmentation with autogenous fat. *Laryngoscope.* 1992;102:495-500.
79. Isshiki N, Morita H, Okamura H, Hiramoto M. Thyroplasty as a new phono-surgical technique. *Acta Otolaryngol (Stockholm).* 1974;78:451-457.
80. Blaugrund S. Laryngeal framework surgery. In: Ford C, Bless D, eds. *Phonosurgery.* New York, NY: Raven Press; 1991:183-200.
81. Isshiki N. Laryngeal framework surgery. *Adv Otolaryngol Head Neck Surg.* 1991;6:37-56.
82. Koufman J. Thyroplasty for vocal fold medialization: an alternative to Teflon injection. *Larygoscope.* 1986;96:726-731.
83. Tucker H. *The Larynx.* New York, NY: Thieme Medical Publishers; 1987.
84. Smith M, Gray S. Laryngeal framework surgery in children. In: Titze I, ed. *Progress Report 5.* Iowa City, Iowa: National Center for Voice and Speech; 1994:91-98.
85. Crumley R. Laryngeal reinnervation techniques. In: Ford C, Bless D, eds. *Phonosurgery.* New York, NY: Raven Press;1991:201-212.
86. McFarlane S, Watterson T, Lewis K, Boone D. Effect of voice therapy facilitation techniques on airflow in unilateral paralysis patients. *Phonoscope.* 1998;1:187-191.
87. Dedo H. Recurrent nerve section for spastic dysphonia. *Ann Otol Rhinol Laryngol.* 1976;85:451-459.
88. Dedo H, Izdebski K. Intermediate results of 306 recurrent laryngeal nerve sections for spastic dysphonia. *Laryngoscope.* 1983;93:9-16.
89. Aronson A, DeSanto G. Adductor spasmodic dysphonia: three years after recurrent laryngeal nerve resection. *Laryngoscope.* 1983;93:1-8.
90. Blitzer A, Brin M. Laryngeal dystonia: A series with botulinum toxin therapy. *Ann Otol Rhinol Laryngol.* 1991;100:85-90.
91. Blitzer A, Brin M, Fahn S, Lovelace R. Localized injections of botulinum toxin for the treatment of focal laryngeal dystonia. *Laryngoscope.* 1988;98:193-197.
92. Ludlow C, Naunton R, Sedory S, Schulz G, Hallett M. Effects of botulinum toxin injections on speech in adductor spasmodic dysphonia. *Neurology.* 1988;38:1220-1225.
93. Ford C, Bless D, Lowery D. Indirect laryngoscopic approach for injection of botulinum toxin in spasmodic dysphonia. *Otolaryngol Head Neck Surg.* 1990;103:752-758.
94. Cooper M. In: Cooper M, ed. *Approaches to Vocal Rehabilitation.* Springfield, Ill: Charles C. Thomas; 1977.
95. Murry T, Woodson G. Combined-modality treatment of adductor spasmodic dysphonia with botulinum toxin and voice therapy. *J Voice.* 1995;9:460-465.

8

The Professional Voice

"The voice so sweet, the words so fair,
As some soft chime had stroked the air;
And though the sound were parted thence,
Still left an echo in the sense."
—*Eupheme*, Samuel Johnson

We have described the laryngeal mechanism in terms of its physical structure and function and have discussed many etiologic factors that may lead to the development of various laryngeal pathologies. We then presented management strategies designed to help patients return the laryngeal mechanism to as near a normal state as possible, yielding improved or normal voice qualities. A large group of individuals are, by the very nature of their occupations, at a greater risk of developing voice problems and laryngeal pathologies. These individuals are directly dependent on vocal communication for their livelihood. They are classified as users of a "professional" voice. The impact of a voice disorder on this population is twofold. Not only does it cause vocal symptoms that are characteristic of the disorder, it also carries with it a high level of emotional strain and anxiety. This anxiety is caused by the disorder's potential impact on the person's reputation, the ability to meet professional commitments, or simply the ability to perform his or her job. These concerns and anxieties add to the actual causes of the voice disorder and must also be addressed in a positive manner within the vocal management program.

The management approach must go beyond the manipulation of inappropriate vocal properties and must involve all aspects of vocal hygiene counseling. The rehabilitation often will require the involvement of a team of professionals. The team may comprise the professional voice user, the otolaryngologist, the voice pathologist, and the professional voice user's teacher of singing, vocal coach, producer, and manager. Successful voice rehabilitation may depend on the abilities of these disciplines to compromise and work together, with the patient's long-term vocal health as the primary consideration. Ideally, the professional voice user will ultimately become responsible for the well-being of his or her own vocal health.

The Professional Voice User

We are all dependent on vocal communication in our everyday lives. Indeed, most people view the loss of voice for even a brief time as a major inconvenience. Those who rely directly on their voices for their livelihoods in a public forum are likely to experience more than an inconvenience with the development of a voice disorder. Voice disorders, whether they are acute or chronic, may threaten, shorten, change, or even end some careers. For example, the singer who develops acute laryngitis on opening night may suffer poor reviews. The stage actor who develops intermittent periods of dysphonia caused by vocal misuse may develop a reputation of unreliability. The effectiveness of a political campaign may be diminished when the politician becomes dysphonic and is unable to project the desired image.

This chapter will focus primarily on the elite vocal performer (singers and actors) for whom a slight alteration in vocal quality can have a devastating effect.[1] There are other professionals including teachers, ministers, lawyers, salespeople, auctioneers, lecturers, and health care providers, to name a few, who fall into a category of professional voice users that when vocal quality is affected, job performance is also affected. Many less "public" professionals are also "at risk" for the development of laryngeal disorders with the same level of social, emotional, and job-threatening anxieties present. Whenever individuals depend on their voices to function successfully in their occupations, they may be considered professional voice users. For many, the care and proper use of the voice may never become an issue. For others, a voice disorder may create real or imagined personal threats. The psychodynamics of vocal management may dictate the success or failure these professionals experience within their professions.

History

The 20th century has benefited from the visionary efforts of G Paul Moore, PhD, Hans von Leden, MD, and Wilber J Gould, MD, in their advancement of the treatment of the professional voice. Their fundamental foundation of building a multidiscipline, combining professionals from art and science, continues to generate national and international collaborative research in the area of voice. From this collaborative effort, several professional conferences on voice are held both nationally and internationally.

These conferences bring together otolaryngologists, speech-language pathologists, voice scientists, physicists, voice teachers, voice coaches, singers, actors, performers, acting teachers, and other professionals interested in the area of voice. They provide information on the most recent advancements in the areas of technology, science, and clinical applications regarding the study of voice. In 1971, New York's Juilliard School of Music hosted the first Voice Foundation Symposium on the Care of the Professional Voice under the direction of W J Gould, MD. This symposium, currently held in Philadelphia under the chairmanship of Robert T Sataloff, MD, presented its 28th conference in 1999. Other conferences held yearly include the Pacific Voice Conference, Medicine in the Vocal Arts-Spoleto Festival, and Canadian Voice Care Conference. In 1980, researchers in the fields of voice science and laryngology held the first of a series of biennial Vocal Fold Physiology conferences. These conferences promoted a global interest in voice care to promote laryngeal research, and brought about the 1st World Voice Congress held in 1995 in Oporto, Portugal, with the 2nd World Voice Congress held in 1998 in São Paulo, Brazil.

Throughout the United States, and in some other countries, otolaryngology offices have adopted the team approach in the treatment of voice disorders. There are otolarygological centers that pride themselves on being providers of voice-care excellence. Besides the otolaryngologist and voice pathologist, a teacher of singing is also on staff. The voice pathologist is licensed to provide voice therapy for the injured voice, and the teacher of singing provides instructions on singing and vocal technique. Although the numbers are few, dual specialization exists where teachers of singing are also certified speech-language pathologists. The American Speech-Language-Hearing Association (ASHA) and National Association of Teachers of Singing (NATS) published a joint statement on voice therapy for singers.[2] In this statement, any member of NATS who has taken the recommended coursework outlined is qualified to work with an otolaryngologist and a speech-language pathologist as a team in remediating diagnosed voice disorders. This professional is precluded from doing voice therapy unless he or she is also licensed and certified as a speech-language pathologist. Likewise, the voice pathologist who works with singers needs to receive instructions in vocal pedagogy and voice performance and should not provide singing instruction unless the voice pathologist is an experienced teacher of singing and has met the requirements of NATS.

The National Association of Teachers of Singing (NATS) was founded in 1944 by the American Academy of Teachers of Singing, the New York Singing Teachers Association, and the Chicago Singing Teachers Guild.[3] This organization has strived to promote the highest standards of singing through teaching and research. The Association's periodical, *Journal of Singing*, is the only professional journal in the United States devoted to singing and the teaching of singing.[4] This journal publishes articles on the art of singing, vocal function, vocal literature, care of the professional voice, and the teaching of singing.

Another organization that serves the professional voice user is the Voice and Speech Trainers Association (VASTA).

Founded in 1986, this organization is dedicated to voice and speech training for the professional voice user in acting and the performing arts. The Association publishes a triannual *VASTA Newsletter*.

Both NATS and VASTA extend an affiliation membership to professionals or groups in related fields interested in the professional voice. Many voice pathologists and otolaryngologists have memberships in both organizations and receive publications and attend conferences to learn current research and training directions in the performing arts.

Because voice pathologists, teachers of singing, and theater trainers all work with the performer and because some of the techniques used are similar, a word of caution is in order. It is critical that we maintain focus within our scope of practice, and respect others' professional boundaries. Treating voice and speech disorders has legal implications and requires a master's degree in speech pathology, as well as a license and certification. Similarly, voice pathologists are not trained to teach singing or acting. Therefore, it is necessary for all professions to work together to achieve the professional goals in vocally rehabilitating the performer. Our collaborative efforts will bring about impressive results and provide the best possible care for performers to use their instrument optimally in speech and singing and maintain a healthy laryngeal mechanism.

The "At-risk" Status

Individuals who use their voices professionally are subject to the development of laryngeal pathologies caused by any of the etiologic factors mentioned in previous chapters. As voice pathologists, we must be acutely aware of the influences of phonotrauma and vocal misuse on the laryngeal system. We cannot assume that the professional voice user understands the relationship of these "at-risk" behaviors and how these behaviors correlate with changes in vocal performance. We find only a few professional voice owners who have even a vague awareness of the anatomy and physiology of the vocal mechanism. Also, although many people do indeed possess "trained" voices for acting, singing, and public speaking, as well as excellent techniques for these functions, other vocal misuses and abuses are often present as primary causes of their vocal difficulties.

Similarities between singers and actors and individuals who are athletes are quite parallel. Athletes, because of the physical nature of their work, are at greater risk than most people for developing muscular and joint injuries. Likewise, because actors and singers are dependent on their voices and, as a rule, demand more from them than the average speaker, they are at greater risk for developing laryngeal pathologies.[5] Despite these similarities, a major difference exists between the management approaches of athletes and professional voice users. The prized athlete generally rests the injury long enough for it to heal and for the possibility of permanent damage to be eliminated. Singers and actors, however, usually minimize the disability to avoid canceling an engagement. They continue using the voice, often risking permanent damage. After all, "The show must go on!"

The less "public" professional voice users behave in the same manner as singers and actors. Educators continue to teach, speech-language pathologists continue to practice, teachers of singing continue to teach, vocal coaches continue to teach acting, salespeople continue to sell, preachers and ministers continue to preach, and receptionists continue to perform their vocal duties. Rather than risk loss of income or damage to their reputations as reliable and productive workers, these individuals meet their vocal demands.

Professional Roles

Successful treatment of voice disorders in the professional voice user relies on a multidisciplinary team to attend to the various vocal needs and the individual's professional and social needs. The team's responsibility is to assist in the prevention, care, and rehabilitation of all types of voice problems. Each team member should have a keen understanding of the pathophysiology of the individual's voice disorder. The key members of the voice care team include the otolaryngologist, voice pathologist, and primary care physician. Other specialists may include the singing teacher, drama coach, psychologist, psychiatrists, neurologist, gastroenterologist, pulmonologist, and occasionally other medical specialties. The composition of the voice care team may differ from individual to individual, depending on the patient's level of vocal usage and demand to return to normal performance. Individuals may react differently to the same type of voice disorder; some are willing to accept immediate treatment, whereas others may elect to go at a slower pace in remediating the problem(s).

The voice care team members treating the professional voice user will depend on the patient's profession and level of vocal usage. The otolaryngologist, voice pathologist, and primary care physician most often provide support for the nonperformance professional. The otolaryngologist evaluates the laryngeal condition and then treats the condition with rest, medication, surgery, or referral. The voice pathologist evaluates the causes of the laryngeal pathology and then establishes a program for the modification or elimination of these causes. The primary care physician continues to treat the patient for other health-related problems that may or may not contribute to the voice disorder.

The professional who uses the voice for stage and singing performances is often subjected to the concerns and influences of others in addition to the otolaryngologist and voice pathologist. These individuals may include the producer of the event, the agent or manager of the performer, and possibly the vocal teacher or coach. Let us examine the roles of each.

The Otolaryngologist

The major role of the otolaryngologist in the treatment of the professional voice is in the physical diagnosis of the laryngeal mechanism to determine the condition and the function of the mechanism at that moment. When presented with a laryngeal pathology in a professional voice user, the otolaryngologist often is asked to "get me through this performance!" When faced with an important performance, such as a one-time audition, opening night, or a one-night stand, it is often possible for the otolaryngologist to administer antiinflammatory steroid medications (Prednisone or similar drugs) and vasoconstrictors that may make it possible for the patient to perform. In making the decision to help a patient make it through the one important performance, it is nonetheless extremely important to balance the risk of further or more permanent damage against the need to perform. The performer must understand that a "quick fix" is possible, but it is not a long-term solution. Administering drugs in these cases is similar to doping a racehorse or an athlete. A short period of voice rest is often recommended after such performances. The performer should be cautious in seeking out a physician who readily prescribes these medications because they usually mask the symptoms and may cause further damage and longer recovery periods. For chronic vocal disorders, there may be a necessity for daily medication, such as those precipitated by laryngopharyngeal reflux or allergies, to maintain a balance. Administration of medication(s) depends on the etiology of the dysphonia. Input from the voice pathologist is paramount to the successful recovery of the performer's voice. Depending on the etiology of the vocal problem, surgery is usually a last resort and performed when the patient has followed through with all presurgical conditioning procedures in voice therapy.

When phonosurgery is performed, great care is taken to preserve the free vibratory vocal fold edge preserving the mucosal wave. As previously mentioned, voice is dependent on respiration, phonation, and resonance. Surgery that alters any one of these components can affect the voice quality of the vocal performer. The surgeon should discuss possible subtle changes with the patient prior to surgery.[6] Postsurgical guidelines, reviewed prior to surgery, must be strictly followed to assure proper healing and recovery. In our practice, minimal recommendations following laryngeal surgery include 7 days of complete vocal rest, 2 liters of water daily, and no caffeine.

The Voice Pathologist

The voice pathologist evaluates all aspects of voice use and production including breath support, phonation, and resonance or (placement) of the voice to determine the causes of the voice disorder. When working with the professional voice user, nonstage voicing habits and the performer's technique need to be assessed separately to determine the etiologic factors that contribute to the voice disorder. These voicing habits may not be apparent during the office evaluation and case history interview. It is useful to obtain tape recordings of the speaker's voice in various settings, set up role-play scenarios, and whenever possible, observe live performances. This need is especially critical with teachers, salespeople, ministers, preachers, politicians, and lecturers. It is essential when working with performers. Inappropriate vocal components that are not heard during the quiet conversational voice used throughout the diagnostic evaluation are often quite evident during public presentations. The voice pathologist "must become familiar with the full range of vocal stressors that may be found in the performance environment."[7(p697)]

Once the causes for the disorder have been identified, however subtle, the impact these causes have on the vocal mechanism must be described in detail to the patient. The voice pathologist must compile all the data collected from patient history, observation, acoustic and aerodynamic testing, videostroboscopy, and the patient's perceptual and physiological sensations to develop a hypothesis of the cause as it relates to respiration, phonation, and resonance. Using pictures, diagrams, and models to describe the laryngeal mechanism and the pathology is extremely helpful for patient understanding. If a copy of the videolaryngostroboscopic evaluation is available, the educational benefits are enormous. Many people who use voice for their livelihoods have little knowledge of the normal structure and function of the laryngeal mechanism. Providing this information is an important role of the voice pathologist. Issues regarding general vocal hygiene should be discussed as they relate to the patient's specific voice disorder. A management plan is then tailored to the patient and is designed to modify or eliminate the causes of the voice disorder.

If pathology is present and begins to resolve, efforts are made to rebuild the patient's vocal confidence. The public voice is gradually reintroduced and tested by the patient for effectiveness. When the laryngeal mechanism is healthy and the patient's confidence has been renewed, the patient is discharged from therapy with periodic recheck times established.

At times, the diagnostic evaluation of a singer will yield no etiologic factors responsible for the development of the voice disorder. When this occurs, a competent vocal coach should be found to evaluate the present singing techniques and modify them as needed to attain a healthy mechanism.

The final goal of voice therapy is not only the return of normal laryngeal structure and function, but also the development of an understanding that the ultimate responsibility for the wellbeing of the laryngeal mechanism rests with the professional voice user. The responsibility does not lie with the otolaryngologist, voice pathologist, the producer, agent, manager, or coach. In spite of the pressures to perform in the presence of vocal difficulties, the owner of the voice must take charge. Decisions regarding whether to perform may be made by honestly answering one question: "Will I compromise the rest of my career by performing tonight?"

When working with performers, it is important for the voice pathologist to understand specific vocabulary with which the performer is familiar and how the vocal problem may result in a physical alteration or limitation of a desired effect. Examples of terms (see the glossary of singing terms at the end of this chapter) include messa di voce, vibrato, passaggio, leggiero, and tessitura to name a few. Voice pathologists are directed to study the science behind the performance in an attempt to understand the working mechanics of each integral part as it relates to the whole system.[8-11] Performers understand imagery and visualization terms (such as focus, lift, placement, mask, dark color, bright color, ring, and buzz), which are used to describe specific artistic outcome of a tone. These terms are difficult to define scientifically but take on an interpretation and meaning within the individual and between the performer and the singing or acting teacher. It may be beneficial for the voice pathologist to learn the "feel" of these terms by taking instructions or observing a master instructor in the performing arts.

The Producer

The producer of a public event has the major responsibility for guaranteeing that the money invested in the performance is secure. The producer is responsible for overseeing the operations of the event and for reacting quickly and positively to any situations that could threaten the event's success. These situations include dealing with the physical and emotional problems and needs of the performers. Keeping in mind that the producer's main concern is the financial success of the event, it is not difficult to understand that this pressure would possibly make the producer less than sympathetic with a performer suffering vocal problems. The inability to perform is a threat not only to the event's success but ultimately the producer's reputation, which is itself ultimately responsible for securing investors for future events. The producer may, therefore, apply great pressure on the performer or the performer's manager or agent to guarantee that the "show must go on."

The Agent or Manager

The agent or manager is responsible for the overall career development of the professional voice user. Career development involves selling the performer's services to producers, developing public relations strategies, deciding on appropriate jobs to accept or reject, scheduling performances, and often handling business affairs.

There is huge competition among a great number of performers for a limited number of parts. Professionals who are good enough or lucky enough to find steady work in the performing arts are usually associated with top managers. These performers often sustain themselves as attractive employees through their own professional reliability. It is the manager's or agent's responsibility to guarantee that his or her clients remain as attractive as possible to those in the hiring positions. The success and the financial gain of the manager or agent are totally dependent on his or her ability to keep clients working. The more clients that work, the more attractive is the manager to other potential clients. Producers will not hire performers who have developed reputations for unreliability. This reputation may develop quickly, especially by performers in the nonstar category. Therefore, we may understand the pressure that the manager or agent may place on a client to perform even in the presence of vocal difficulties. This pressure to perform is not an indictment of producers, managers, or agents, but simply a statement of the reality of competing interests.

Clinical Pathways

A number of disciplines are involved with the voice care team. How can all of the disciplines work together, and who should address what problems when the professional has a voice disorder? There is no set protocol for providing care for the professional voice user. Nonetheless, the key personnel providing care for the professional voice user include the otolaryngologist, voice pathologist, and vocal pedagogue. Let us look at some possibilities.

Otolaryngology-Voice Pathology-Voice Pedagogy

Referrals to the otolaryngologist come from many sources. There are self-referrals; but more often, referrals come from family practitioners. The chief complaint is dysphonia with hoarseness, although, the individual may be referred for complaints of a "lump" sensation in the throat, dysphagia, sinus drainage, allergies, ear problems, throat discomfort, cough, airway problems, or possible neurological involvement. Other medical disciplines also refer directly to the otolaryngologist. The otolaryngologist diagnoses and medically treats the individual if warranted. The otolaryngologist refers to the voice pathologist for evaluation. The voice pathologist works to:

- reeducate the individual on vocal hygiene
- provide vocal exercises designed to balance the subsystems of voice production
- provide vocal exercises to promote an open front focus using diaphragmatic breath support
- provide exercises to reduce muscular tension
- design regimens to eliminate all phonotrauma behaviors and vocal misues
- provide continued support in counseling the patient regarding reflux precautions if needed.

Voice therapy is recommended prior to removal of any mass lesions that may have developed from improper or phonotraumatic vocal techniques. If therapy does not occur prior to surgical removal of a lesion(s) and the patient is unaware of the possible etiology of the dysphonia, the likelihood of recurrence is much greater.[12,13] During vocal rehabilitation with the voice pathologist, the performer should be working with the voice teacher or vocal coach. Often the individual has altered vocal technique in response to the dysphonia. It is necessary for the performer to learn or relearn to use a healthy technique that will reduce or eliminate the chances of future vocal problems.

Voice Pedagogy-Otolaryngologist-Voice Pathology

When working closely with the professional voice user, the teacher of singing or vocal coach may detect subtle perceptual changes or possible limitations in the voice. The performer may have acute or chronic vocal problems. Some of the symptoms may include increased effort to initiate voicing, difficulty sustaining voice (especially on softer tones), an increase in recovery time, loss of vocal range, vocal fatigue or pain after performance, and unsteady passaggio. The referral to the otolaryngologist may come directly from the teacher of singing or vocal coach. Once assessed by the otolaryngologist, the individual is then referred to the voice pathologist to interpret and describe stroboscopic findings. The findings may indicate a muscle tension dysphonia. Voice therapy then would be recommended to focus on a return to a healthy laryngeal function in both speech and singing.

Voice Pedagogy-Voice Pathology-Otolaryngology

Over the last 20 years, teachers of singing and vocal coaches have worked closely with trained speech-language pathologists who have specialized in the area of voice, particularly if a voice lab is within the same city or in one nearby. Some voice labs offer stroboscopic screenings for freshman vocal or theatrical majors to serve as a baseline. In most voice labs throughout the United States, the voice pathologist performs the videolaryngostroboscopic examination, interprets the findings, and reviews these results with the otolaryngologist. By establishing these close professional working relationships, the teacher of singing or vocal coach may refer directly to the voice pathologist when the performer is having vocal problems. Often, the individuals have not seen an otolaryngologist; therefore, medical referral would then come from the voice pathologist.

Otolaryngology-Voice Pedagogy

The performer may be on the road, traveling to different cities, when a vocal problem develops. An otolaryngologist may see the performer and treat the problem medically if needed. The performer's problem may be with vocal technique or style. Performers generally study or have studied with a teacher of singing or vocal coach. It would be appropriate for the otolaryngologist to refer back to the voice pedagogue to address issues of technique; changes in style, repertoire or environmental conditions; and to evaluate preexisting conditions that are or have been troublesome for the individual. The voice pedagogue can offer suggestions on vocal rehearsals, vocal use, and vocal warm-ups.

Voice Pathologist-Voice Pedagogy

The performer may have worked or is currently working with a voice pathologist for vocal rehabilitation and wants to return to performing. Once the underlying condition that caused or contributed to the dysphonia improves, it is appropriate for the voice pathologist to refer to the voice pedagogue for assessment of the singing or acting voice. This is recommended to prevent future injury to the voice during performance.

Common Etiologic Factors

Personality Factors

Intense, volatile, excitable, emotional, neurotic, anxious, temperamental, moody, intemperate, vain, and unstable are all terms that Punt used when describing the personalities of professional actors and singers.[14] Although these personality attributes also have been described as necessary for the successful artist, a person's emotional or mental state will have an effect on vocal production. Weiner supported this view when he stated that the human voice is one of the most accurate and sensitive indicators of the state of a personality; it tends to mirror what is happening in a person's life.[15(p67)]

Punt further suggested that the direct relationship between emotions and voice quality by observing that in times of extreme stress, even the trained voice user will project emotional problems into the voice.[14] The vocal mechanism may even be perfectly healthy and free of visible pathology, but its precision of movement may be adversely affected by the state of mind and the emotions of the owner of the voice.

Many of these personality factors are also present in many "unartistic" professional voice users. For example, salespeople are often described as hard driving, intense, and fast talking. Ministers may be subjected to emotional strain by the personal needs and problems of congregational members. Physicians may be under stress by the demands of patients and their families and the huge responsibility of controlling their health and well-being, such as when dealing closely with death. Educators and lecturers may be intense or even anxious about their teaching responsibilities. They may also be worried about receiving good evaluations to secure their jobs or promotions. In short, inherent personality characteristics, which are to some extent demanded of professional voice users, along with the anxieties and stresses created by the various professional challenges, may all contribute to the development of a voice disorder.

Phonotrauma

Individuals who use their voices professionally are subject to the same vocal misuses and phonotraumatic behaviors as those found in the general speaking public. The overall effect that phonotraumatic behaviors have on the livelihood of the professional voice user is more detrimental. For example, the laryngeal changes associated with shouting at a football or basketball game would not be the same for the professional and nonprofessional voice users. Let us speculate that a mild edema and erythema developed resulting in a mild-to-moderate dysphonia. The nonprofessional voice user would be able to return to work the next day with no ill effect on job performance, whereas the professional voice user may suffer the consequences of a missed performance, a lost sale, an inadequate public appeal, and so forth.

Another factor associated with phonotrauma and professional voice users is the unique, itinerant lifestyle they live. Inherent in the lifestyles of many public "performers" are periods of socializing and other extraneous activities that may contribute to vocal hyperfunction. These activities may include talking over noise in the hustle and bustle of the backstage area following a performance, loud talking during postperformance dinners and parties, or unusual vocal demands created by frequent appearances that take place in noisy public forums for promotional purposes.

Phonotrauma and vocal misuse behaviors may also occur during performances. Many singers and actors have highly trained voices, but others may be guilty of using inappropriate vocal techniques. These inappropriate uses of the vocal components may be present while singing musical parts not suited to the artist's voice, while using poor respiratory support for a particular role, or while singing or speaking with an improper tone focus. Although loud singing and stage shouting need not be vocally abusive, they often create vocal problems in the untrained voice. When these activities do cause vocal problems, the difficulties usually are the result of a lack of abdominal and diaphragmatic breath support, the use of hard glottal attacks, and a general constriction of the upper vocal tract. Training to promote an open front focus using abdominal and diaphragmatic breath support in the speaking voice is beneficial for the singer, actor, and nonprofessional voice user.

By the nature of their acting roles, actors often work in less than optimal conditions on stage. Some theaters are designed with appropriate acoustics, whereas others place more demands on the human voice. Volatile or emotional character portrayals can be potentially harmful even to the trained "vocal athlete." Many are requested to scream, cry, shriek, cough, gasp, and so forth, in addition to competing with various accompanying background music, noises, and sounds. Costumes and makeup may place added restrictions, creating limited mobility and requiring more demand on the voice.[16]

Assessment of vocal technique by a trained acting-voice trainer on body alignment, body tension, breath support, relaxation, and isolation of the articulators, forward placement, and presentation style is essential to develop and maintain a healthy acting voice. The actor must be aware and note areas of body tension, such as locked knees, clenched jaw, relaxed abdominal breathing, and proper alignment of the head being balanced over a lengthened and relaxed neck and spine. A projected voice should be produced with relaxed articulators and a forward resonating focus, connecting the breath through the vocal tract without muscular tension.[17]

Another potential form of vocal abuse in the singer is the use of a singing technique known as belting. Belting is often used in theatrical shows for projection of the voice. The belted singing voice is produced at a high-intensity level with strong vocal fold adduction. As long as the respiratory effort is adequate to support the voice and the supraglottic structures are not constricted, belting is not abusive. Vocal problems occur when the respiratory effort is inadequate for the high-intensity level causing constriction of the entire upper airway. Numerous popular singers have constructed successful careers using this form of singing, but many others have suffered harsh vocal consequences as a result of this form of laryngeal hyperfunction.

After a big performance, voice rest or vocal naps (short periods of no talking throughout the day) over a 2- or 3-day period is recommended to allow for healing. Longevity of the voice may depend on the need to incorporate a vocal recovery period and take time for tissue regeneration.[18]

Phonotrauma may also be related to environmental conditions in which the performer works. For example, the classical singer may be forced to compete with an overly enthusiastic and loud orchestra in a hall with limited or poor acoustics and a musty back stage area. Rock singers often compete with the high-intensity levels of their own heavily amplified electronic instruments. Other entertainers sing or perform in small clubs with dense ambient smoke and must compete with noisy patrons and poor amplification. Actors compete with various special effects, such as smoke and background noises. Considering the environments in which many professionals are asked to perform, it is surprising that more voice disorders do not occur.

Other less "public" professional voice users have their own forms of vocal abuse. Examples include:

- teachers who shout during playground, cafeteria, or bus duty
- salespeople who often hold business meetings or make sales presentations over lunch in noisy restaurants
- ministers who give sermons at the top of their loudness range without the aid of a microphone
- politicians who present frequently in various surroundings without the use of a microphone.

Many salespeople use a pseudo-authoritative voice with greater vocal effort. Continued use of this hyperfunctional voice will often lead to laryngeal pathology.

In concluding this section on phonotrauma and the professional voice user, it is strongly suggested that the voice pathologist consider the obvious when evaluating these patients. Common vocal behaviors can contribute to voice problems in any speakers, including professional speakers. Shouting at children, pets, or during sporting events, talking loudly to a hard-of-hearing relative, constant throat clearing, persistent coughing, grunting during exercise such as weight lifting, prolonged talking; abusive laughter, and shouting in anger: All of these behaviors are just as likely to occur in the professional as in the nonprofessional voice user.

Drugs

Side effects of many medications can be detrimental to the professional voice user.[19] Many factors (such as age, gender, body composition, metabolism, and concurrent administration of other medications) can influence a person's response to a medication. Some individuals are very sensitive to minimum dosing levels; therefore, finding the correct dosage for the performer is critical to prevent or reduce possible side effects that may affect the voice.[20,21] There are a number of prescription medicines and over-the-counter agents that can adversely affect the voice.[21,22] (See also Chapter 4.)

Recreational drugs, such as alcohol, cigarettes, marijuana, and cocaine, have significant adverse effects on voice production. All of these agents are irritating to the respiratory tract and larynx and may contribute to the development of voice disorders. Some of the reasons given by professional voice users for using these abusive agents include:

- stress and pressures of auditions and subsequent rejection
- stress of giving performances that will always please the audiences
- tight schedules that yield minimal time for relaxation
- difficult personal relationships
- individual emotional conflicts.

In addition to these reasons, it is fair to say that our culture has influenced the use of alcohol and "recreational" drugs not only in this population, but also in the general population.

Alcohol is abusive both as a local oral and laryngeal irritant and as a vasodilator of the mucosal lining of the larynx. The effect of vasodilatation is drying of the mucous membrane that increases the likelihood of vocal fold hemorrhage during phonation. Excessive consumption of alcohol may lead to a chronic dysphonia, which has been commonly described as a "gin" or "whiskey" voice.[23] Caffeine is also a vasodilator and has a dehydrating effect on the mucosal membrane. It is found in products such as coffee, tea, soda, chocolate, and prescription and nonprescription drugs. Excessive caffeine intake can lead to thick, sticky mucus that accumulates on the true vocal fold surface. Thick mucus on the vocal folds can lead to chronic habitual throat clearing or coughing. Cigarette and marijuana smoke are both irritants of the respiratory tract and larynx. Both types of smoke dry out the mucosal lining of the larynx, causing mild edema and erythema. This laryngeal condition causes an increased sensitivity that often creates excessive coughing, which is also vocally abusive. Cocaine is also a local irritant that produces changes in the nasal, pharyngeal, and laryngeal mucosal linings.

Hydration

Hydration is extremely important for optimal mucosal wave vibration and performance of the entire laryngeal system. Systemic tissue hydration is necessary for the three subsystems of voice to work efficiently and without effort to produce voice. The body functions optimally when it is adequately hydrated. Dehydration causes depletion of moisture content at the cellular level, and systemic dehydration can augment the problem. We can use the late Dr Van Lawrence's axiom, "sing wet and pee pale" as a rule of thumb in monitoring one's degree of internal systemic hydration. For adults, two liters of water is recommended for adequate daily consumption.

Verdolini-Marston et al [24] manipulated conditions of hydration (no-treatment, hydrated, and slightly dehydrated) and found phonation threshold pressure, especially for higher pitches, decreased in the hydrated condition. Highest phonation threshold pressures were found for the dry condition, especially at low pitches. Hydration is also an important ingredient for treatment of nodules and polyps during therapy, with greater improvement seen following hydration.[25] The inverse relation between phonatory effort and hydration levels, especially for high pitches, was observed in a double blind, placebo-controlled study.[26] Increased perturbation measures were recorded following inhalation of dry air.[27] These studies support the clinical findings of a relationship between hydration and vocal performance and relative humidity and vocal performance.

Common Pathologies

The professional voice user may be susceptible to developing all types of laryngeal pathologies, but functional pathologies are most likely to occur because of improper or excessive use of voice. These common pathologies include acute and chronic noninfectious laryngitis, vocal nodules, vocal fold polyps, contact ulcers or granulomas, gastroesophageal reflux disease, laryngeal fatigue, vocal fold cysts, and vascular pathologies.

Acute and Chronic Noninfectious Laryngitis

On examining the causes of all laryngeal pathologies in the professional voice user, it is most important to determine whether the cause is long-standing and frequently occurring or simply an acute occurrence. Acute noninfectious laryngitis is usually the result of an unusual, short-term period of vocal misuse. It may result from shouting, vocal enthusiasm at a sporting event, singing out of the optimum range, or consuming an unusual amount of alcohol, caffeine, and cigarettes in a short period of time.

During acute laryngitis, the vocal folds usually have a dull pink color or a thickened, sticky mucous lining. The major symptoms may vary from mild to a severe dysphonia characterized by hoarseness, lowered pitch, and impairment in the vocal range. Singers with acute laryngitis demonstrate difficulty in achieving the upper parts of their ranges, especially at low-intensity levels.

Treatments for acute laryngitis include elimination or modification of the causes, steam inhalation, and short-term voice rest when possible. Voice rest permits the laryngeal muscles and the mucosal lining to rebound from the acute abuse. Continued speaking or singing in the presence of the pathology may lead to more serious pathologies, such as submucosal hemorrhages or nodules.

Chronic abuse or misuse of the laryngeal mechanism may lead to the development of chronic noninfectious laryngitis. This laryngeal pathology is usually indicative of a long history of vocal difficulties. The vocal characteristics of the chronic condition are similar to acute laryngitis; the dysphonic quality is more permanent and resistive to change. The long-term voice misuse causes a drying of the mucous membrane and a more persistent voice fatigue than does the acute condition.

Typical treatment for both acute and chronic laryngitis involves a short period of vocal rest or incorporation of vocal "naps" throughout the day, followed by identification and modification of the causative factors. When a performance or presentation cannot be postponed, it is possible for the otolaryngologist to prepare the patient for the performance with the use of laryngeal spray solutions or corticosteroids that diminish laryngeal sensitivity and reduce congestion and edema. This treatment is usually considered if a period of vocal rest is available after the performance.[14] Because of the high risk of more serious laryngeal damage, this treatment is only used when it is absolutely necessary that the patient perform.

The effects of a dysphonic voice quality caused by noninfectious chronic laryngitis may have serious implications on the livelihoods of some individuals. Others, however, have used their voice disorders to their advantage by developing distinctive vocal characteristics. More often, the long-term vocal effects of chronic laryngitis lead to the premature end of a performance career or a reduction in earning capabilities.

Vocal Nodules

To the professional voice user, one of the most frightening of all laryngeal pathologies, and the bane of all professionals singers, is vocal nodules. We suspect that this fear is present mainly because nodules are one of the most common and most discussed pathologies even among people with a relative naivete regarding voice disorders. Indeed, it is not unusual for even the most trained professional singer to develop small bilateral nodules during particularly forceful singing.

The voice symptoms of vocal nodules are variable depending on their size, duration of existence, and mechanical effects on phonation. Efforts to produce normal phonation in the presence of nodules leads to forceful methods of phonation causing voice fatigue and often an inappropriate constriction of the supraglottic structures. Higher tones are most adversely affected, especially when produced at lower intensity levels. Glottal closure is generally hourglass in shape, causing airflow leak. Phonation breaks, breathiness, decreased frequency range, and decreased maximum sustained phonation usually occur when nodules are of moderate size or larger. Fibrous nodules create greater stiffness in vibration with decreased amplitude of vibration and mucosal wave.

The treatment of vocal nodules again involves identification and modification of their causes. Along with traditional vocal hygiene counseling, much emphasis is placed on patient education and counseling regarding the impact of nodules on the patient's career. Often, the anxiety level expressed by the patient as a result of the pathology is much higher than the pathology warrants. With the patient's complete cooperation, nodules often may be resolved quickly and effectively with minimal career interruption. Frankly, it is often much easier to modify the causes of vocal nodules than to reverse the long-standing causes of chronic laryngitis.

The voice diagnostic examination may occasionally fail to identify any possible causes for the development of vocal nodules, especially in singers. When causes cannot be identified, evaluation of the singing technique by a competent vocal coach is appropriate. It is not the voice pathologist's role to evaluate artistic techniques or abilities. If the vocal coach or singing teacher finds the technique faulty, then voice lessons designed to improve vocal technique are advised.

Vocal nodules occur more often in the untrained singing voice than in the classically trained voice. Some pop and rock singers have capitalized on dysphonic voice qualities; others agonize over their inability to produce adequate phonation. Resolution of the nodules through traditional voice therapy along with vocal training becomes essential for many untrained singers who wish to continue their careers. Although voice therapy is not long term (approximately 3 months or less), the patient must often sacrifice some performance time to restore voice quality. However, it is better to sacrifice a little time for concentrated voice training to resolve the problem than to continue the vocal struggles. A little time taken now may help to ensure a long career. The alternative may be no career at all.

Peppard et al[28] compared singers and nonsingers with vocal fold nodules to control groups of singers and nonsingers and found the trained singers without nodules to perform superiorly in all tasks. The singers with nodules were found to have smaller nodules with less impairment of vibratory function and less severe vocal symptoms than their nonsinging counterparts. The singers with nodules also performed better on frequency range and maximum phonation time tasks, compared with the nonsingers with nodules, but not as well as normal singers. Singers with vocal problems probably tend to seek evaluation sooner because their vocal demands would show a diminution in performance

Surgery is occasionally recommended for the excision of vocal nodules, but as a rule of thumb, surgery should be avoided on professionals' vocal folds if at all possible. Although the physical risks of the surgery may be minimal, the psychological effects could be most damaging. Some patients are reluctant to return to full vocal use for fear of redeveloping the laryngeal pathology. Their fear is often so strong that even though the laryngeal mechanisms are normal, the patients will not use full voice. Of course, this fear jeopardizes their careers. Vocal fold surgery performed without strong counseling from the surgeon or voice pathologist is not advised. Even when surgery is performed, the causes of the pathology must be modified to reduce the possibility of recurrence, and the patient must also follow a plan for successful return to normal phonation.

Contact Ulcers and Granulomas

Contact ulcers occur most commonly in male public speakers, teachers, sales representatives, politicians, and actors. Contact ulcers can result from a grinding, hammering action of the vocal processes of the arytenoid cartilages. These actions occur during the repeated use of a loud, low-pitched, pseudo-authoritative voice, which is often used to project a desired masculine or authority image. The mild-to-moderate dysphonia that is a result of slowly developing granulomas is characterized by a low pitch and huskiness. Other factors also associated with the development of contact ulcers involve cigarette smoking, excessive alcohol and caffeine consumption, and reflux of stomach acids into the posterior laryngeal area. Contact ulcers are most effectively treated by retraining the appropriate use of the vocal components of pitch and loudness. Reduction or elimination of alcohol, caffeine, and smoking is also strongly advised. If reflux is the cause of contact ulcers and granulomas, then an antireflux regimen with medical management is recommended. These patients will need to be monitored closely until the resolution of the pathology.

Gastroesophageal Reflux Disease (GERD) and Laryngopharyngeal Reflux (LPR)

Probably the most underdiagnosed and most common gastrointestinal problem that affects professional voice users is gastroesophageal reflux disease. Incidence of 7% to 10% of the population has been reported in the literature.[29] Professional and nonprofessional voice users are prone to many of the precipitating factors that promote reflux. See listed symptoms and precipitating factors in Chapter 4. Many singers or actors prefer to eat a minimal amount of food prior to a performance. They may then eat a larger meal after the performance, late in the evening. Some individuals may over-eat and then go to bed with a full stomach. When in a reclined body position, the larynx, esophagus, and stomach are on the same plane, and the gastric contents from the stomach may reflux all the way to the posterior laryngeal area. Foods that reportedly promote reflux include coffee (caffeinated or decaffeinated), sodas, chocolate, high-fat foods, citrus beverages, tomato products, spicy foods, and alcohol. Smoking and weight gain also have been shown to increase reflux. Other contributing factors include stress and poor sleep habits.

Possible physiological etiologies of gastroesophageal reflux include a hiatal hernia, lower esophageal sphincter dysfunction, and esophageal dysmotility. Individuals complain of heartburn and acid regurgitation and report a burning or bitter taste in the throat. Some patients will report a sensation of a feeling of a "lump" in the throat or present with symptoms of chronic cough (nonproductive), hoarseness, chronic throat clearing with little mucus production, and chest pain or discomfort. Singers report any of the above symptoms but may experience difficulty singing higher notes or have a decrease in their frequency range. Others may report a history of chronic laryngitis. It is also noted that prevalence of acid reflux has been implicated in the pathogenesis of vocal fold nodules[30] as well as posterior laryngitis,[31-33] subglottic stenosis,[34] and contact ulcer and granuloma.[35]

Physical examination of the larynx may show erythematous arytenoids,[36] small contact ulcerations, or granuloma in the vocal process area. The most commonly observed changes involve a thickening or mounding of tissue (pachydermia), an opalescence coloration to the tissue in the interarytenoid space, or both. A cobblestone appearance to the tissue in the posterior laryngeal area may occur directly superior to the esophageal inlet. The true vocal folds may appear edematous and erythematous. The amplitude of vibration and mucosal wave can range from mildly to severely decreased.

Treatment includes dietary restrictions (avoiding foods that are acidic or are irritants) and behavioral lifestyle changes. Lifestyle changes involve weight reduction (if necessary), avoidance of overeating or eating late at night (not within 3-4 hours of bedtime), smoking cessation, elevating the head of the bed or use of a wedge-shaped pillow, and taking an antacid between meals and before bedtime. Patients are strongly advised to follow these restrictions in addition to taking their prescribed medicine as directed by the physician. If a conservative approach is not effective in treatment (approximately 3-month trial), additional medical tests may be ordered. These may include ambulatory 24-hour double probe pH monitoring to measure frequency and duration of gastric reflux into the esophagus, barium esophagram with fluoroscopy, or direct endoscopy. If patients report pain in the substernal area (region of the lower esophageal sphincter), a gastroenterological workup may be necessary.

The combination of medical, dietary, and lifestyle changes in conjunction with voice therapy is highly successful in the treatment of laryngopharyngeal reflux.[37] Voice therapy is beneficial to ensure easy onset of phonation when speaking. Retraining singing habits to eliminate initial hard onsets during singing may also need to be addressed. Recommending the use of an amplification device is also helpful to increase vocal volume and avoid overadduction of the vocal folds.

Vocal Fatigue

As reported in Chapter 4, it is possible that pathological conditions of the larynx, voice misuse, or voice overuse will lead to vocal fatigue. The singer or actor with symptoms of vocal fatigue will complain about a lack of consistency in the quality of the vocal output, decreased endurance, loss of frequency and intensity control, and complaints of effortful, unstable, and ineffective voice production. In both the speaker and the singer, discomfort and muscular aching in the laryngeal area are often present.

Theories about the existence of laryngeal muscle fatigue have been reported for many years, giving rise to the term laryngeal myasthenia. As stated in Chapter 4, this term reflects the sensations of tiredness that the patient reports following vocalization. Punt[14] attempted to categorize what he described as a muscular disorder of the larynx into three groups: acute, subacute, and chronic myasthenia.

Acute myasthenia was described as being caused by a brief period of severe vocal misuse and abuse. Edema and erythema of the mucosal lining of the vocal folds may also accompany the myasthenia. Subacute myasthenia was described as having many causes. Punt[14] suggested these causes include long-term vocal misuse, emotional difficulties, coughing, throat clearing, and overwork of the voice. He also suggested that the lack of preseason vocal training could lead to subacute myasthenia. This would be comparable to the football player who puts on the pads and equipment and takes part in a full-scale scrimmage the first day of training camp. More than likely the player would experience muscle strain, soreness, or even a pulled leg muscle. Because the larynx is also a muscular system, Punt hypothesized that attempting to sing or act without proper conditioning after an extended layoff would cause a subacute weakness. Chronic myasthenia was described as having the same causes as the subacute type. The difference was in the length of time that the causes were present. In chronic myasthenia, the voice user continues the same improper vocal habits over many years, creating the possibility of a more permanent laryngeal muscle weakness, which is also more resistant to change.

Discussion of laryngeal pathologies typically focuses on what the eye can see. The presence or absence of mucosal change or growths is described. The discussion of laryngeal fatigue attempts to describe the changes in the balance of the three subsystems of voice production: respiration, phonation, and resonance. Evaluation of this disorder is therefore limited to the patient's history, as well as laryngeal videostroboscopy. Vibratory patterns of the vocal folds as observed through stroboscopy will often demonstrate underlying vocal incoordination through the observance of out-of-phase vibrations and incomplete glottic closure,[38] as well as high airflow rates and decreased maximum phonation times.[39] In the case of laryngeal fatigue, the underlying causes of the disorder (ie, imbalance of the voice subsystems), not the apparent vocal symptoms, must be treated. The voice user must understand that the voice mechanism requires daily care. It must be trained, warmed up, cooled down, and kept in shape in much the same manner as the legs of a dancer or the arm of a baseball pitcher.

Treatment of voice fatigue in the professional voice user involves identification of the underlying causes and then modification or elimination of those causes. The voice pathologist may choose to initiate direct Vocal Function Exercises for balancing the three subsystems of voice production, Resonant Voice Therapy, or both to promote an open frontal focus (see Chapter 7). When significant progress has been made in improving voice production, the patient may be reintroduced to professional voice use.

Vocal Fold Hemorrhage and Vascular Pathologies

Vocal fold hemorrhages result from a rupture of a blood vessel within the vocal fold. Hemorrhages can be caused by internal or external laryngeal trauma. A sudden vocal quality change is the most common symptom; however, a more permanent dysphonia may result if submucosal scarring develops following the resolution of the hematoma.[40] Professional singers may observe immediate changes with a reduction in pitch range or a development of an "edge" to the voice. As the blood disperses into the submucosal tissue, it creates a mass effect, causing a decrease in amplitude and mucosal wave. Unilateral and bilateral hemorrhages can result.[41] Other professional voice users may note progressive hoarseness over a period of days, vocal fatigue, or both.

Professional voice users may be more susceptible to vocal injury secondary to vocal demand and strain placed on the voice. They also may seek medical treatment immediately because they feel and hear even a slight aberrant vocal change that may not be apparent to others. Hemorrhages result from harsh coughing;

throat clearing; sneezing; yelling; forceful singing; shearing effect from an existing mass lesion such as a cyst, or vascular insults; inflammatory changes; and blunt external injury to the larynx. Increased risks are greater in individuals who use aspirin, ibuprofen, or other medications that alter blood clotting abilities.[40] Other risk factors that have been associated with vocal fold hemorrhage involve hormonal influences. Hormonal imbalances among women including abnormal menstrual cycles, use of estrogen supplements, gynecological surgery, and use of birth control pills,[42] as well anecdotal reported premenstrual and early menstrual hormonal changes,[24] have influenced the development of vocal fold hemorrhages.

Treatment for recovery from a vocal fold hemorrhage is complete vocal rest for 1 week. Singers are advised to significantly reduce voice use and seek medical advice if a sudden quality change occurs during a performance. Individuals can often return to their prehemorrhagic vocal quality if early diagnosis is made and the person is compliant with absolute voice rest. Limited use of the speaking voice may resume 1 to 2 weeks following complete voice rest. Routine voice therapy and singing lessons are recommended following resolution of the hemorrhage to address the phonotraumatic behaviors that caused the problem and to address maladaptive compensatory behaviors that may be present secondary to the injury. For full recovery, singers may be restricted from singing for 6 weeks.[40,43] Hemorrhages that result from the presence of a mass lesion take longer to heal and recover. Although rare, sometimes a hemorrhage needs evacuation of the hematoma, especially when enlarged vessels are involved.[44]

Several vascular lesions other than vocal fold hemorrhages can present problems for professional voice users (Figure 8-1). These include:

- vascular dilatation arising form a thickened capillary located on the vibratory edge or on the superior surface of the true vocal folds (Figure 8-2)
- capillary ectasia, which is a varicose dilation of the capillaries of the vocal fold (Figure 8-3)
- hemangioma presenting as a purplish red, firm mass that can be either sessile or pedunculated

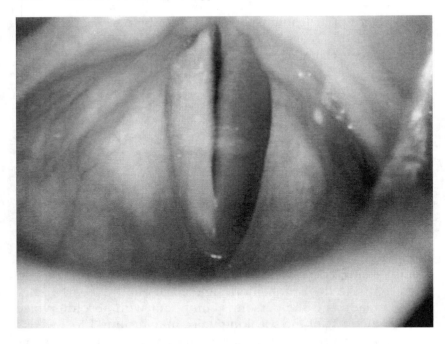

Figure 8-1. Hemorrhage of the left vocal fold during phonation. Reprinted with permission from Abitbol.[44]

Singers may not have any vocal problems if small capillary ectasia exists on the superior surface of the true focal folds away from the vibrating free edge; however, larger capillary ectasia and hemangioma may have significant effects on the vocal quality. Videostroboscopy is an essential tool for distinguishing the vascular lesion(s) and necessary for developing a plan of treatment. Abitbol[44] reported that most of the patients treated with capillary ectasia were female professional singers who were involved with increased strain and hormonal problems

> A 22-year-old singer had been experiencing vocal difficulties for several months. Her chief complaints were inability to consistently sing the high notes in her range and increased breathiness when singing higher notes. She complained of not being able to hold the higher notes as long in duration as compared with the lower notes. Her range was becoming narrower. Longer warm-ups were needed, and

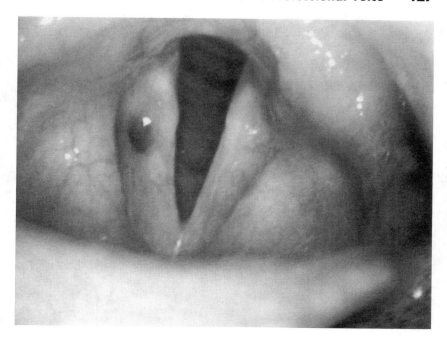

Figure 8-2. Angioma of the superior surface of the right vocal fold. Reprinted with permission from Abitbol.[44]

she was having difficulty singing softly and initiating a tone. She complained of a feeling of increased mucus and vocal fatigue with use. A videostroboscopic examination revealed a questionable right intracordal cyst with accompanying capillary ectasia. Increased edema and erythema was observed bilaterally with contralateral nodular tissue thickening. Mucus started to accumulate on the vocal fold surface after sustained phonation. A posterior glottal chink was observed for sustained lower pitches, whereas an hourglass glottal closure was observed for sustained higher pitches. Under simulated slow-motion stroboscopy, the amplitude of vibration was moderately decreased on the right and mildly to moderately decreased on the left. The mucosal wave was moderately to severely decreased on the right and mildly to moderately decreased on the left. An open phase predominated during the vibratory cycle, and the symmetry of vibration was irregular during the initiation and ending of phonation, as well as during changes in pitch and loudness.

Because of the increased edema and erythema and uncertainty of a possible underlying cyst, the otolaryngologist and voice pathologist

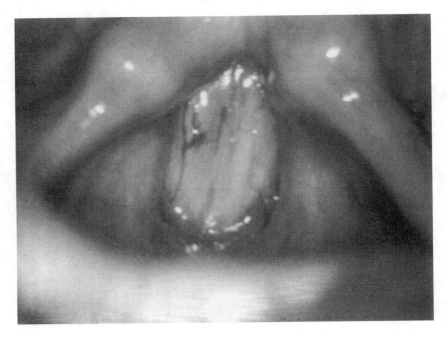

Figure 8-3. Microvarices: ectasia on the right vocal fold. Reprinted with permission from Abitbol.[44]

recommended a 4- to 5-week period of trial voice therapy with a repeat videostroboscopy in 5 weeks. The individual was enrolled in voice therapy consisting of a hydration program, vocal hygiene counseling including no singing, Resonant Vocal Therapy, and Vocal Function Exercises. A repeat videostrobe was performed the 5th week following the initiation of therapy. Results showed that with no edema and erythema present, an intracordal cyst was evident with prominent capillary ectasia and feeder vessel to the area of the cyst. The contralateral nodular thickness was significantly reduced in size. The individual was taken into surgery for a microlaryngoscopy to remove the right true vocal fold cyst and for superficial laser vaporization of the dilated vessel. Great care was taken not to disrupt the vibrating free edge of the vocal fold.

The individual was placed on 7 days of complete voice rest following surgery with a strict hydration program of drinking at least 2 liters of water daily. Voice therapy resumed 1 week following surgery with light humming and Resonant Voice Therapy. Conservative voice use was recommended for the 2nd week following surgery. The individual was reintroduced to the Vocal Function Exercises the second week following surgery. She started vocal lessons the 4th week following surgery. This was in addition to seeing the voice pathologist. She started back singing 6 weeks following surgery.

Supportive Training and Techniques

Throughout the years, a number of philosophical techniques have been written about and presented to focus on effective and efficient use of coordinated movements. These include:

- The Alexander Technique
- The Linklater Method
- The Feldenkrais Method®
- The Lessac System

Trained instructors have continued to pass these techniques to others throughout the decades. Many vocal teachers and vocal coaches, as well as performers, have been trained in these techniques. The underlying philosophical concept is based on establishing a balance and integration between the mind and body that permits physiologic freedom of movement during performance. The term "movement" is used in a generic sense and encompasses everything people do. These techniques incorporate auditory, visual, and kinesthetic awareness to attain self-discovery of freedom of movement. Increasing one's awareness of what facilitates beneficial and natural movement on a conscious level is paramount to influence changes at all levels. Only after a conscious level of self-discovery of ease of total function can one achieve a state of unconscious acts of repetition that will allow for effortless performance. In a performer it is the coordinated and integrated movement of the emotional, physical, and artistic demands on the voice in synchrony that must be met. Professionals have refined movements that appear effortless and natural to their audiences. The following are general descriptions of these techniques.

Alexander Technique

Frederick Matthias Alexander (1869-1955) of Australia was a professional Shakespearean actor. During his career, he repeatedly developed laryngitis while performing. He wrote of "gasping" and "sucking in air," and his breathing became audible during his recitations. Despite medical treatment and vocal training, nothing helped. He sought to self-analyze his technique of delivery. While practicing in front of a mirror, he discovered that increased muscular tension contributed to his vocal problems. Throughout the years, he discovered that proper alignment of the head, neck, and torso was critical to every body activity. From his work, he developed a hands-on teaching method that promoted balance, support, and coordination through freedom of movement. He began teaching his method to singers and actors in London in the 1890s. This technique has helped instrumentalists, dancers, singers, actors, and athletes. It can be incorporated into all facets of one's life.[45]

The Alexander Technique focuses on developing awareness and consciously controlling bodily movements to allow for integration and coordination of the mind and body to perform activities without effort and muscular tension. Alexander believed that habituated maladaptive habits limited and impaired coordinated movement and postural patterns and even impeded learning. These unconscious habits alter sensory feedback and change perceptions and feelings, which affect people both physically and mentally in everything they do. Alexander's "respiratory re-education" focuses on proper body alignment and coordination of breathing and vocalization with ease. For additional reading on the development of the technique and Alexander's self-discoveries, the reader is directed to the text *Alexander Technique: The Essential Writings of F. Matthias Alexander.*[46]

One learns the mind-body integration of whole patterns of coordinated movement and body alignment through the guidance of certified instructors. Hands-on guidance helps the individual experience the freedom of a more natural movement without the interference of maladaptive habituated patterning, thus allowing for sensory internalization of ease of coordinated movement.

Certified instructors of the Alexander Technique in the United States can be obtained through two professional organizations: North American Society for the Teachers of the Alexander Technique or Alexander Technique International.

The Linklater Method

Actress Kristin Linklater trained and studied under Iris Warren at the London Academy of Music and Dramatic Art in England. In 1963, she came to the United States and has since trained numerous teachers, actors, directors, and public speakers. Liberating our "natural" voices minus tension and habituated patterns is the basic premise of her designed approach. It is assumed that all individuals have a voice capable of performance through a two-to-four octave natural pitch range. It is also assumed that as humans, we have physiological tensions and psychological inhibitory responses that impair the ability of the natural voice to perform.

Emphasis on mind-body unity through physical awareness and relaxation unravels the habitual patterns that impede the natural voice. Linklater stated, "breath and sound must always be connected to thought and feeling so that the two processes work simultaneously to activate and release inner impulses and to dissolve physical blocks."[47(p. 2)] Her method incorporates combining imagery and imagination to achieve a sound that is produced freely under any conditions. Emphasis is placed on awareness of postural alignment, breath support, relaxation of the articulators, resonance to enhance vocal range, and bridging the voice to acting "speaking the text."[47]

The Feldenkrais Method®

Moshe Feldenkrais (1904-1984), born in Russia, held mechanical and electrical engineering degrees, as well as a doctor of science in physics from the Sorbonne in Paris. He had an interest in athletics and earned a black belt in judo. Suffering from a serious knee injury, which lead him to study human anatomy, psychology, and physiology, he developed a method of self-aware coordinated mind-body exercises. A type of supportive therapy, the individual becomes aware of his or her own movement and functioning, including habituated tensions and rigidity, and learns new ways of coordinated patterning that enhances overall efficiency and improves muscular function with greater effectiveness. One aims to achieve movement with minimal effort and maximum efficiency.

There are two modalities to learning in the Feldenkrais Method: Functional Integration® and Awareness Through Movement.®[48-50] Functional Integration involves noninvasive, hands-on body manipulations performed while sitting, standing, or lying down. These body manipulations help the individual learn and feel appropriate movements through tactile and kinesthetic input that are inhibitory and increase overall bodily functioning. Once internalized, the individual can focus attention to habituated tense movement and cognitively change positioning to the newly acquired neuromuscular patterning that is free of tension and rigidity.

Awareness Through Movement involves verbal instruction of sequential movements in basic body positions of sitting, standing, or lying on the floor. The instructor focuses on self-awareness through sensations and how to achieve improved motor functioning with comfort and ease and abandon habitual patterns. The goal is to improve flexibility and coordination in all movement.

The Lessac System

Arthur Lessac studied at the Eastman School of Music in Rochester, New York, and is a professor emeritus of Theatre at the State University of New York at Binghamton. Renowned both as an actor and as a singer, his method strives to cultivate awareness or attention in coordinating mind and body. The performer must "physically experience the feeling while at the very same time behaviorally feeling the experience."[51(p1)] Training focuses on kinesthetic awareness where the performer is requested to physically feel and cognitively process vocal sounds replacing habituated behaviors.

According to Lessac,[51] there are four concepts that are essential for the performer. These include: (1) body esthetics,

(2) inner harmonic sensing, (3) organic instructions, and (4) the "familiar event" principle. Body esthetics focuses on sensations and expanding awareness such as bodily feelings or sounds of being open, flowing, and rhythmic versus closed, turbulent, or rigid. Internal bodily processing provided with integration from the five senses of hearing, feeling, tasting, seeing, and smelling, creates an intrinsic harmonious feeling. It is through inner harmonic sensing (like a 6th sense) that performers develop intrasensitivity when engaged in a bodily activity. Organic instructions refer to the performer being in conscious control of the body and mind as to not inhibit freedom of movement. The last step is finding a number of familiar events that are pleasing and can be imaged to evoke a body action that is performed naturally without effort.

Lessac's method of producing voice requires awareness of the anatomy and the ability to produce a natural forward vowel without facial, oral, and neck tension. Tonal production relies on an awareness of a buzz or ring vibration felt on the alveolar ridge, in the nasal area, and in the forehead with effortless projection of the tone. Consonants are viewed as musical instruments. Playing the consonant, one should feel its vibrations and range. Finally, one adds meaning to each consonant and then applies that meaning to speech with emotional feelings.

Summary

This chapter serves as an overview of the professional voice user and is not meant to be all-inclusive. In the last decade, we have witnessed a strong interest in interdisciplinary research and training at the institutions that combine medicine, science, and the arts. As a result of the collaborative efforts among these disciplines, a plethora of research articles, books, videotapes, compact discs, and audiotapes are available resources for us all to use. As we proceed into the 21st century, we must continue to recognize the importance of a multidisciplinary team in providing the best care possible for the individual with vocal problems.

Glossary of
Terms Used in Singing

Allegro: quick, fast

Crescendo: gradually increasing in volume

Decrescendo: reduction in volume

Diminuendo: lessening the tone from loud to soft

Fortissimo: as loud as possible

Glissando: "gliding" to include all possible pitches between the initial and final pitch sounded

Legato: smooth and connected quality, with no noticeable interruption between the notes

Mezza voce: "half voice"; singing softly with breath support

Messa di voce: gradual swelling and diminishing of the voice (crescendo and diminuendo on a sustained tone)

Passaggio: break between vocal registers

Pianissimo: very soft

Portamento: a continuous gliding from one note to another including all intervening tones

Singer's formant: a high spectrum peak occurring between 2.3 and 3.5 kHz; a "ring" that is heard in a voice.

Overtone: partial higher than the fundamental

Vibrato: regular fluctuation in pitch, timbre, intensity, or a combination of the three

References

1. Koufman J, Isaccson G. The spectrum of vocal dysfunction In: Koufman J, Isaccson G, eds. *The Otolaryngologic Clinics of North America: Voice Disorders.* Philadelphia, Pa: WB Saunders; 1991:985-988.
2. American Speech-Language-Hearing Association. The role of the speech-language pathologist and teacher of singing in remediation of singers with voice disorders.) *ASHA.* 1993;35:63.
3. Westerman JG. What's in a name? *J Singing.* 1996;53:1-2.
4. McKinney J. Something old – something new. *J Singing.* 1997;53:1-2.
5. Khambato A. Laryngeal disorders in singers and other voice users. In: Ballantyne J, Groves J, eds. *Scott Brown's Diseases of the Ear, Nose, and Throat, Vol 4: Throat.* 4th ed. London, England: Butterworths; 1979.

6. Irving RM, Epstein R, Harries MLL. Care of the professional voice. *Clin Otolaryngol.* 1997;22:202-205.

7. Wilder C N. Speech-language pathology and the professional voice user: an overview. In: Sataloff RT, ed. *Professional Voice: The Science and Art of Clinical Care.* 2nd ed. San Diego, Calif: Singular Publishing Group; 1997: 695-698.

8. Sundberg J. *The Science of the Singing Voice.* Dekalb, Ill: Northern Illinois University Press; 1987.

9. DeJonckere PH, Hirano M, Sundberg J. *Vibrato.* San Diego, Calif: Singular Publishing Group; 1995.

10. Titze I. *Principles of Voice Production.* Englewood Cliffs, NJ: Prentice Hall; 1994.

11. Vennard W. *Singing: The Mechanism and the Technic.* New York, NY: Carl Fischer; 1968.

12. Lancer M, Syder D, Jones AS, Le Bortillier A. The outcome of different management patterns for vocal cord nodules. *J Laryngol Otol.* 1988;102:423-427.

13. Murry T, Woodson GE. A comparison of three methods for the management of vocal fold nodules. *J Voice.* 1992;6:271-276.

14. Punt N. *The Singer's and Actor's Throat: The Vocal Mechanism of the Professional Voice User and Its Care and Health in Disease.* 3rd ed. London, England: William Heinemann Medical Books; 1979.

15. Weiner H. Medical problems and treatment: panel discussion. In: Lawrence V, ed. *Transcripts of the 7th Symposium on Care of the Professional Voice Part III: Medical/Surgical Therapy.* New York, NY: The Voice Foundation; 1978.

16. Raphael BN. Special considerations relating to members of the acting profession. In: Sataloff RT, ed. *Professional Voice: The Science and Art of Clinical Care.* 2nd ed. San Diego, Calif: Singular Publishing Group; 1997:203-205.

17. Freed SL, Raphael BN, Sataloff RT. The role of the acting-voice trainer in medical care of professional voice users In: Sataloff RT, ed. *Professional Voice: The Science and Art of Clinical Care.* 2nd ed. San Diego, Calif: Singular Publishing Group; 1997:765-774.

18. Titze I. A few thoughts about longevity in singing. *NATS J.* 1994;50:36-38.

19. Martin FG. Drugs and vocal function. *J Voice.* 1988;2:338-344.

20. Sataloff RT, Lawrence VL, Hawkshaw M, Rosen DC. Medications and their effects on the voice. In: Benninger MS, Jacobson BH, Johnson AF, eds. *Vocal Arts Medicine: The Care and Prevention of Professional Voice Disorders.* New York, NY: Thieme Medical Publishers; 1994:216-225.

21. Sataloff RT, Hawkshaw M, Rosen DC. Medications: effects and side effects in professional voice users. In: Sataloff RT, ed. *Professional Voice: The Science and Art of Clinical Care.* 2nd ed. San Diego, Calif: Singular Publishing Group Inc; 1997:457-469.

22. Nair G, Sataloff RT. Vocal pharmacology: introducing the subject at Drew University. *J Singing.* 1999;55:53-63.

23. Sataloff R. *Professional Voice: The Science and Art of Clinical Care.* New York, NY: Raven Press; 1991:Chap 5.

24. Verdolini-Marston K, Titze IR, Druker DG. Changes in phonation threshold pressure with induced conditions of hydration. *J Voice.* 1990;4:142-151.

25. Verdolini-Marston K, Sandage M, Titze I. Effect of hydration treatments on laryngeal nodules and polyps and related voice measures. *J Voice.* 1994;8:30-47.

26. Verdolini K, Titze IR, Fennell A. Dependence of phonatory effort on hydration level. *J Speech Hear Res.* 1994;37:1001-1007.

27. Hemler RJB, Wieneke GH, Dejonckere PH. The effect of relative humidity of inhaled air on acoustic parameters of voice in normal subjects. *J Voice.* 1997;11:295-300.

28. Peppard RC, Bless DM, Milenkovic P. Comparison of young adult singers and nonsingers with vocal nodules. *J Voice.* 1988;2:250-260.

29. Nebel L, Forbes M, Castell D. Symptomatic gastroesophageal reflux: incidence and precipitating factors. *Am J Dig Dis.* 1976;21:953-956.

30. Kuhn J, Toohill RJ, Ulualp SO, Kulpa J, Hofmann C, Arndorfer R, Shaker R. Pharyngeal acid reflux events in patients with vocal cord nodules. *Laryngoscope.* 1998;108:1146-1149.

31. Shaker R, Milbrath M, Ren J, Toohill RJ, Hogan WJ, Li Q, Hofmann CL. Esophagopharyngeal distribution of refluxed gastric acid in patients with reflux laryngitis. *Gastroenterololgy.* 1995;109:1575-1582.

32. Koufman JA. The otolaryngologic manifestations of gastroesophageal reflux disease GERD: a clinical investigation of 225 patients using ambulatory 24 hour pH monitoring and an experimental investigation of the role of acid and pepsin in the development of laryngeal injury. *Laryngoscope.* 1991;101(suppl 53):1-78.

33. Jacob P, Kahrilas PJ, Herzon G. Proximal esophageal pH-metry in patients with reflux laryngitis. *Gastroenterology.* 1991;100:305-310.

34. Toohill RJ, Jindal JR, Gastroesophageal reflux as a cause of idiopathic subglottic stenosis. *Operative Tech Otolaryngol – Head Neck Surg.* 1997;8:149-152.

35. Ohman L, Olfsson J, Tibbling I, Ericsson G. Esophageal dysfunction in patients with contact ulcer of the larynx. *Ann Otol Rhinol Laryngol.* 1983;92:228-230.

36. Lumpkin SMM, Bishop S, Katz P. Chronic dysphonia secondary to gastroesophageal reflux disease GERD: diagnosis using simultaneous dual-probe prolonged pH monitoring. *J Voice.* 1989;3:351-355.

37. Ross J, Noordzji JP, Woo P. 1988 Voice disorders in patients with suspected laryngo-pharyngeal reflux disease. *J Voice.* 1988;12:84-88.

38. Stemple JC, Stanley J, Lee L. Objective measures of voice production in normal subjects following prolonged voice use. *J Voice.* 1995;9:127-133.

39. Eustace CS, Stemple JC, Lee L. Objective measures of voice production in patients complaining of laryngeal fatigue. *J Voice.* 1996;10:146-154.

40. Spiegel JR, Sataloff RT, Hawkshaw M, Caputo Rosen D. Vocal fold hemorrhage. In: Sataloff RT, ed. *Professional Voice: The Science and Art of Clinical Care.* 2nd ed. San Diego Calif: Singular Publishing Group; 1997:541-554.

41. Abitbol J. Vocal cord hemorrhages. *J Voice.* 1988;2:261-266.

42. Lin PT, Stern JC, Gould WJ. Risk factors and management of vocal cord hemorrhages: an experience with 44 cases. *J Voice.* 1991;5:74-77.

43. Sataloff RT. Vocal fold hemorrhage: diagnosis and treatment. *NATS J.* 1995;51:45-48.

44. Abitbol J. *Atlas of Laser Voice Surgery.* San Diego, Calif: Singular Publishing Group; 1995.

45. Conable B, Conable W. *How to Learn the Alexander Technique: A Manual for Students.* Columbus, Ohio: Andover Press; 1995.

46. Alexander FM. *Alexander Technique: The Essential Writings of F Matthias Alexander.* New York, NY; Carol Publishing Group; 1995.

47. Linklater K. *Freeing the Natural Voice.* New York, NY: Drama Book Publishers; 1976.

48. Rywerant Y. *The Feldenkrais Method: Teaching by Handling.* New Canaan, Conn: Keats Publishing; 1983.

49. Feldenkrais M. *Body and Mature Behavior.* New York, NY: International Universities Press; 1970.

50. Feldenkrais M. *Awareness Through Movement.* NewYork, NY: Harper Row; 1972.

51. Lessac A. *The Use and Training of the Human Voice: A Bio-Dynamic Approach to Vocal Life.* Mountain View, Calif: Mayfield Publishing; 1997.

9

Rehabilitation of the Laryngectomized Patient

Total rehabilitation of the laryngectomized patient involves inter-action between a number of specialists from a multidisciplinary team. The diagnosis of laryngeal cancer has a significant impact on the patient's emotional and physical health. Multimodality treatment including chemotherapy, radiation, surgery, and reha-bilitation involves various health professionals participating in the patient's progression of care. A primary participant on the team is the voice pathologist. The voice pathologist's role goes beyond basic speech retraining approaches to include both patient and family counseling. This chapter will discuss:

- methods of voice restoration for the laryngectomized patient
- physical changes following surgery
- emotional needs of the patient and significant others
- social adjustments that must also be considered for total rehabilitation.

Incidence of Laryngeal Cancer

The Surveillance Research Program of the American Cancer Society's Department of Epidemiology and Surveillance annually compiles and reports cancer incidence, mortality, and survival data for the United States and around the world.[1] Cancer statistics are also published in the journal *CA-A Cancer Journal for Clinicians*. Head and neck cancer is the sixth most common form of cancer worldwide, with oral cancer being the most common site and laryngeal cancer the second most common site within the head and neck region.[2] Laryngeal cancers make up less than 1% of all cancers and around 6% of all cancers of the respiratory system. Squamous cell carcinomas comprise 90% of head and neck cancers. Fifty-six percent of squamous cell carcinomas of the larynx occur in the glottal region, with 31% in the supraglottic larynx and approximately 1% in the subglottic larynx.[3]

The American Cancer Society estimates that 10 600 new cases of laryngeal cancer (8600 for males and 2000 for females) will occur each year in the United States.[4] The total number of estimated deaths in the United States from laryngeal cancer in 1999 was reported to be 4200 (3300 males and 900 females). The 5-year survival rate of patients with laryngeal cancer has varied little in the last 20 years. Shah et al[3] looked at 16 213 patients with laryngeal cancer and found a 5-year survival rate of 75%. Advance laryngeal disease (Stage III or IV) among these patients demonstrated less than 40% survival.

Annual global estimated figures on laryngeal cancer are 136 000 new cases and 73 500 deaths. Worldwide laryngeal cancer occurs mostly in men, with a greater male-to-female ratio (almost 7:1) than for any other site.

Etiology

The primary carcinogens for laryngeal cancer appear to be inhaled cigarette, pipe, and cigar smoke. The sites at greatest risk for developing cancer from smoking are anatomical areas that have direct exposure to the irritants. Risks of developing laryngeal carcinoma will vary depending on daily consumption, type, and manner of tobacco use.[5] A synergistic effect between tobacco use and large amounts of alcohol consumption has been reported. Alcohol appears to potentiate the cancer-causing effect of tobacco smoke, creating a significantly higher risk than if each were used alone.[6] Alcohol and tobacco consistently have been implicated as being carcinogenic, but laryngeal cancer may certainly develop in their absence.

Symptoms of Laryngeal Cancer

Cancer is the uncontrolled, rapid growth of malignant cells. As cancer cells grow and divide, they accumulate and form tumors destroying and invading normal tissue. Cancer is a pathological diagnosis and is classified by the body part in which it develops. Cancer cells can also spread to other parts of the body traveling through the bloodstream or lymphatic system. Metastasis is the spread of cancer from a primary tumor to a new site. For example, if laryngeal cancer spreads to the lymph glands in the neck, the primary site is still the larynx, with metastasis to the neck. Early identification of laryngeal carcinoma increases the chance that malignancy will remain localized and thus less difficult to treat.

The larynx can be divided into three regions: supraglottis, glottis, and subglottis. The **supraglottis** is composed of the lingual and laryngeal area of the epiglottis, laryngeal aspect of the aryepiglottic folds, arytenoids, and the ventricular folds. The **glottis** is composed of the superior and inferior surfaces of the true vocal folds, which includes the anterior and posterior commissures. The **subglottis** is composed of the inferior region of the glottis extending to the lower margin of the cricoid cartilage. The area surrounding the larynx is referred to as the **hypopharynx** and includes the pharyngoesophageal junction, right and left pyriform sinuses, lateral and posterior hypopharyngeal walls, and the postcricoid region.

Cancer can arise in any of these three regions, but symptoms vary depending on the origin of cancer development. Laryngeal cancers that form on the vocal folds (glottis) are often detected early because of the mass effect that interrupts the vibration of the vocal folds. Hoarseness is the most common symptom when lesions involve the true vocal folds. Vocal fold lesions can cause a change in vocal pitch and, if large enough, breathing problems (dyspnea) and audible breathing (stridor). Persistent hoarseness may motivate an individual to see a physician because of a fear of "throat" cancer; however, the fear of cancer may also elicit the opposite reaction, a refusal to seek medical evaluation. Because hoarseness is one of the seven warning signals of possible cancer as listed by the American Cancer Society,[4] individuals should seek a medical evaluation if hoarseness extends beyond a 2-week period.

Cancers that originate in the supraglottis, subglottis, or hypopharyngeal areas are usually discovered at later stages because the symptoms are more vague. When the vocal folds are not involved, the lesion may present with many symptoms including:

- lump-in-the-throat feeling
- persistent throat clearing
- persistent coughing
- sense of discomfort in the throat
- persistent sore throat
- difficulty breathing
- burning sensation when swallowing
- difficulty swallowing or pain when swallowing
- referred pain from the larynx to the ear
- unexplained weight loss.

In later stages, the malignancy will cause difficulty swallowing and breathing with the eventual appearance of hoarseness.[7] If the malignancy progresses beyond the confines of the larynx, it is likely to metastasize to the lymphatic system and appear as a lump on the neck. Pain is rarely reported until the later stages of the disease.

Medical Evaluation

An indirect mirror laryngoscopy performed by an otolaryngologist is the first step in evaluating the presence of laryngeal cancer. The otolaryngologist assesses the laryngeal structures, vocal fold mobility, tissue coloration, and presence of pathology. Elicitation of the gag reflex or the inability to sustain the vowel /i/ for a given period of time may create an abbreviated view of the laryngeal structures when using mirror laryngoscopy. Fiberoptic endoscopy instrumentation gives the examiner longer imaging capabilities. When the endoscopy instrumentation is coupled to a video camera, VCR, and monitor, a complete visual examination can be documented and reviewed. Endoscopy examinations can be performed with either a flexible or rigid scope. A flexible nasendoscopy is performed by passing the endoscope through one of the patient's nares. Once the scope is positioned to view the true vocal folds, the patient is requested to perform a number of various speech tasks including abductory and adductory phonatory tasks to assess vocal fold mobility.

Rigid endoscopy with stroboscopy is performed with the endoscope positioned in the mouth as far back as the oropharynx. The true vocal folds and laryngeal structures are thus magnified, allowing for visualization of any tissue change. Stroboscopic images showing changes in the true vocal fold mucosal lining may indicate precancerous lesions or carcinoma in situ. Nonvibratory segments may indicate a more invasive lesion.

Noninvasive imaging techniques, which include computed tomography (CT) scanning or magnetic resonance imaging (MRI), are performed to view the laryngeal structures to determine the exact location and extent of the lesion, presence or absence of regional lymph node metastasis, and presence or absence of distant metastases.

If a malignant lesion is suspected based on the laryngeal examination and case history of the patient, a direct laryngoscopy is performed to biopsy the lesion(s). A biopsy involves excising small samples of tissue under suspicion and evaluating them microscopically to determine the cell type. The most common occurring type of laryngeal cancer is squamous cell. The otolaryngologist will also note the location and extent of the lesion. All microscopic, visual, and X-ray information is analyzed, and the appropriate treatments are planned. Treatment may include radiation therapy, chemotherapy, surgery, or combination of these.

Staging and TNM Classification

Laryngeal cancer is classified using the tumor-node-metastasis **(TNM)** system (Table 9-1). The clinical staging of cancer was developed with the underlying premise that cancers of similar histology or site of origin share similar patterns of growth and metastasis. **TNM** staging is a clinical decision made by the physician after a physical examination and may be augmented by additional information obtained from radiographic and endoscopic examinations, surgical exploration and biopsy.[8] In describing the anatomic extent of the lesion, **T** refers to features of tumor size, location, and extent of spread into surrounding tissues; **N** identifies the absence or presence and extent of the regional lymph node metastasis; and **M** refers to the absence or presence of distant metastasis. The numbers assigned to the **TNM** classification system refer to the extent of the tumor. Laryngeal cancer is also described using another stage grouping that gives information about the severity of tumor, lymph nodes, and metastasis. The stage is described using Roman numerals from I to IV. The higher numbers indicate more metastasis to the surrounding neck tissue and are associated with more advanced disease. A patient with a clinical classification of Stage IV, T4 N1 M0 has a large tumor with metastasis to the lymph nodes but no distant spread of the disease.

This clinical classification system assists the physician in planning treatment, serves as a prognostic indicator, facilitates communication among treatment centers, and serves as a baseline to compare the results of treatment.

Treatment Options for Laryngeal Cancer

Conservation

Attempts to establish a curative treatment for laryngeal carcinoma date back to the late 1800s. In 1876, Billroth performed the first total laryngectomy in the treatment of laryngeal carcinoma. Surgery thus remained the treatment modality until the advent of fractionated external beam radiation in the early 1920s.

Table 9-1. The TNM Classification System

Primary Tumor (T)

TX: Cannot be staged (information not available)

TO: No evidence of tumor

Tis: Carcinoma is situ. The cancer cells are limited to the epithelium, without invasion into the connective tissue of the larynx.

Supraglottis

The T stage of the cancer of the supraglottis is based on how many subsites are involved and how far outside the larynx the cancer has spread. The five subsites of the supraglottic part of the larynx are the:

- ventricular folds
- arytenoids
- suprahyoid epiglottis
- infrahyoid epiglottis
- aryepiglottic folds (laryngeal aspect).

T1 Tumor is limited to one subsite of the supraglottis with normal vocal cord mobility

T2 Tumor invades the mucosa of more than one adjacent subsite of the supraglottis or glottis or region outside the supraglottis (eg, mucosa of base of tongue, vallecula, medial wall of pyriform sinus) with normal vocal cord mobility

T3 Tumor is limited to the larynx with vocal cord fixation and/or invades any of the following: postcricoid area, pre-epiglottic tissues

T4 Tumor invades through thyroid cartilage and/or extends into soft tissues of the neck, thyroid, and/or esophagus

Glottis

T1 Tumor is limited to the vocal cord(s) and may involve anterior or posterior commissure with normal vocal cord mobility
    T1a Tumor is limited to one vocal cord
    T1b Tumor involves both vocal cords

T2 Tumor extends to the supraglottis and/or subglottis and/or with impaired vocal cord mobility

T3 Tumor limited to larynx with vocal cord fixation

T4 Tumor invades the thyroid cartilage and/or extends to tissues beyond the larynx (eg, trachea, soft tissues of neck, including thyroid, pharynx)

(continued)

Table 9-1. *(continued)*

Subglottis

T1 Tumor limited to the subglottis

T2 Tumor extends to the vocal cord(s) with normal or impaired mobility

T3 Tumor limited to the larynx with vocal cord fixation

T4 Tumor invades through cricoid or thyroid cartilage and/or extends to other tissues beyond the larynx (eg, trachea, soft tissues of neck, including thyroid, esophagus)

Regional Lymph Nodes (N)

NX Regional lymph nodes cannot be assessed

N0 No regional lymph node metastasis

N1 Metastasis in a single ipsilateral lymph node, 3 cm or less in greatest dimension

N2 Metastasis in a single ipsilateral lymph node, more than 3 cm but not more than 6 cm in greatest dimension; or in multiple ipsilateral lymph nodes, none more than 6 cm in greatest dimension, or in bilateral or contralateral lymph nodes, none more than 6 cm in greatest dimension
    N2a Metastasis in a single ipsilateral lymph node more than 3 cm but not more than 6 cm in greatest dimension
    N2b Metastasis in multiple ipsilateral lymph nodes, none more than 6 cm in greatest dimension
    N2c Metastasis in bilateral or contralateral lymph nodes, none more than 6 cm in greatest dimension

N3 Metastasis in a lymph node more than 6 cm in greatest dimension

Distant Metastasis (M)

MX Distant metastasis cannot be assessed

M0 No distant metastasis

M1 Distant metastasis

STAGE GROUPING

Stage 0	Tis	N0	M0
Stage I	T1	N0	M0 *(continued)*

Table 9-1. *(continued)*

STAGE GROUPING *(continued)*

Stage II	T2	N0	M0
Stage III	T3	N0	M0
	T1	N1	M0
	T2	N1	M0
	T3	N1	M0
Stage IVA	T4	N0	M0
	T4	N1	M0
	Any T	N2	M0
Stage IVB	Any T	N3	M0
Stage IVC	Any T	Any N	M1

Since that time, histological refinements permitted better understanding of the lymphatic system and metastases in the larynx, which brought about conservation treatments.[9]

Radiation Therapy

When a lesion is found to be isolated to a specific location and is in the early stages of laryngeal cancer, radiation therapy (also referred to as radiotherapy) is the most definitive treatment. In more advanced stages of laryngeal carcinoma, radiation therapy can be used for either definitive or adjuvant (additional) treatment.

Radiation therapy involves the use of high-energy rays or particles directed to a marked treatment field targeting the tumor site and surrounding tissue. Generally, radiotherapy treatments to the head and neck area are administered in the form of an external beam rather than interstitially (within tissues). Radiotherapy affects all cells, both normal and cancerous, within the area being radiated. The objective of radiation therapy is to administer the maximum dosage (fractions) allowable for destruction of the tumor without irreversibly damaging surrounding healthy structures and tissue. A limiting factor in dosage administration of radiation is normal tissue reaction to the radiation.[10]

Schemes of administering radiation have changed in the past few years with the advancement of newer technology and three-dimensional reconstruction of the tumor site. Conventional accelerated radiotherapy involves approximately 6000 cGy in 25 to 30 fractions of radiation administered daily over a 6- to 7-week period to a specified field. Newer radiotherapy procedures, such as hyper-fractionated acceleration, is administered twice a day. Intensity-modulated radiotherapy delivers higher than conventional dosing to the tumor site with less administered to the adjacent surrounding normal tissues thus preserving function. Less damage to surrounding tissue is advantageous to a patient. For example, with conventional accelerated radiotherapy, a patient may have permanent xerostoma (dry mouth) caused by destruction of the parotid gland. With intensity-modulated radiotherapy, the parotids are preserved, thus maintaining a better quality of life without laryngeal dryness.[10]

Radiation therapy may also be administered as an adjuvant treatment before or after surgery. When surgery is required to excise a malignant lesion, the surgeon may choose to "shrink" the lesion with radiation therapy prior to surgery. Following surgery, radiation may be used to destroy any cancerous cells that were not detected and removed at the time of surgery. Generally, individuals who have radical neck dissections to remove metastatic lymph nodes at the time of a total laryngectomy will undergo radiation treatments following surgery. Patients obtain the best results with postoperative radiation therapy if treatments begin within 6 weeks following surgery and end within 100 days of surgery.[11,12] Radiation therapy can also be used to palliate symptoms, such as pain caused by metastases.

Most patients experience various side effects as a result of radiation therapy. Some of these specific to laryngeal cancer include difficulty swallowing, diminished taste, skin irritation, tissue swelling, tissue hardening, possible breathing problems secondary to increased edema, decreased salivary flow, dry mouth, sore throat, tiredness, and nausea. If an individual receives radiation without surgery, the treatments may also cause increased hoarseness. All of these side effects may progressively worsen as the treatments progress and gradually subside when they are completed. The healing process following surgery appears to progress more rapidly when the patient has not undergone radiation therapy prior to surgery.

Surgery

Total laryngectomy involves the surgical excision of the entire cartilaginous larynx including the epiglottis, its inferior and superior muscular and membranous attachments, the hyoid bone, the extrinsic strap muscles; it may include the upper two or three tracheal rings as well. If the cancer cells have metastasized to the cervical lymph nodes, surgery will include a radical neck dissection that may be performed on the right, left, or both sides of the neck. A radical neck dissection involves excision of the lymph nodes, associated veins, the accessory nerve, and other involved neck muscles.

The biological function of the larynx is to serve as a valve to protect the trachea and lungs from aspiration of swallowed liquids and solids (Figure 9-1). After laryngeal excision, the original pulmonary airway cannot be protected or maintained. Thus, the trachea is redirected and sutured to the external neck area just above the notch of the sternum. This opening in the neck is called a stoma. The stoma serves as the point of air exchange with the atmosphere. There no longer remains a connection between the trachea and the pharynx, nose, and mouth (Figure 9-2).

The esophagus remains intact during the total laryngectomy. Because of the previous attachment of the larynx and the pharynx, the anterior pharyngeal walls must be joined and sutured together with the hypopharynx and then sutured to the upper esophagus. When the pharynx is sutured to the base of the tongue, the oral-pharyngeal-esophageal track is completed. The passage of liquids and foods remains the same as before the surgery.

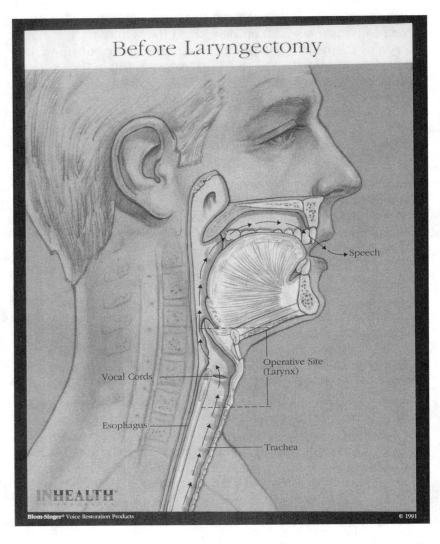

Figure 9-1. Larynx before laryngectomy. (Photo courtesy of InHealth Technologies.)

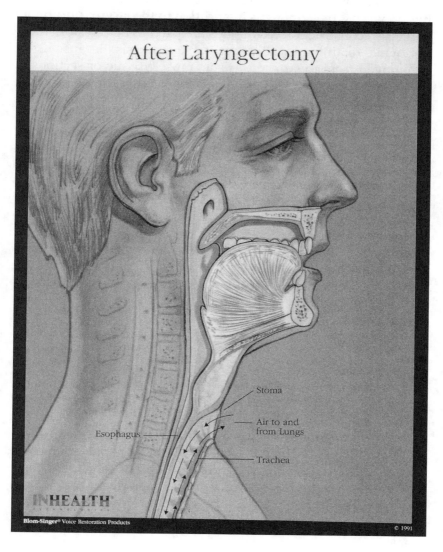

Figure 9-2. After laryngectomy. (Photo courtesy of InHealth Technologies.)

Methods of Reconstruction

When cancer involves other structures such as the pharynx, hypopharynx, or esophagus in addition to the larynx, additional surgical reconstruction techniques are used to help restore function while retaining socially acceptable cosmesis. Because tissue is removed from the cancerous site, muscle tissue or sections of the alimentary tract can be used to reconstruct the defect. This gives support and protection to the head and neck area where the tissue was resected. The factors that account for the success of tissue transfer are preradiation or postradiation treatments, revascularization, and nutritional status of the individual. Reattachment of the microvessels of the flap to the remaining tissue is important to prevent necrosis. Radiation and poor nutritional intake are negative indicators for tissue transfer. The type of reconstruction depends on the location and extent of tissue resection and presents a challenge in restoring the physiologic requirements for swallowing and voice production. Each reconstruction technique has both merits and disadvantages for voice restoration.[13] The following is a discussion of some of the methods of reconstruction.

Myocutaneous Flaps

The pectoralis major (taken from the chest) myocutaneous flap has been used to reconstruct the pharynx and provide protection of the carotid following radical neck dissection.[14,15] Because it is highly vascularized and easily accessible for reconstruction, the pectoralis muscle is commonly used as a regional flap for reconstruction. Voice production is generally functional, but not equal to tracheoesophageal voice (use of a voice prostheis) production following a total laryngectomy. These patients are also subject to tissue changes that may occur from wound healing and radiation treatments.

Free Flaps

A free flap is tissue removed from a donor site and placed into the recipient site using microvascular anastomosis (connecting the vessels). One donor site that is often used for pharyngoesophageal reconstruction is the radial forearm.[16] The radial forearm flap is much thinner with less bulk compared to the pectoralis muscle flap. It has excellent vascularity and is not adversely affected by postoperative radiation. Although radial forearm flaps used in reconstruction of the laryngopharynx tend to be stiffer in comparison to pharyngeal mucosa, patients can achieve acceptable and functional voicing with a voice prosthesis.[13]

Jejunal Free Flap

A portion of the jejunum (second portion of the small intestine) can be used to replace a laryngopharyngectomy defect. Because of discoordination of the intrinsic jejunal peristalsis and increased mucus production, individuals may develop swallowing problems.[17] Voicing is characterized by a wet, gurgly, hypotonic, soft quality with decreased intensity and generally poor quality. Sustained voicing is decreased secondary to the hypotonicity of the tissue.

Gastric Pull-up

When removing the entire esophagus, a gastric pull-up can be performed that involves the transposition of the entire stomach.[13] Usually patients need to eat smaller meals and more frequently. Voice restoration can be performed as a secondary procedure however, the resulting voice is characterized by a wet quality with decreased volume.

Patients undergoing flap reconstruction surgery may experience difficulty swallowing. A videoflouroscopy study can be informative for assessing the patency of the reconstructed area during swallowing and for voicing. If the reconstructed area is narrowed, the patient may undergo dilation of the lumen. When an individual with reconstruction has a voice prosthesis for communication purposes but is not able to produce voice after a reasonable amount of training, the voice pathologist needs to investigate and introduce other methods of communication to provide the patient with functional speech.

Chemotherapy

Chemotherapy is the administration of anticancer drugs intravenously or by mouth. The cytotoxic drugs are systemically delivered via the circulatory system to the individual cells, killing or changing the cancerous cells and inhibiting tumor growth. The two most common cytotoxic drugs that are used in the treatment of head and neck carcinomas are cisplatin (alkylating agent) and 5-fluorouracil (5-FU) (antimetabolites). Alkylating agents are drugs that react chemically and damage the DNA in the cell nucleus preventing the cell from dividing and growing. Antimetabolites damage cells by interfering with the production of DNA preventing essential nutrients to the cells' normal growth process.[18] Other chemotherapy agents are currently being tested for laryngeal and hypopharyngeal carcinomas. These drugs can be administered separately or in combination with other treatments.

Studies have shown that chemotherapy concurrent with radiation therapy may have promising long-term effects; however, researchers are currently conducting studies to determine the best regimens for treatment of advanced carcinoma in the head and neck patient. Chemotherapy is also used for palliative measures in unresectable cancers of individuals where radiation treatments, surgery, or both have failed to control tumor growth. It also has been used for patients who have been unable to undergo surgery because of other health concerns.

Side effects from chemotherapy may include nausea, vomiting, fatigue, hair loss, sores in the mouth, weakened immunity system, bleeding, bruising, allergic reactions, and damage to other internal organs including the kidneys, heart, lungs, liver, and nervous system. Individuals undergoing chemotherapy must have frequent blood tests to monitor blood counts. With the advancement of antinausea medications, most individuals can tolerate chemotherapy. During treatment, it is advised that patients eat frequent small meals, hydrate with water, and avoid alcoholic and caffeinated beverages, aspirin, and exposure to known infections and viruses. Not all individuals experience side effects from chemotherapy. Side effects are usually dependent on the type of drug administered, the amount given, and the duration of the treatment. Most side effects stop after treatment is completed.

Treatment Research for The 21st Century

Treatment of laryngeal carcinoma is continuing to expand and develop in promising ways. Researchers are closely studing the p53 tumor suppressor gene located on chromosome 17, known to contribute to the aggressiveness of tumor growth in head and neck cancers. It has been found that patients exhibiting high levels of p53 and low levels of ki-67 have return of cancer following radiation treatments.[19] As research becomes more refined, these biological markers will provide us with a more specific prognostic indicator and will help to determine the best treatment regimen available to address individual head and neck cancers.

Otolaryngologist Dr Marshall Strome made history in January 1998, at the Cleveland Clinic Foundation, when he performed the first successful laryngeal transplant in recent history. The patient was a 40-year-old male whose larynx was partially destroyed in a 1978 motorcycle accident. Three anatomical structures, the pharynx, larynx, and thyroid gland, were transplanted into the recipient. To date, although vocal fold movement is guarded and the patient still breathes from a tracheostoma, he is able to produce voice, protect his airway, and swallow functionally.[20]

Organ transplantation offers hope in the future as microsurgical techniques become more refined in harvesting from the donor and transplanting into the recipient. Advancements in immunosuppressant drugs will reduce the potential of tissue rejection and decrease the chances of infection. Although laryngeal transplantation may be years away for laryngeal cancer survivors, medical research will continue to proceed forward offering hope for patients in the 21st century.

Need for Follow-up Treatment

Individuals treated for laryngeal cancer are at risk for developing recurrences or new cancers in the head and neck area. Physicians must closely follow these individuals after treatment. Recurrent cancers are likely to return within the first 2 years after initial treatment. It is important for the otolaryngologist to follow the patient on a monthly basis during the 1st year, bimonthly visits the 2nd year, quarterly visits the 3rd year, and 6-month follow-ups the 4th and 5th years. When the patient remains free of cancer after 5 years from the initial date of diagnosis, yearly visits are generally recommended.

Following treatment, the patient is advised to immediately report any new symptoms to the otolaryngologist to rule out possible recurrences. The voice pathologist must also be keenly aware of any physical changes or patient-reported symptoms that may be signs of recurrences or metastatic disease. These changes should be shared immediately with the otolaryngologist. The following case illustrates the importance of this medical follow up.

An 83-year-old gentleman who communicated using tracheoesophageal speech came to the clinic with difficulty talking. A new, small, raised and irritated area was visible on the left of the patient's stoma. Also, he reported a recent weight loss. Both the weight loss and the unusual appearing tissue were suspicious. The physician was notified, and a biopsy was performed. The result of the biopsy was recurrent squamous cell carcinoma, and the patient underwent chemotherapy. Several months following chemotherapy, the site of the lesion remained free of disease.

Multidisciplinary Rehabilitation Team

Rehabilitation of the total laryngectomized individual involves many different professionals. A multidisciplinary team approach is essential to serve the medical, psychological, communication, and social needs of the patient and family. In medical settings where a number of total laryngectomees are treated each year, it is possible to form such a team from existing professional personnel. The interaction of the multidisciplinary team involves evaluating treatment options and the total needs of the patient and the family. These needs may include treatment modalities, preconsultation and preparing the individual for surgery, providing support and educational training through the hospital stay, planning for discharge support, and planning actions to meet future needs. The primary goal is to return the patient to as normal a lifestyle and quality of life as possible.

Surgeon

The surgeon serves as the primary case manager and is responsible for diagnosis of the disease, treatment planning, and the entire medical management of the patient. The surgeon informs the patient of the medical condition and details the implications of the surgery and subsequent medical treatments. He or she makes referrals to other medical team members regarding treatment options. Referral to other medical personnel is important to help the patient obtain all necessary information regarding the various treatment modalities. When necessary, the surgeon also makes referrals to other appropriate team members.

Plastic and Reconstructive Surgeon

A plastic and reconstructive surgeon may also join the surgical team. In some settings when surgery involves removal of structures such as the pharynx, hypopharynx, or esophagus in addition to a total laryngectomy, the plastic and reconstructive surgeon uses microvascular surgery to repair these defects by removing healthy muscle or skin from other parts of the body and reconstructing the tissue.

Radiation Oncologist

The radiation oncologist studies the stage of the tumor and the involvement of surrounding tissue, as well as uninvolved critical structures to determine if radiation therapy would be an acceptable definitive treatment option for the patient. If radiotherapy is selected, the radiation oncologist plans the type, chooses the treatment schema, and calculates optimal dosage levels that will irradiate the tumor and spread of the disease while preserving function.

Oncologist

The oncologist specializes in the treatment of cancer through the administration of chemotherapy. The oncologist reviews the tumor type and selects a chemotherapeutic regimen including the chemical agents, dosage levels, and treatment schedules. If a patient qualifies to be in a clinical research trial, the oncologist manages the protocol to be followed.

Speech-language Pathologist

The speech-language pathologist is directly responsible for evaluating and providing for the patient's short-term and long-term communication needs, as well as management of swallowing if needed. Intervention occurs throughout the individual's treatment of the disease including pretreatment consultation. The initial speech pathology consultation with the patient may include family members and or close friends. It is an informational-educational session discussing issues related to changes in speech and alternate forms of communication (should the patient undergo surgical removal of the larynx). Management of swallowing problems is also discussed as needed in the course of treatment and the patient is assured of intervention if needed. For alaryngeal speech therapy the patient is seen postoperatively by the speech-language pathologist to address communication needs, swallowing issues, and voice restoration. (A complete description of the speech-language pathologist's role follows in the section "The Role of Speech Pathology.")

Oncology Nurse

The oncology nurse is an essential member of the multidisciplinary team in the rehabilitation of the laryngectomized patient during the patient's hospitalization. Beyond the day-to-day care and moral support provided by the nurse, the nurse is responsible for teaching the patient and family the skills necessary for independent stoma care, including use of a suctioning machine. The nurse helps the patient understand and accept the new experience of breathing through the stoma and often-uncomfortable experience of coughing and sneezing from the stoma. Stoma hygiene is important and the tasks of caring for the respiratory system must be learned prior to hospital discharge. The patient is educated and trained to care for a stoma vent or possible tracheostomy tube as needed. The nurse also serves in a supportive role for the hospitalized patient undergoing chemotherapy for the treatment of laryngeal carcinoma.

Dietitian

Patients respond better to surgery and heal more rapidly when they are in good nutritional health. The dietitian is responsible for evaluating the nutritional needs of each patient and correcting nutritional imbalances. Because of the social habits of some patients and presurgical swallowing problems experienced by others, many patients who undergo a total laryngectomy do not maintain adequate nutritional health. Occasionally, surgery is not scheduled until the patient's nutritional level can be improved. This improvement may involve supplementing food intake with high nutrients, which may be taken orally or in an intravenous solution. Following surgery, the dietitian monitors caloric intake and determines the nutritional requirements necessary for the patient to gain and maintain an adequate weight. The patient and family are also advised of the proper eating habits necessary upon discharge. If the patient receives radiation, chemotherapy, or both, the dietitian also monitors the patient's weight and nutritional intake.

Radiologist

The radiologist interprets the results of the chest X ray, CT, or MRI tests and aids the surgeon in planning the most appropriate treatment approach.

Physical Therapist

Patients who undergo total laryngectomy with radical neck dissection may require the services of a physical therapist. Surgical trauma and excision of neck and shoulder muscles and the spinal accessory nerve will often limit the patient's ability to freely move the arm, shoulder, and neck of the dissected side. The physical therapist designs and implements therapy programs based upon the physical disabilities created by the surgery.

Dentist or Prosthodontist

Radiation-induced oral mucosal tissue changes may include stomatitis, xerostomia, tissue necrosis, hypogeusia (taste change), and trismus. These conditions affect both the patient's oral sensations and oral function. A pretreatment dental examination with prophylaxis for patients receiving radiation therapy is recommended. The dentist evaluates the condition of the mouth and teeth documenting baseline conditions and possible risk factors prior to treatment. If extensive decay or poor dentition is present, dental extraction or repair is recommended to prevent further complications secondary to radiation. If the teeth are in good condition, the dentist will recommend a preventive program. Preradiation dental cleaning is recommended to reduce bacterial infections. To reduce any radiation-induced oral problems, the dentist may prescribe daily fluoride treatments and instructions on proper brushing and flossing. Check-ups are recommended during radiation treatments if problems arise, 2 months following treatment, and then every 6 months.

A prosthodontic evaluation prior to radiation treatment assures proper fitting or adjustment to dentures and or prosthetic devices. Devices may need adjustments to prevent sliding or friction against tissue to alleviate possible irritation. Dentures and appliances are removed during treatments. Following completion of radiation therapy and when appropriate, patients who have undergone dental extractions can be fitted for dentures or prosthetic appliances to help with chewing and speech.

Psychologist

The psychologist provides extended patient and family counseling as needed. The laryngectomized patient is required to make many emotional and social adjustments. The psychologist helps the patient deal with such issues as potential death, serious illness, disfigurement, anger, postoperative depression, changing family roles, self-image, and sexuality.

Audiologist

Hearing acuity and presbycusis may need to be addressed in this population. Hearing sensitivity may change following a laryngectomy.[21] It is also possible that normal eustachian tube functioning may be impaired by surgery, subsequent radiation therapy, or both, causing middle ear dysfunction. The audiologist is responsible for evaluating the auditory condition of the laryngectomized patient and recommending amplification when appropriate. Hearing loss may impede the patient's speech monitoring during the rehabilitation process.[22,23]

In addition to testing the patient, audiological evaluation of the spouse or companion is strongly recommended.[24] Successful rehabilitation may be limited if the spouse is not able to hear the patient's speech efforts adequately.

The Laryngectomized Visitor

An important team member is the nonprofessional who has experienced the patient's situation and has adjusted to it well. The laryngectomized visitor who has learned to speak well may lift the patient's spirits and provide the motivation for successful recovery and rehabilitation. It is also recommended that the visitor's spouse meet with the patient's spouse. Spouse-to-spouse support is often just as valuable as patient-to-patient support.

Special Concerns of the Laryngectomized Patient

The ultimate goal of a total laryngectomy is to "cure" the patient of cancer through surgical excision of the malignancy. Because of the ability to isolate and excise the cancer through laryngeal excision, cancer of the larynx is one of the most curable forms of cancer when the disease is identified early. The results of the surgery leave the patient with the major problem of reestablishing oral communication. The patient must also address several other physical, psychological, and social concerns. If the patient is to live a quality life, the ability to make the appropriate adjustments is as important as reestablishing speech. Let us consider some of these concerns.

Communication

Only one part of oral communication is missing following a total laryngectomy: a sound generator. The patient's language and cognitive abilities, as well as the ability to articulate, remain intact. Although implications of the loss of voice have been explained well to the patient, the impact is often not fully realized until the patient awakens from the anesthesia and automatically tries to speak. The realization is even more dramatic later when the patient attempts to express his or her feelings and needs and is constrained by cumbersome writing or unintelligible articulation and mouthing of words and phrases. Most people take for granted the ability to speak because speaking is an automatic act. If the speaking ability is withdrawn or impaired, one quickly realizes the profound loss of this expressive communication modality.

The laryngectomized individual is soon confronted with communication deprivation. There is a distinct difference in communicating to make one's needs known (such as, hunger, thirst, yes, no, bathroom, etc) and communicating complex thoughts, feelings, and actions. The initial forms of communication for the laryngectomized patient are usually writing and mouthing words. Writing is slow and laborious for both the patient and the reader, and not all patients can write. Mouthing words is effective only if the patient's articulation is excellent and if the listener has the ability to understand speech without sound. Often patients have many thoughts that they would like to express but, because of the effort to communicate, do not try to do so. If this situation is allowed to continue, the patient will soon become isolated.

It is in the patient's best interest to reestablish some form of oral communication as soon as possible. This goal may be accomplished soon after surgery, while still hospitalized, with the use of an artificial larynx. A longstanding negative bias against early use of an artificial larynx prevailed for years based on the worry that the patient would develop a dependency on the device and would therefore not be as likely to develop other forms of alaryngeal speech. Currently, clinicians understand that early oral communication is essential and that withholding an available means of communication is more likely to disrupt the rehabilitation process.

The early days following surgery are usually quite traumatic for the patient and the family. Providing an effective means of communication will ease this trauma. Other forms of communication can be explored as soon as the patient is medically and physically healed and released by the physician.

Physical Concerns

Respiration

Another concern of the laryngectomized patient is adjustment to breathing through the stoma. Prior to surgery, normal respiratory exchange had the advantages of the nose. The nose is essentially an air treatment center. Before reaching the lungs, the air is filtered by the hairs in the nose, humidified by the mucous membrane of the nose and pharynx, and warmed along the entire upper respiratory tract. The laryngectomized patient no longer has advantages of a natural filtering, moistening, and warming air treatment system. Without a substitute, untreated air is inhaled directly into the trachea and lungs. The laryngectomee is subjected to the atmospheric conditions whether the air is dry or humidified. Dry air causes increased mucous buildup with thicker secretions and decreased ciliary function. Humidified air helps thin the secretions and also reduces the amount of secretions.

Passive heat and moisture exchange (HME) stoma air-filtering systems are available for the laryngectomee. These specially designed filters are placed over the stoma by peristomal adhesion and serve to compensate for the loss of upper airway function.[25-28] Air is exchanged through the filter. Inhaled air is filtered and humidified by the natural moisture in the material created by the condensation from the exhalations and warmed by the warmth of the material. This warm, filtered, moist, air exchange reduces the amount of mucus and the likelihood for mucous to become encrusted and build up in the bronchial pathways.

Warming and filtering the air also decreases coughing. Commercially available heat and moisture exchangers include:

- InHealth Blom-Singer® HumidiFilter System (Figure 9-3,A)
- Free Vent (Figure 9-3,B)
- Provox® Stomafilter (Figure 9-3,C)
- Stom-Vent2™ (Figure 9-3,D)

Selection of an HME may be dependent on daily cost, as well as fixation of the device to the stoma.[29]

Stoma covers (Figure 9-4) are worn directly over the stoma. A stoma cover is made of porous material, either cloth or foam. Stoma covers provide a protective function, as well as improve the cosmetic appearance of the neck. The exchange of air through the material of the stoma cover aids to warm and add moisture when breathing. Stoma covers protect the airway by filtering out dust, fumes, insects, and other foreign matter. The laryngectomized patient should also consider wearing stoma covers for cosmetic reasons. The general population is likely to

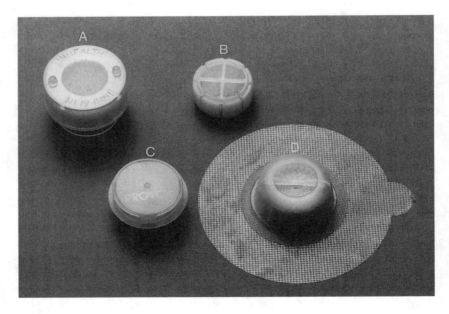

Figure 9-3. Four heat and moisture exchangers used in the laryngectomized patient.

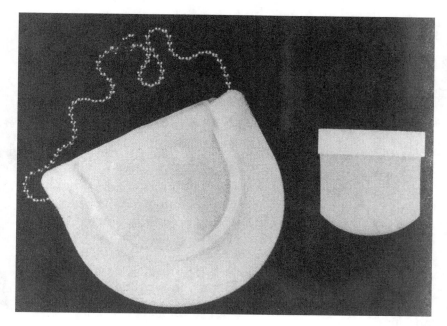

Figure 9-4. Stoma covers.

be uncomfortable around laryngectomized patients with an uncovered stoma in full view. This accommodation is part of the patient's social adjustment and acceptance. There are health benefits, too. Covering the stoma is especially beneficial in cold weather and when the air is dry. Use of a room humidifier is recommended following surgery to lessen irritation of the lining of the trachea through drying.[30]

Coughing and Sneezing

Breathing is only one of the respiratory functions of the stoma. Laryngectomized patients also cough and sneeze through the stoma. These patients need to be reminded to cover the stoma instead of the mouth when coughing, otherwise the discharged mucus is expelled into the air or on others.

Another concern is the "runny" nose. Posterior drainage and swallowing remain intact, but because the respiratory connection between the nose and the lungs no longer exists, no mechanism prevents drainage through the nose. The laryngec-tomized patient must either wipe or use the small amount of intraoral pressure to blow the nose free of mucus. A tissue or handkerchief should be available at all times.

Tracheal Tubes and Tracheostoma Vents

Concerns regarding the stoma also include the use and care of the tracheal tubes and tracheostoma vents (Figure 9-5). At the time of surgery, a tracheal tube may be inserted in the stoma as a means of keeping it open and maintaining the air passage. As the tissue shrinks during the healing process, the tube maintains the integrity of the stoma, preventing a reduction in its size. Generally the patient does not need a tracheal tube; however, if after several days the stoma starts to shrink, the physician may insert a tracheostoma vent to prevent further stenosis. Tra-cheostoma vents are manufactured in various diameter sizes and lengths.

As mentioned previously, it is important for the patient to assume independent care of the stoma that includes cleaning the

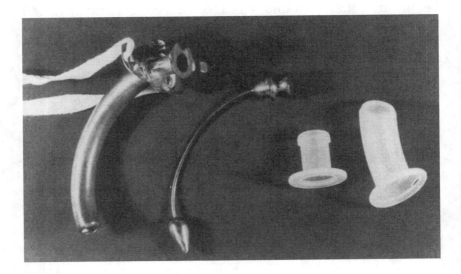

Figure 9-5. Tracheal tube and stoma vents.

tracheal tube or vent. Following surgery, most patients secrete and cough thick mucus plugs. These plugs hinder air exchange, making breathing difficult. Care of the stoma and tracheal tube involves removing the inner tube (cannula) for washing, removing dried mucus from the stoma with a long handle tweezers, and suctioning accumulated mucous secretions from the trachea with a suction machine.[31] Mild soap and water can be used to clean the tracheostoma vent. Patients are taught to inhale a small amount of commercially prepared saline solution into the stoma to thin out thick secretions to make it easier to suction or expel. Regular stoma care maintains an open airway and prevents irritating mucous crusts from forming on the skin around the stoma.

As healing progresses, most patients are able to reduce gradually and eventually eliminate the use of a tracheal tube or stoma vent. Some patients are required to wear a tracheostoma vent 24 hours per day to prevent stoma stenosis; others maintain an adequate stoma size by wearing a vent only several hours per day. The tracheostoma vent can be fenestrated (opened) to accommodate the voice prosthesis for tracheoesophageal speech.

Swallowing

Generally, swallowing is not affected following a total laryngectomy. If a tracheoesophageal puncture was performed as part of the primary procedure, the patient is fed through the catheter that is directed down the esophagus via the TEP. Usually the patient is permitted to start taking clear liquids orally on the 7th day following surgery. This is assuming normal healing has taken place and no fistulas have developed that would delay oral feeds. A bedside swallowing evaluation by the speech-language pathologist assesses labial, lingual, and palatal range of movement and makes recommendations regarding the consistency of food intake. A modified barium swallow examination is performed to assess the oral, pharyngeal, and esophageal phase of swallowing should a patient develop swallowing problems. Some patients will develop esophageal narrowing secondary to wound healing, and radiation therapy, or both, which creates a feeling of food sticking in the throat. Esophageal dilatations will improve swallowing for these patients.

Smell and Taste

Two other related physical changes with which the laryngectomized patient is concerned are changes in smell and taste. Because the patient can no longer inhale air through the nose, the ability to smell is impaired. There is actually no impairment in the olfactory organ itself; the odor is simply not able to reach the organ to be sensed. A patient who happens to be in an area with an intense odor such as fresh paint, gasoline, or smoke, may be aware of the odor as it permeates the nasal cavity. Otherwise, the inability to inhale air through the nose greatly limits this sense.

Diedrich and Youngstrom[22] reported that 31% of the laryngectomized patients they studied reported a diminished ability to taste. Because taste is greatly influenced by the ability to smell,[32] the act of eating may often be reduced to simply a necessity. Some patients report that this may be attributed to their adjustment to the loss of smell because this sense is related to taste. Although smell and taste are impaired, maintaining good nutritional intake is paramount.

Safety

Safety issues related to breathing through the stoma are real concerns of the laryngectomized patient and family. In the event of accident or illness, emergency medical personnel must be alerted that the patient is a neck breather so appropriate medical aid may be administered. This may include mouth-to-stoma resuscitation or administration of oxygen via the stoma. *First Aid for (Neck-Breathers) Laryngectomees* is a helpful pamphlet that provides explicit instructions for resuscitation. It is available from the International Association of Laryngectomees.[33] Patients are strongly advised to wear medical alert bracelets, carry an emergency identification card, and place emergency identification cards on the windshields of their car and in an obvious location in their homes (Figure 9-6). The laryngectomized patient should

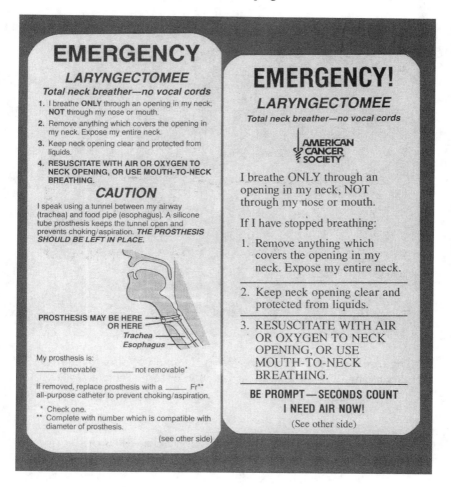

Figure 9-6. Safety cards. (Photo by Rick Berkey, St. Elizabeth Medical Center, Dayton, Ohio.)

inform the medical emergency personnel who service the area in which they live of the surgical alterations including first aid procedures for neck breathers.

Activities related to water, such as bathing, fishing, and swimming, are important to discuss with the patient. Safety around water is of the utmost importance. Bathing and showering may present special problems for the patient. A special rubber shower collar (Figure 9-7) is available as a safety aid for this

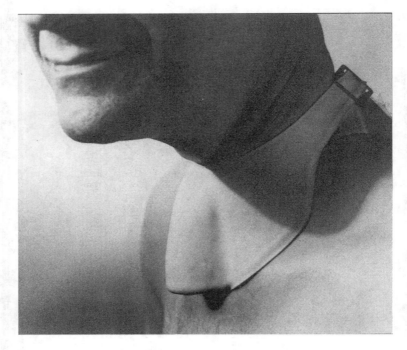

Figure 9-7. Shower collar. (From "Helping Words for the Laryngectomee," International Association of Laryngectomees.)

purpose. The collar fits tightly around the neck to deflect water from entering the stoma. Holes on the underside of the collar permit safe air exchange. This device is recommended for patients who prefer to take showers.[34]

Water sports require their own forms of caution and safety. Those who want to continue swimming as a hobby are advised to seek special training.[30] A Larkel (modified snorkel) is a device that allows the laryngectomee to safely swim. Special training is required to learn to use this device. Without training, this activity is extremely dangerous for the patient and is not advisable. Fishing from the bank or dock requires caution. The patient should only fish where there is easy access to the water and where the footing is stable. Boating is also potentially dangerous. The laryngectomized patient is cautioned to limit boating activities to stable crafts. A superior quality life vest should be worn, and extreme caution should be maintained at all times.

Lifting

One of the biological functions of the larynx is to allow pulmonary air to be trapped within the lungs when the vocal folds are held in complete adduction, making it easier to lift objects. The laryngectomized patient can no longer regulate the larynx to build thoracic air pressure. Theoretically, lifting should be difficult for the laryngectomee. In Diedrich and Youngstrom's survey of patients, they found that 45% of their patients reported no difficulty lifting, 42% reported some difficulty, and 13% reported great difficulty.[22] The majority of the surveyed patients had not experienced problems with lifting. Laryngectomees who usually have problems have undergone radical neck dissection and experience related neck, shoulder, and arm movement problems.

Psychosocial Concerns

The laryngectomized patient may have many psychological adjustments to make. In an excellent review of the basic psychological stages of patients, Gardner described adjustments that were made preoperatively, immediately postoperatively, and upon reentering the familiar environment.[31] These adjustments focused on the patient's reaction to the disease, the physical changes as a result of the surgery, self-concept based on the feeling of adequacy and appearance, and emotional reactions related to the physical and psychological changes.

When told that they have cancer of the larynx, it is not unusual for patients to be more concerned about the disease than about the ramifications of surgery. To many individuals, cancer is synonymous with death.[35] Sometimes patients often do not hear the complete explanation of the disease and its treatment as provided by the physician. All patients eventually must deal with reality, and the patient must move toward understanding the surgery and its consequences.

The Laryngectomized Speaker's Source Book, published by the International Association of Laryngectomees (IAL), provides an excellent description of the fears and concerns of the patient.[36] (The IAL is an international teaching and support group composed of and operated by laryngectomized individuals.) It describes fears related to the operation such as taking the anesthetic, fear of pain following surgery, fear of mutilation, and fear of not being able to speak.

The immediate postoperative period may be a time of considerable frustration. Many patients experience acute physical stress; worries about health, families and finances; and uncertainties about the future. The concept of being a "whole" person may also arise. The reaction of some patients is to resign themselves to being cared for by others, to becoming dependent. Those who make the appropriate adjustments work through these difficulties and maintain their presurgical independence. All of these concerns and frustrations are compounded by the inability to communicate feelings adequately because of limited nonverbal means.

As the patient returns to a normal environment, many family and social issues must be resolved. It is quite possible, especially in the typical age group that temporary role reversals occur during the hospitalization and rehabilitation period. Husbands may take over the domestic roles of their wives, or wives may play the traditional male roles of the family. When role reversals take place, it is necessary for the family to evaluate relationships and either to maintain new role distributions or return to the previous roles.

Personal and sexual relationships may also be affected by the laryngectomy. Individuals with strong interpersonal relationships and positive self-images will seldom experience difficulties or sexual disorientation. Following surgery, however, some patients experience less than adequate self-images and often need psychological counseling to work through these problems.

Blood and Blood[37] found that the laryngectomized patient who spoke openly and candidly about his or her disability and rehabilitation process was more socially accepted than the patient who was reticent or acted embarrassed about the situation. Therefore, the well-adjusted patient may find more success in attempting to return to the previous work setting. Indeed, many patients, even those who require skilled oral communication such as managers, business people, and salespeople, have successfully returned to their jobs and careers. When patients are not able to meet previous job requirements because of physical or communication deficits, job retraining or employment changes may be required. The various state rehabilitation commissions may be helpful in training patients for new employment opportunities. Some patients choose early retirement following laryngectomy surgery.

Attitudes that people have regarding cancer have become more sophisticated with increased understanding of the disease. Nonetheless, we have experienced some patients, spouses, family members, and employers who have operated with the belief that "cancer is contagious." If present, the serious misconception must be carefully dispelled in order for the rehabilitation program to be successful.

Speech Rehabilitation Alternatives

The goal of the speech rehabilitation program following total laryngectomy is to achieve the most effective speech possible for the individual speaker in terms of age, gender, and dialect. As we have discussed, there are three options available to the total laryngectomy patient:

- artificial larynx
- esophageal speech
- surgical prosthetics

No categorical statements concerning the "best" approach can be made. Each option must be weighed and evaluated against each patient's own set of circumstances. The deciding factor is based on which method is the most effective for the individual patient. Watterson and McFarlane advocate learning two modes of communication, one to serve as the primary mode of speaking and the other to use as a backup.[38]

Artificial Larynges

Pneumatic Artificial Larynx

Historically, the development of artificial larynges dates back to 1859.[39] Throughout the years, two major types of artificial larynges have emerged, pneumatic and electronic, with the electronic being the most widely used of the two types. Although seldom used in the United States, the Memacon and Tokyo pneumatic artificial larynges (Figure 9-8) are still available for purchase.[38] The pneumatic larynx utilizes pulmonary air as its power source. A cuff that contains a reed or a membrane fits over the stoma. As the patient expels air for speech, a flexible rubber or plastic tube placed into the patient's mouth transmits the vibration from the membrane. The patient articulates as the sound is produced. Loudness variations occur as the air pressure levels change during breathing for speech. Sound quality from the pneumatic larynges may be more pleasing than the electromechanical devices. There is no electronic noise or buzzing sound with the pneumatic device. The major disadvantage of the pneumatic instruments is the presence of the tube in the mouth that may interfere with articulation and eventually collect saliva or moisture condensation within the tube or on the diaphragm. The cuff, as well, may become clogged with mucus. This device does require the use of one hand for placement of the cuff over the stoma.

Electronic Artificial Larynges

There are three types of electronic artificial larynges, neck-type devices (Figure 9-9), oral devices (Figure 9-10), and intraoral devices (Figure 9-11). All electronic larynges are battery-powered sound generators. Some of the devices operate using 9-volt alkaline batteries and others use rechargeable batteries. These devices may differ in size, weight, quality of sound, ability to control pitch and volume, appearance, type of batteries needed, and durability. There are a number of battery-operated electronic artificial larynges that are commercially available for purchase.

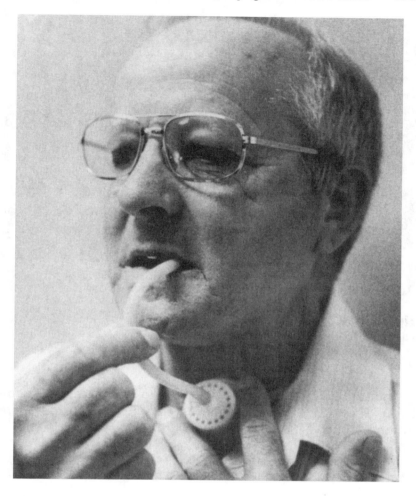

Figure 9-8. Pneumatic artifical larynx.

Neck-type Devices

The neck-type artificial larynges are the most popular of the ala-ryngeal devices. The sound source is a diaphragm in the head of the instrument that is set into vibration when the speaker acti-vates the device by depressing a button. The speaker operates the neck-type artificial larynges by placing the head of the device firmly against the neck or cheek allowing for the sound to

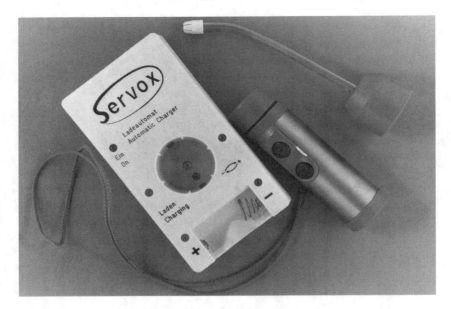

Figure 9-9. Servox artificial larynges. (Photo by Rick Berkey, St. Elizabeth Medical Center, Dayton, Ohio.)

be transmitted through the tissues and into the oral cavity (Figure 9-12). They currently range in cost and relative quality from around $230 to $600. The electronic devices permit variations in volume and pitch through manipulation of switch controls.

Oral Devices

Oral artificial larynges, such as a Cooper-Rand (Figure 9–10) or P.O. Vox, generate sound in a small transducer and transmit the sound through a plastic sound conduction tube. The speaker places the plastic tube, which is attached to the tone generator, approximately 1 to 1½ inches in the mouth on top of the tongue. The plastic tube can either enter the mouth at midline or from the corner of the mouth with the tube entering at a diagonal. The speaker is instructed to coordinate the activation of the sound generator and speech simultaneously. Practice should incorporate the use of natural pauses and reducing rate of speech to improve intelligibility.

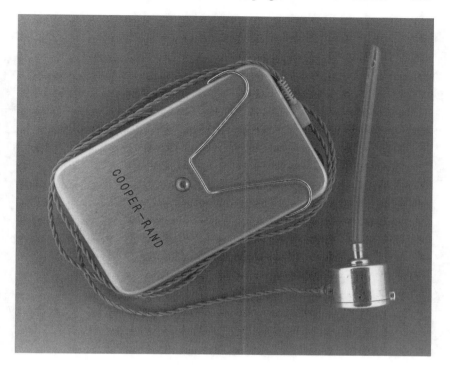

Figure 9-10. Cooper-Rand intraoral artificial larynx. (Photo by Rick Berkey, St. Elizabeth Medical Center, Dayton, Ohio.)

Most neck-type devices can be converted into an oral device by affixing a rubber or plastic adapter onto the head of the electrolarynx. The plastic conduction tube is then inserted into the center of the adapter for sound to be transmitted through it. An oral artificial device is ideal for patients who experience extensive scar tissue or edema of the neck preventing sound to adequately transfer through the tissues when using a neck-type electrolarynx. This type of device can be effectively used immediately following surgery to communicate with the hospital staff and family members. As with the pneumatic device, the disadvantage involves the oral tube's interference with articulation and collection of saliva within the tube.

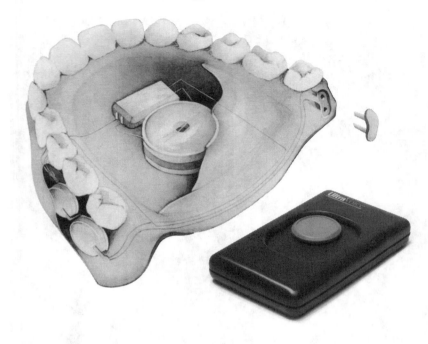

Figure 9-11. Ultravoice intraoral device.

Intraoral Devices

The Ultravoice (Figure 9-11) is a remote-control-operated device that can be custom built into an upper denture or an orthodontic retainer. It consists of an oral unit that is mounted into the acrylic denture, a hand-held remote control unit, and a charging unit that charges both the oral and hand-held component simultaneously. By using the hand-held unit, the patient has control over the activation of the device, as well as pitch and loudness. This device is individually customized, as maxillary impressions must be taken to fit the patient properly. This device is costly; however, it may be the only one that some patients can use. Training involves slowing down the rate of speech and coordinating the activation of the hand-held device and initiation of oral speech articulation simultaneously. The patient controls pitch and loudness by moving a button on the hand-held unit. The patient may need therapy for incorporating pitch inflections

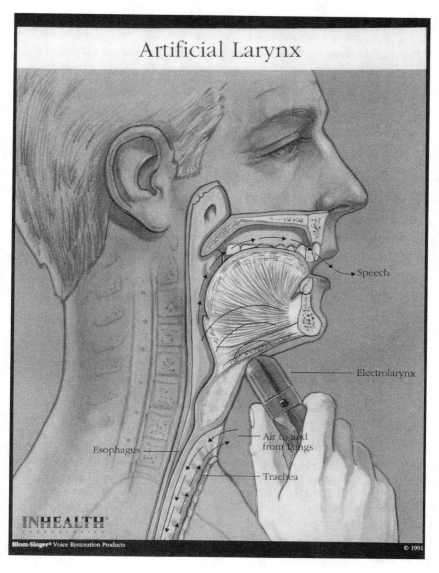

Figure 9-12. Representation of speech being produced with a neck-type artificial larynx. (Photo courtesy of InHealth Technologies.)

and volume control during conversational speech. Consider the following case history:

A 66-year-old gentleman was evaluated by the otolaryngologist following a several month history of persistent hoarseness. He did not complain of any hemoptysis, shortness of breath, or dysphagia. He quit smoking 2 years prior to the evaluation and had a history of smoking two packs of cigarettes per day for 40 years. Videolaryngostroboscopic examination revealed the presence of a whitish granular lesion involving the anterior aspect of the right true vocal fold. Vocal fold mobility was normal bilaterally. The otolaryngologist revealed no evidence of lymphadenopathy. A microlaryngoscopy with biopsy confirmed squamous cell carcinoma and was staged a T1a lesion. The patient was evaluated by the radiation oncologist and elected to receive radiation therapy. He received 6750 rads over a 2-month period with resolution of the malignancy.

Fourteen months after receiving radiation treatments, an enlarged left cervical mass appeared. Biopsy revealed metastatic squamous cell carcinoma. All available options were presented to this patient including a total laryngectomy, radiation and chemotherapy, and a combination of surgery and radiation therapy. The patient did not want to loose his larynx and opted for the radical neck dissection and partial laryngectomy with follow-up radiation therapy. The patient underwent a right anterolateral partial laryngectomy with a left radical neck dissection and additional 9000 rads of radiation therapy. After completion of radiation therapy, this patient presented with significant radiation mucositis involving the oral cavity, pharynx, and hypopharynx. He also experienced pain when swallowing and difficulty swallowing. Secondary to radionecrosis of the larynx 7 months following the second series of radiation treatments, the patient underwent a total laryngectomy with a tracheoesophageal puncture and reconstruction of pectoralis major myocutaneous flap.

The patient was seen for his initial voice prosthesis fitting 7 weeks following his surgery. This patient experienced a slow course of healing secondary to the previous radiation treatments. The patient was initially fitted with a 3.0-cm voice prosthesis. He achieved short bursts of voicing on vowels. The patient was also fitted with a tracheostoma vent secondary to stoma stenosis. Because of his inability to produce voicing 2 months following his second round of radiation treatments, an insufflation test was administered. Voicing was weak and inconsistent with ability to sustain vowels for approximately 1 second. Alternative methods of voicing were initiated. A neck type electrolarynx failed because of poor sound transfer into the oral cavity secondary to the neck tissue hardening from the radiation treatments. An oral adapter was place onto the head of the electrolarynx. The patient was trained using the oral device; however, intelligibility was minimal at best. Three esophagrams over a 7-month period revealed gradual narrowing and finally stenosis of the cervical esophagus. Esophageal dilatations were performed to dilate the esophagus for swallowing. Secondary to poor healing, the otolaryngologist did not advise performing a myotomy. Although the patient was trained to use the oral adapter to speak, it was not adequate for communication purposes. Because the patient was edentulous and had to get a new set of dentures made, it was recommended that he try the intraoral device. Although all modes of alaryngeal speech were tried with this individual, the intraoral device was the most effective and provided the best intelligibility for this individual given his complicated recovery period. This patient has remained cancer-free 2 years following his total laryngectomy.

Treatment Considerations for Artificial Larynges

The following are suggestions when instructing the patient to use an artificial larynx for communication. Some patients will quickly master the art of using the device; whereas others may require several sessions of speech therapy as well as following through on structured home exercises. The following is a discussion of various factors that affect speech intelligibility using artificial larynges.

Articulation. Instruct the patient to slightly overarticulate words without over-exaggerating oral movements. Patients who articulate with little oral movement are difficult to understand when using an artificial larynx. Teaching patients to over-articulate slightly will help open the vocal tract to improve resonance of the sound. Teach patients to enhance their articulation by instructing them to use the intraoral air for the articulation of voiceless consonants.

Placement. The speech-language pathologist should experiment with various placements around the neck area for the best possible sound transfer into the oral cavity. While the patient is asked to count, the speech-language pathologist moves the electrolarynx around the neck area, finding the place on the neck that transmits the clearest and loudest sound into the oral cavity. All patients have a particular site that serves to transmit the sound with the greatest amount of energy into the oral cavity. The difference in sound between this placement and other placement sites should be demonstrated. The best placement site is usually under the mandible and slightly off midline of the neck.

The vibrating head of the artificial larynx should be directed toward the oral cavity to enhance vocal tract resonance. The patient's cheek may be the best placement especially if the neck tissue is dense or hardened from radiation treatments.

Larynx-to-skin Seal.   Instruct the patient to place the head of the artificial larynx against the palm of the hand to demonstrate acquiring a seal without sound leakage. This technique will help the patient to understand how to manipulate the sound generator control. Success in using the neck device electrolarynx is proper placement of the vibrating head sealed firmly against the skin to prevent noise leakage from the device. Speech intelligibility is markedly affected if the device is not flush to the skin.

Developing Conversational Speech.   Once the "spot" is found for the best sound transfer, request that the patient practice finding this area quickly and precisely with consistency. Using the mirror will help the patient locate the area, as will marking the site with a piece of tape. Counting, reading short phrases and sentences, and responding to questions can serve as practice material both in therapy and practicing at home. Expand quickly into conversational speech. As the patient becomes consistent with placement and appropriate sound generation when reading phrases and sentences, advance to the conversational level. Patients will have a tendency to talk in a monotonous, robotlike speech. Demonstrate and insist on the use of normal phrasing, with appropriate cessation of sound for natural pauses, and with normal rate. The initiation and ending of speech must be coordinated with the activation and deactivation of the sound generator respectively.

Coordination of Movements.   Teach the patient to remove the artificial larynx from the neck when not speaking. Patients are likely to fall into the habit of leaving the device positioned on or near the neck during conversational speech. The flow of the conversation can be much improved if the patient places the artificial larynx on the neck only when he or she wants to talk. This serves as a natural signal to the other speakers, much as when we take a deep breath prior to speaking during conversation, that the patient has something to say.

Stoma Noise. Following surgery, the laryngectomized patient breathes through the stoma. If air is forced through the stoma, either during inhalation or exhalation, a noise can be heard that is referred to as "stoma noise." This stoma noise can interfere with the patient's intelligibility of speech and become annoying for the listener. Rapid muscular contraction of the thoracic or abdominal muscles may result in increased air turbulence at the level of the stoma. If you ask the patient to whisper or speak with increased loudness, much stoma noise will be produced. To help eliminate or reduce the amount of stoma noise, teach the patient to mouth, not whisper, the words. The patient should practice reading phrases by just mouthing the words and at the same time monitoring the amount of stoma noise being heard.

The patient who has mastered these steps should be encouraged to discontinue nonoral means of communication. Usually, patients agree to this transition with little argument because oral communication is much more flexible and expansive. The patient will continue to improve simply by using the artificial larynx in all speaking situations. As a final means of demonstrating its effectiveness, the voice pathologist should consider talking to the patient on the telephone during a therapy session to assess telephone intelligibility. The 60 to 80 Hz tone generated by the artificial larynx is carried well over the telephone. Using the artificial larynx on the telephone reopens another avenue of communication for the patient.

Esophageal Speech

An artificial larynx provides the patient with a new, external source of sound vibration. Esophageal voice utilizes the patient's remaining anatomical structures to provide a new, internal source for sound generation. These vibrating structures are the cricopharyngeus muscle of the upper esophagus and the middle and inferior pharyngeal constrictor muscles. When used for sound generation, these structures collectively are termed the pharyngoesophageal, or PE segment. The PE segment lies approximately at the level of C-5 (Figure 9-13).

To generate sound, the PE segment needs a power source. Because the patient can no longer inhale air into the nose and

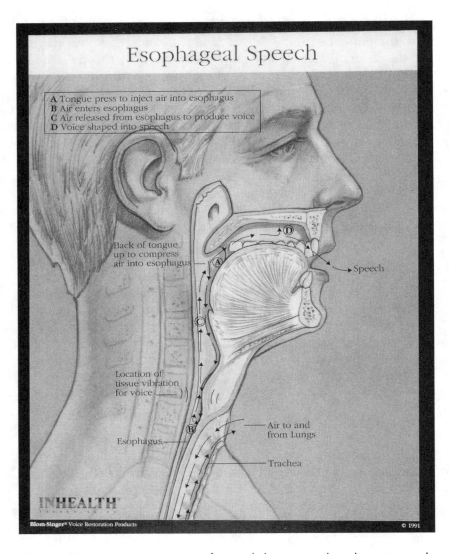

Figure 9-13. Representation of speech being produced using esophageal speech. (Photo courtesy of InHealth Technologies.)

mouth, another air source must be found. This source is simply the atmospheric air that is always present in the oral and nasal cavities. With training, patients can be taught to place this ambient air into the upper esophagus, which serves as an air reservoir, and then expel this air vibrating the PE segment and surrounding tissues. When the patient articulates using this sound for voice, esophageal speech is produced. Fluent esophageal speech depends on the rapid intake and release of air from the esophagus.

A number of factors seem to influence the success of learning esophageal speech including physiological and psychological factors.[40] Proficient esophageal speakers appear to possess the anatomical structure necessary to produce esophageal vibration and display a high degree of individual motivation to focus on dedicated daily practice, accept small incremental improvement throughout the learning process as well as setbacks, and remain positive and relaxed throughout therapy.

The first step in developing esophageal speech is learning how to place air into the upper esophagus. The two major methods of air intake are the **injection** (positive pressure approach) and the **inhalation** (negative pressure approach) methods. The injection method includes **glossopharyngeal press** and **plosive injection**. These methods are described by a number of individuals.[6,22,41-43] These techniques of esophageal speech production are based on how the PE segment opens to allow for air intake and then expels the air during voicing.

Inhalation Method

The inhalation method uses a rapid expansion of the thoracic cavity during inspiration to draw ambient air into the esophagus. The esophagus is in a state of negative pressure, and as air is inhaled into the lungs, the intraesophageal pressure drops even further, below atmosphere. Therefore, air from the oral and pharyngeal cavities can be drawn passively into the esophagus. Air pressure in these two locations becomes equalized momentarily, just after the ambient air is drawn into the esophagus.[43] Instructions to the patient may include the following:

■ Demonstrate the expansion of the thoracic cavity using a diagram. This demonstration will make the patient aware of how the normal respiratory system works. As the cavity expands, air is drawn into the lungs; as it contracts, the air is expelled.

■ Explain to the patient that as the thoracic cavity expands, so does the diameter of the esophagus. As the esophagus expands, the increased area is filled with ambient air. This air can then be expelled to produce vibration of the PE segment.

■ The patient is then asked to close his or her mouth and to take air into the stoma through a quick, sharp inhalation. This inhalation may be enhanced by momentarily covering the stoma with the hand. It may be helpful to have the patient imagine that he or she is sniffing through the nose.[22] The patient should then attempt to expel the air by saying "ah." The subsequent decrease in thoracic size will force the air out of the esophagus if esophageal insufflation has occurred. Continue this procedure until sound is produced.

Injection Method

The injection method of air intake is achieved by compressing the intraoral air into the esophagus with assistance from the tongue or lips and sometimes the cheeks. There are two types of injection. The first type is air injection by tongue pumping, which is also referred to as a **glossopharyngeal press** or a glossal press.[22] Instructions to the patient for teaching this method may include the following:

■ Tell the patient to open his or her mouth and "bite off" a piece of air. This action and imagery helps the patient feel the ambient air from one point to another. It also helps to increase the air pressure in the back of the oral cavity.

■ At the end of the "bite," the patient is instructed to close the lips to seal the oral cavity. At the same time, with the tongue tip pushing against the alveolus, the middle section of the tongue should pump the air against both the hard and soft palates. This action will cause the base of the tongue to move backward in a rocking motion, pushing the air into the upper esophagus. In using the glossopharyn-

geal press, the patient may feel the tongue moving posteriorly and actually making contact with the pharyngeal wall.
Once the patient learns this method of air intake, the lips
can either be slightly open or closed since the tongue serves
to pump the air into the esophagus.

■ The patient should feel and perhaps hear the air as it is
forced past the PE segment and into the esophagus. When
the air passes the segment, an attempt should be made to
expel the air by saying "ah."

The **consonant injection** method of air intake is the second type of injection of air into the esophagus. This method
uses the natural intraoral air pressures created by plosive and
fricative sounds to inject air into the esophagus. Instructions to
the patient for teaching this method may include the following:

■ Ask the patient to produce voiceless consonants (such as
/t/, /k/, /p/, and /sk/) one at a time in quick succession.
The consonants should be made firmly with exaggerated
oral movement to encourage airflow into the esophagus.
This rapid repetition of the consonants, especially a tongue-
tip alveolar stop, fricative or a bilabial, as well as tongue
positioning facilitates build up of air pressure in the esophagus. Production of the consonants forces the air pressure
in the esophagus with the result of almost immediate
expulsion and sound production. Discourage any stoma
noise or sounds made by the tongue and palatal-pharyn-
geal contact.

■ When the esophageal sound is produced consistently utilizing the consonants, add consonant-vowel combinations
to the practice regimen. This will force a lengthening of the
esophageal sound.

■ Constantly add new consonant-vowel combinations, expanding the patient's repertoire of sounds on which injection can take place.

■ Finally, attempt to drop the consonant and have the
patient inject the air using the tongue for production of the
vowel only.

Although the inhalation and injection methods are of primary interest, a swallow method has also been advocated.[44]
Using this method, the patient is asked simply to open and close

the mouth and to swallow air. The underlying theory of this method is that a normal swallow produces relaxation of the cricopharyngeus thus allowing air to enter the esophagus. Using this method, the patient is encouraged to swallow air to produce voice. The swallow method of air injection is the least efficient and may be taught as a last resort. One of the problems with this method is that if the swallowed air reaches the stomach, it cannot be readily expelled.

The therapist should encourage practice of the method easiest for the patient to inject air into the esophagus. Often, the most effective approach is a combination of approaches. Indeed, Isshiki and Snidecor reported that most esophageal speakers actually do use a combination of injection techniques.[45] Perhaps the simplest approach is to ask the patient, "Can you burp on purpose?" It is surprising how many patients can inject air and burp before the therapy program begins. Therefore, before beginning a long explanation of air injection, just ask!

Once the patient can place air consistently into the upper esophagus, by whatever method, much time should be spent practicing single-syllable words. A solid foundation for conversational esophageal speech must be laid at the single-syllable level. All vowel-consonant and consonant-vowel combinations should be practiced and drilled until the percentage of successful intelligible productions is at least at a 90% level. Lengthening the vowels in the single-syllable productions will prepare the patient to move on to two-syllable words.

From two-syllable words, it is possible to start building phrases. Phrase work may continue from two-syllable phrases through eight-syllable phrases produced on one air injection. The average length of a conversational phrase is approximately seven syllables.

It is important for the patient to inject the air into the esophagus as smoothly as possible and to expel the air producing voicing with minimal effort. Berlin listed four training objectives in establishing proficient esophageal speech.[46,47] These objectives may be quantified by the patient and clinician during the training process.

■ **Skill 1:** The ability to phonate reliably on demand. Proficient esophageal speakers are able to produce phonation 100% of the time.

■ **Skill 2:** The second skill is to achieve a short latency between air injection into the esophagus and phonation. A stopwatch is used to measure the latency period. When the patient signals the clinician that he or she initiated the air injection into the esophagus, the clinician starts the stopwatch and then stops the stopwatch when the clinician hears vocalization. Proficient esophageal speakers are able to maintain a short latency, ranging between 0.2 to 0.6 seconds between air injection and phonation. Because the laryngectomee's esophageal air capacity ranges from 40 to 80 cubic centimeters (cc) of air,[48] which is much less than the vital capacity of lungs in healthy adults, frequent reinflation of the esophagus must take place while the patient is talking. Thus, it is important for the patient to quickly inflate the esophagus and expel the air during conversational speech.

■ **Skill 3:** The third skill is to maintain an adequate duration of phonation. A stopwatch is also required to record the maximum sustained duration of the vowel /a/ on one air intake. Good esophageal speakers are able to sustain /a/ for 2.4 to 3.6 seconds.

■ **Skill 4:** The fourth skill is the ability to sustain phonation during articulation. This skill refers to the number of times the syllable /da/ can be repeated on one air intake without consciously reinjecting air into the esophagus. Proficient esophageal speakers are able to phonate 8 to 10 syllables per air intake.

Several factors are monitored and modified throughout the phrase building process. These include stoma noise, air "klunking" noise (caused by forceful air injections), eye blinking, and other unnecessary facial expressions or grimaces. Loudness, inflection, and phrasing exercises are also practiced in treatment to increase overall speech naturalness.

Proficient esophageal speech is a learned process that requires much work and dedication to be mastered. Motivation, desire, and vigor are essential factors that must be present for successful voice development to occur.[49] Patients who do not make a positive commitment or who are unwilling to devote sufficient time to the process are not likely to do well. Other factors that may have a negative influence on the successful development of esophageal voice include postradiation fibrosis, pharyngeal scarring, esophageal stenosis, recurring suture line fistulas, and defects in neural innervation.[50] Sloane, Griffin, and O'Dwyer[51] found that anatomic differences in the reconstructed PE segment had a profound effect in the acquisition of esophageal speech. They used the Blom-Singer esophageal insufflation test (described later in this chapter), combined with videofluroscopy, to assess the PE segment during esophageal speech and found hypotonicity, hypertonicity, PE spasm, and stricture of the reconstructed pharynx to affect the dynamics of esophageal speech.

Surgical Prosthetics

Another option for speech rehabilitation following a total laryngectomy is the use of a surgical prosthesis. The possible reestablishment of voice through laryngeal reconstruction and prosthetic surgery has long been recognized. Reports dating as far back as 1874 detail the results of voicing achieved either through the spontaneous creation of a tracheoesophageal (TE) fistula or through the creation of planned TE shunts.[52-54] In their excellent article, Blom and Singer[55] presented the history of the attempts to restore voicing through various laryngeal reconstruction techniques, shunt surgeries, and surgical prostheses (also see[56-63]).

The primary goal of all the shunt-type surgeries was to effectively channel pulmonary air into the esophagus where the air could set the pharyngoesophageal segment into vibration for the production of voice. Although several of these procedures were successful in meeting this goal, two major problems seemed to persist with these techniques: aspiration of saliva, liquids, and foods into the trachea through the fistula and breakdown or stenosis of the shunts.[59]

Singer and Blom developed the tracheoesophageal puncture (TEP) voice restoration technique to solve these problems. In this 15- to 20-minute surgical procedure, a fistula is created between the trachea and the esophagus in the superior border of the stoma. The tracheoesophageal puncture can be performed as a primary (at the time of surgery) or secondary surgical voice restoration procedure.[64,65] Following the puncture, a 14 French [Fr] balloon catheter is directed downward through the fistula from the trachea and into the esophagus.[65,66] Approximately 5 cc of water is injected into the catheter balloon to weight down the distal end, keeping it from extruding. The proximal end of the catheter is capped and secured to the neck with tape or a suture. Freeman and Hamaker[64] recommend using a Silastic-coated tube because it has less tissue reactivity compared with latex rubber catheters. The catheter can serve as a feeding tube following a primary laryngectomy or a myotomy at the time of the tracheo-esophageal puncture.

The tracheoesophageal puncture creates a fistula between the posterior wall of the trachea and the anterior wall of the esophagus for the insertion of a voice prosthesis. The voice prosthesis is a one-way valve made of medically high-grade silicone. Once inserted into the tracheoesophageal puncture, the voice prosthesis prevents aspiration during swallowing and fistula stenosis. The one-way valve permits pulmonary air to enter the esophagus when the stoma is occluded while the patient exhales. The valve opens under positive pressure as the air enters the esophagus and closes by elastic recoil. It does not permit a reverse flow of saliva or liquids into the trachea. The voice prosthesis is cylindrical in shape with a neck strap(s) that is taped to the skin of the neck to keep it in place. At the distal end, a slit, hinged, or ball valve is placed in the esophagus. An anterior opening at the proximal end allows pulmonary air to flow through the voice prosthesis and permits internal cleaning. The prosthesis is securely retained in the fistula by a flexible "retention collar" that holds the prosthesis in place by gripping the inside of the esophageal wall to prevent dislodgment (Figure 9-14).

The length of the voice prosthesis ranges in size from 6 mm (1.4 cm) to 28 mm (3.6 cm). The most commonly used diameter of voice prostheses is a 16 French; however, a 20 French diameter voice prosthesis is also available.

There are several manufacturers of voice prostheses. InHealth Technologies manufactures three styles of Blom-Singer voice prostheses, which include the Duckbill, Low Pressure, and Indwelling Low Pressure prostheses (Figure 9-15 A, B, C). Bivona Medical Technologies manufactures the Duckbill, Ultra Low™ Resistance, and the Bivona-Colorado™ Voice Prosthesis (Figure 9-16 A, B, C). The Provox® 2 Indwelling Voice Prosthesis is distributed through Bivona Medical Technologies (Figure 9-17). The

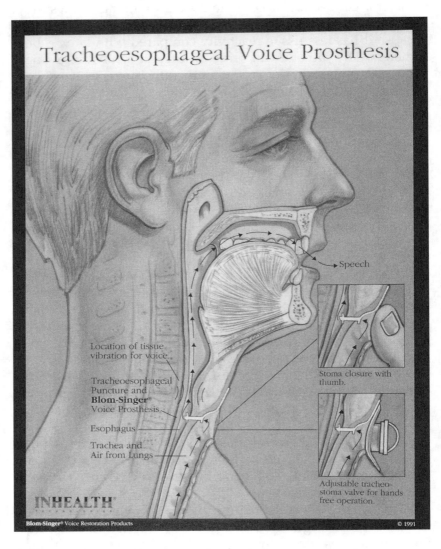

Figure 9-14. Representation of speech being produced using a tracheoesophageal voice prosthesis. (Photo courtesy of InHealth Technologies.)

492

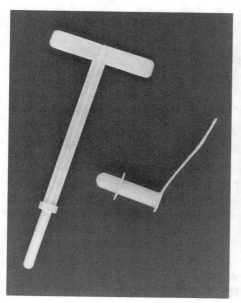

A

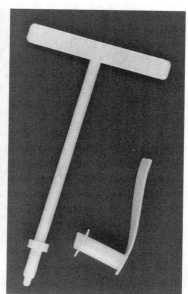

B

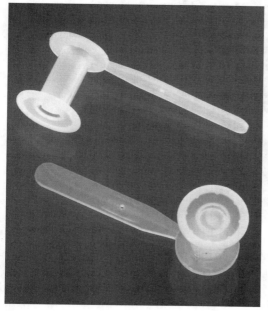

C

Figure 9-15 A. Blom-Singer Duckbill Voice Prosthesis. (Photos by Rick Berkey, St. Elizabeth Medical Center, Dayton, Ohio.) **B.** Blom-Singer Low Pressure Voice Prosthesis. **C.** Blom-Singer InDwelling Low Pressure Voice Prosthesis. (Photo courtesy of InHealth Technologies.)

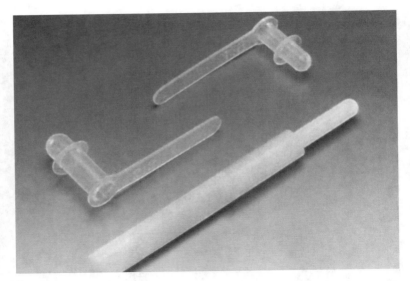

A

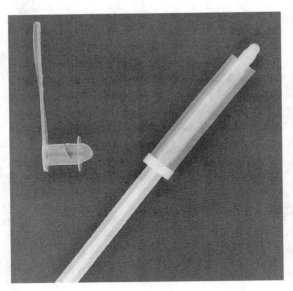

B

Figure 9-16 A. Bivona Duckbill Voice Prosthesis. (Photo courtesy of Bivona Medical Technologies.) **B.** Bivona Ultra Low™ Resistance Voice Prosthesis. (Photo by Rick Berkey, St. Elizabeth Medical Center, Dayton, Ohio.) *(continued)*

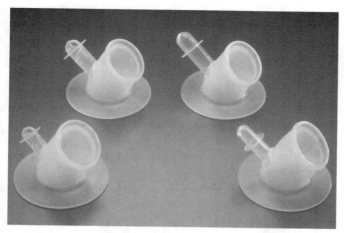

Figure 9-16. *(continued)* **C.** Bivona™ Colorado Voice Prosthesis.

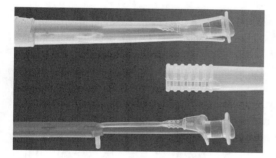

Figure 9-17. Provox® 2 Indwelling Voice Prosthesis.

VoiceMaster® Indwelling low-resistance voice prosthesis is manufactured by enterMed from The Netherlands (Figure 9-18).

When a patient is using a voice prosthesis, the stoma may be occluded manually with a thumb or a finger, or it may be occluded by a tracheostoma valve. The tracheostoma valve has component parts. A housing collar is taped and glued around the stoma. A valve is inserted into the housing collar. When the patient develops sufficient pulmonary air pressure to produce speech, the valve will close, occluding the stoma and directing the air into the voice prosthesis.

The success rate for achieving tracheoesophageal speech is high, although some have reported the possibility of long-term

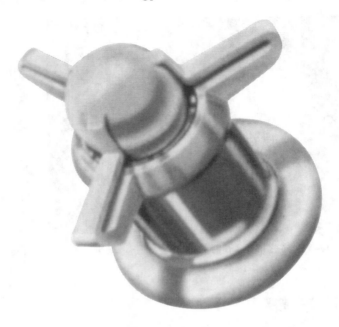

Figure 9-18. VoiceMaster prosthesis. (Photo courtesy of Entermed b.v., PO Box 236, Woerden, The Netherlands.)

problems and complications.[67,68] It has been our experience, however, that if patients are well prepared and properly trained, most total laryngectomy patients can be successful users of this form of communication. Let us examine the speech-language pathologist's role with surgical prosthetics.

Role of the Speech-Language Pathologist and Surgical Prosthetics

The role of the speech-language pathologist who works with surgical prosthetics is multidimensional and includes the following:

- aiding the surgeon in evaluating the patient's suitability to use the voice prosthesis as a form of communication
- sizing and fitting the prosthesis
- teaching the patient to fit and care for the prosthesis
- maximizing the patient's ability to communicate while using the prosthesis
- fitting the tracheostoma valve.

Specialized training is required when working with laryngectomees. The American Speech-Language-Hearing Association has published approved guidelines for "Evaluation and Treatment for Tracheoesophageal Fistulization/Puncture."[69] A number of workshops and seminars are available for the speech-language pathologist throughout the year for basic training, as well as for acquiring information on the latest procedures and techniques. The International Center for Post-Laryngectomy Voice Restoration in Indianapolis, Indiana, offers monthly courses and the International Association of Laryngectomees Voice Rehabilitation Institute offers a yearly 5-day training conference. A number of voice institutes also offer courses in laryngectomy rehabilitation. Postings are listed in the ASHA Leader.

Patient Evaluation

Although most laryngectomized patients may be candidates for surgical prosthetics, certain social situations and medical and physical conditions may decrease the chances for long-term successful use.

For example, patient motivation is important. At times, the family may be more motivated than the patient for the patient to attempt this form of communication. In most cases, however, the patient must be capable of and interested in caring for the prosthesis. Andrews et al listed a number of characteristics necessary for patient selection.[68] These include the following:

- motivation and mental stability
- adequate understanding of the anatomy and the mechanics of the prosthesis
- adequate manual dexterity and visual acuity to care for the stoma and the prosthesis
- no significant hypopharyngeal stenosis
- speech production with esophageal insufflation via a properly positioned esophageal catheter
- adequate pulmonary reserve
- stoma of adequate depth and diameter to accept the prosthesis without airway compromise

Singer and Blom reported that chronic pulmonary disease, diabetes, and alcoholism have not presented significant problems.[61] Our experience has not been positive with patients who have chronic drinking problems. Alcohol abuse has also been found to be a major deterrent in the production of efficient voice, as well as personal care of the tracheoesophageal puncture.[67,70,71]

Cricopharyngeal spasm[72,73] and pharyngeal constrictor hypertonicity[74] have been implicated as reasons for failure to utilize the voice prosthesis successfully. An esophageal air insufflation test, a procedure described by Blom et al[75] informs the speech-language pathologist, surgeon, or both of the ability of the PE segment to vibrate. In this procedure a marked 14 Fr. catheter is inserted transnasally into the upper esophagus to approximately the 25-cm marker. Inserting the catheter to this point ensures the tip of the catheter to be at the approximate level of the cervical esophagus near the proposed tracheoesophageal puncture. A tracheostoma tape housing with an adapter is attached to the peristomal skin. The patient is instructed to open and relax the jaw for the production of the vowel /a/ and to inhale deeply and sustain the vowel for as long as possible while the examiner or patient occludes the stoma adaptor to redirect the air into the esophagus. With this self-insufflation test, the patient should be able to sustain phonation without interruption of the sound for 10 to 15 seconds and produce fluent speech when counting or saying sentences.

If the patient's sound production is strained or exhibits esophageal spasms, the patient may be a candidate for a surgical procedure or Botulinum neurotoxin injections to allow for the PE segment to vibrate. The air insufflation test is valuable for successful patient selection. This test indicates in advance those patients who are likely to experience esophageal spasms post-surgically. If the spasm does occur, the patient is prepared for this possibility. A manometer has also been used to record pressure changes in the esophagus.[75,76] Yetiser et al[77] found insufflation testing was 43% accurate and manometric measurements 86% accurate in evaluating and predicting patients who would develop esophageal speech or tracheoesophageal speech. Techniques for management of pharyngeal constrictor hypertonicity include secondary and primary pharyngeal constrictor muscle myotomy, pharyngeal neurectomy, Botulinum toxin injections, and Cheesman technique.[78] Instead of a surgical approach to treatment of spasms or hypertonicity of the laryngectomized pharynx, unilateral chemical denervation of the pharyngeal constrictor muscles with Botulinum neurotoxin type A has proven to be successful in eliminating muscle spasms.[79,80] A myotomy involves cutting muscle fibers of the pharyngeal constrictures to prevent esophageal spasms when voicing. Pharyngeal neurectomy is resection of all branches in the nerve plexus to eliminate hypertonicity or spasms. The Chessman technique involves surgical closure of the pharyngeal constrictors to reduce hypertonicity and esophageal spasms.[78]

A trial injection of lidocaine into the pharyngoesophageal segment is a prognostic indicator for successful TEP speech prior to Botulinum neurotoxin injections for esophageal spasms. If the patient has a positive response to the lidocaine block demonstrating decreased phonatory effort and no spasms, percutaneous botulinum neurotoxin type A injections under EMG guidance is administered at three separate sites to the cricopharyngeus.[81] Some patients may need repeated injections to help relax the PE segment. Botulinum neurotoxin injections along with voice therapy may facilitate TEP speech and maintain controlled relaxation of the PE segment during speaking, therefore repeated injections may not be necessary.

Patient Fitting

To prevent the risk of disease transmission from blood-borne pathogens, the speech-language pathologist must follow Universal Precautions when fitting a voice prosthesis. These precautions can be reviewed in the "Centers for Disease Control Morbidity and Mortality Weekly Report"[82] or in ASHA's "Aids/HIV Update,"[83] or the guidelines for "Evaluation and Treatment for Tracheoesophageal Fistulization/Puncture."[69]

When the tracheoesophageal puncture is surgically created, the surgeon will place a size 14 Fr balloon catheter through the puncture and direct it into the distal esophagus. If the tracheoesophageal puncture is created as a secondary procedure, prosthesis sizing and fitting may take place approximately 36 to

48 hours after the fistulization. The fistula site must be healed before the voice prosthesis is inserted, otherwise there may be a delay in fitting the patient. If the patient undergoes a tracheo-esophageal puncture as part of the primary laryngectomy, prosthesis sizing and fitting may be delayed for 3 weeks or until the patient's surgical incisions show adequate healing.

The Blom-Singer Duckbill Voice Prostheses and Low Pressure Voice Prostheses are available in nine sizes ranging in length from 6 mm (1.4 cm) to 28 mm (3.6 cm). The Blom-Singer InDwelling Low Pressure Voice Prostheses come in eight lengths ranging from 6 mm (1.4 cm) to 25 mm (3.3 cm). There are eight sizes available in the Bivona Duckbill Voice Prostheses ranging from 1.4 cm to 3.3 cm in length. The Bivona Ultra™ Resistance Voice Prostheses come in seven varying lengths ranging from 1.4 cm to 3.0 cm. Five lengths ranging from 4.5 mm to 12.5 mm are available in the Provox® Indwelling Voice Prostheses. The VoiceMaster® is available in 4 sizes ranging from 8 mm to 10 mm.

At the time of fitting, the speech-language pathologist will measure the tracheoesophageal lumen for the most appropriate size. For the comfort of the patient, it is important for the clinician to give an overview of the entire fitting process and then explain each step in detail so that no surprises are incurred.[84] The following steps may be taken during the initial voice prosthesis fitting process:

- Clean the stoma area of mucus and any encrusted material using hydrogen peroxide applied with cotton applicators and wipe with 4 x 4 gauze.
- Remove any sutures that are holding the catheter in place.
- Slowly but deliberately remove the catheter from the puncture. In case of an inflated balloon catheter, the residual air or water must be withdrawn using a standard 10-cc syringe before the catheter is removed. Before removing the catheter, instruct the patient to refrain from swallowing to prevent saliva from flowing through the TEP.
- Replace the catheter with a French 16 soft red rubber catheter (when using a catheter, make sure the larger end is knotted or capped to prevent leaking of fluids through the catheter) or a Blom-Singer tracheoesophageal puncture dilator (Figure 9-19). The patient can use either device to plug the puncture when cleaning. It is strongly recommended to teach the patient to always keep the puncture

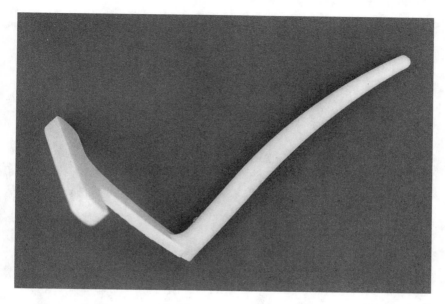

Figure 9-19. Blom-Singer Tracheoesophageal Puncture Dilator. (Photo by Rick Berkey, St. Elizabeth Medical Center, Dayton, Ohio.)

stented with a catheter, dilator, or voice prosthesis. Teach the patient to insert the catheter or dilator in the unlikely event the voice prosthesis ever comes out.

■ Control any mucus from the stoma, the oral cavity, and the nose that was produced when the catheter was removed.

■ With the catheter removed and the puncture unstented, the phonatory mechanism can be tested with the least resistance to airflow. Ask the patient to take a breath. Occlude the stoma with your thumb or finger while the patient slowly exhales saying the vowel /a/. This gives the speech-language pathologist a subjective idea of the ease or difficulty with which the patient can produce voice. If the patient demonstrates much difficulty, then it is possible that internal edema is still present. It may also be an indication of esophageal spasm. If no voicing is produced, one should continue with the sizing and fitting procedure and have the patient return to your office in a week to work on voicing.

■ Place a sizing device (Figure 9-20) into the puncture as far as it will go. The sizing device is essentially a dummy voice prosthesis that has incremental markings and numbers that

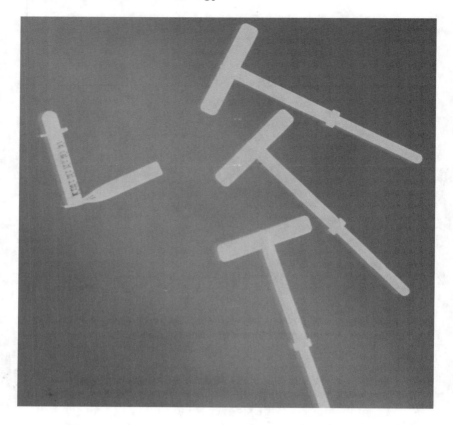

Figure 9-20. Blom-Singer Voice Prosthesis Sizer.

correspond to the various lengths of manufactured prostheses. When the sizing device is completely inserted you may feel the end of the device touch the posterior pharyngeal wall or go down into the esophagus. The patient can usually indicate when he or she feels the sizer against the posterior pharyngeal wall. Gently pull the sizer out until the retention collar grasps the inside of the anterior wall of the esophagus. Look at the number on the sizer that can be seen on the outside of the puncture. Choose the size prosthesis that corresponds to that number. If the size is between numbers, choose the longer prosthesis. It is best to oversize initially. If the prosthesis is sized too short, the fistula will begin to stenose at the anterior wall of the esophagus, preventing airflow through the prosthesis. The speech-language pathologist should allow for a small amount of "play" (forward-backward movement) when the patient swallows.

▪ Remove the sizing device and insert the correct sized voice prosthesis into the puncture using the insertion tool. Make sure you follow the angle of the puncture and firmly push the prosthesis until you feel or hear the retention collar "pop" into the esophagus. Hold the outer flange and gently remove the insertion tool by rotating and pulling it forward. When the insertion tool has been removed, check the seating of the prosthesis by tugging gently on the flange. The prosthesis should hold firmly in place. Tape the flange to the neck. After the prosthesis is fitted, ask the patient to inhale. Occlude the stoma with your thumb or finger while the patient exhales gently sustaining the vowel /a/. If the prosthesis is sized correctly, the diverted air will cause the PE segment to vibrate. The patient must, however, increase the air pressure greater than when voice was produced without the prosthesis in place.

▪ Check to make sure there is no leaking of fluids either around or through the voice prosthesis by having the patient drink water. If leaking is noted around the prosthesis, allow more time for the fistula to seal around the prosthesis. A new or different prosthesis should be inserted if leaking is noted through the prosthesis.

▪ The patient should be taught to occlude the stoma with his or her own thumb or finger and to produce voice independently. Start with sustained vowels then words such as counting. Speech material should be provided and the patient encouraged to practice frequently throughout the day.

▪ Teach the patient or significant other to clean the voice prosthesis without removing it. Mucus and crusts can be softened by using cotton applicators dipped in hydrogen peroxide applied to the anterior opening of the prosthesis. Using a long forceps, these crusts can then be removed.

▪ Schedule the patient to be seen back in the office a few days after the initial voice prosthesis fitting to learn independent care.

Independent Care

When the patient is seen for the second visit, the speech-language pathologist begins to teach the patient and significant other to remove, clean, and reinsert the prosthesis. The prosthesis should by removed for cleaning as needed. Some patients may choose to do so weekly, and others may choose to leave the prosthesis in place for several weeks. Cleaning is preferably accomplished at the same time the patient does the stoma care using adequate lighting and in front of a mirror. To remove the prosthesis, the patient is instructed to firmly grasp the flange and pull forward. When the prosthesis is removed, a size 16 French catheter or a tracheoesophageal puncture dilator is immediately inserted into the fistula to prevent aspiration and stenosis. The prosthesis is cleaned according to the instructions given by the manufacturer. Care should be taken not to violate the slit valve end of the tube. Solvents or petroleum-based cleaning products should not be used because they might damage the silicone.

Patients may also clean the voice prosthesis without removing the device from the tracheoesophageal puncture by using the Blom-Singer Flushing Pipette (Figure 9-21). The Blom-Singer Flushing Pipette is a plastic tapered tube with a bulb on one end. The patient is instructed to fill the pipette with water and position the device into the voice prosthesis until it abuts against the stopper on the stem of the pipette. Once properly positioned, the patient quickly squeezes the bulb on the pipette to inject the water through the prosthesis flushing out any debris

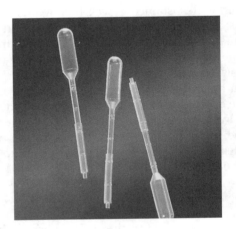

Figure 9-21. Blom-Singer flushing pipette.

that may have accumulated inside the prosthesis. The debris is flushed into the esophagus. Removing the prosthesis for cleaning is recommended if a large mucus plug is contained within the prosthesis.

Instructions for fitting the voice prosthesis include:

■ Check the slit valve or flapper valve to make sure the edges are not stuck together. Place the tip of the insertion tool into the open end of the voice prosthesis. Avoid squeezing or damaging the slit valve at the tip of the prosthesis.

■ Place a small amount of oil-free, water-soluble lubricant (such as Surgi-Lube) on the tip of the prosthesis. Place the tip of the voice prosthesis in the fistula with the neck strap pointed upwards. Firmly insert until the circular retention collar can be felt to "snap" open within the esophagus. (Insertion or removal of the prosthesis occasionally causes slight bleeding at the fistula. Persistent bleeding should be brought to the attention of the physician.)

■ Place a finger against the flange and gently withdraw the insertion tool from the fully inserted prosthesis.

■ Apply a small strip of hypoallergenic adhesive tape over the flange to secure it to the neck to prevent movement or accidental dislodgment.

The low-pressure voice prosthesis has a recessed valve and a low profile tip making insertion more difficult to insert into the fistula. An easier method of insertion for the Blom-Singer Low Pressure Voice Prosthesis is using the Blom-Singer Gel Cap Insertion System (Figure 9-22 A, B). The gel cap provides a smooth, rounded shape to the tip by folding the retention collar in a forward position inside the cap making insertion of the prosthesis less traumatic to the surrounding tissue. The gel cap is designed to dissolve inside the esophagus within minutes after insertion. After the voice prosthesis is correctly placed in the tracheoesophageal puncture, the patient should hold the prosthesis in place with the inserter tool for at least 3 minutes, allowing time for the gel cap to dissolve and the retention collar to unfold. Explicit instructions in applying the gel cap are provided by the manufacturer.

In 1995, the Blom-Singer InDwelling Low Pressure Voice Prosthesis (Figure 9-15 C) was introduced for patients who are unable or resist changing the Low Pressure Voice Prosthesis

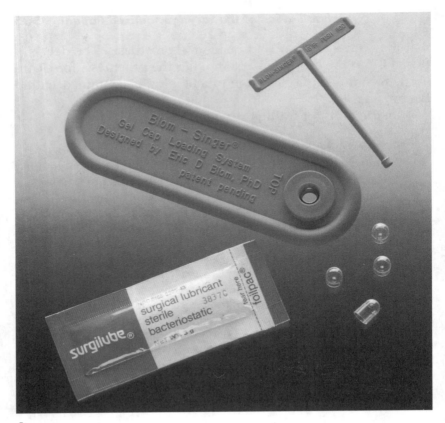

A

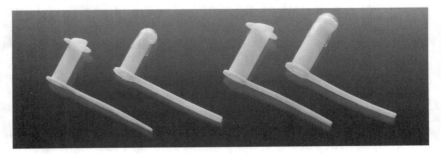

B

Figure 9-22 A. Blom-Singer Gel Cap Insertion System. **B.** Example of gel cap on low pressure voice prosthesis. (Photos courtesy of InHealth Technologies.)

506

every 2 to 3 days as recommended.[85] The Blom-Singer In-Dwelling Low Pressure Voice Prosthesis is a 20 Fr prosthesis inserted and removed by a physician or a trained speech-language pathologist. Inserting the prosthesis requires using the gel cap (as previously described). It is available in lengths ranging from 6 mm to 25 mm.

A Fr 22 tracheoesophageal puncture dilator is inserted into the fistula to slightly dilate the opening. The dilator is removed and the voice prosthesis is inserted with the neck strap pointed upwards. After insertion, the voice prosthesis is held into position for at least 3 minutes allowing the gel cap to dissolve and the retention collar to unfold within the esophagus. Check to make sure the prosthesis is secured by rotating the prosthesis 360°. Once the prosthesis is correctly placed, the voice prosthesis strap is detached from the safety peg on the inserter. If the prosthesis does not rotate freely, an A-P radiographic examination of the tracheostoma is recommended to confirm if the retention collar is positioned within the esophagus.[84]

The InDwelling Voice Prosthesis may be worn until it ceases to function correctly or begins to leak. A hemostat is used to remove the prosthesis by grasping the outer rim of the device pulling gently and firmly until the prosthesis is completely removed. Once removed, a Fr 22 tracheostoma dilator is inserted into the puncture. Keep the dilator in the tracheoesophageal lumen for at least 5 minutes before inserting a new prosthesis. The InDwelling Low Pressure Voice Prosthesis can be cleaned without removal by using the flushing pipettes.

The Blom-Singer Voice Prosthesis is available from International Healthcare Technologies (1110 Mark Avenue, Carpinteria, CA 93013-2918; 805-684-9337 or 800-477-5969). The Bivona Voice Prosthesis is available from Bivona Medical Technologies (5700 W. 23rd Ave., Gary, IN 46406; 219-989-9150 or 800-348-6064).

Maximizing Communication

Once fit with the prosthesis, some patients readily occlude the stoma and speak with excellent phrasing and inflection, similar to their prelaryngectomy speech patterns. Other patients may need instruction in occluding the stoma and to coordinate proper breath control for phrasing and articulation. Patients who have used esophageal voice prior to surgical prosthetics may have to work on eliminating the habit of injecting air into the esophagus. The result of the use of a surgical prosthesis is a superior esophageal voice.

Tracheostoma Valve

The tracheostoma valve is a device designed for laryngectomees who have undergone a tracheoesophageal puncture and communicate with various types of voice prosthesis. The use of this valve obviates the need to manually occlude the stoma for speech production, thus freeing both hands. The Blom-Singer Adjustable Tracheostoma Valve (Figure 9-23) is available from InHealth Technologies and the Bivona Tracheostoma Valve (Figure 9-24) and Bivona Tracheostoma Valve II (Figure 9-25)

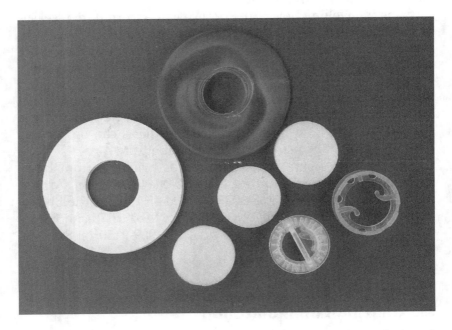

Figure 9-23. Blom-Singer Adjustable Tracheostoma Valve with Humidifilter. (Photo by Rick Berkey, St. Elizabeth Medical Center, Dayton, Ohio.)

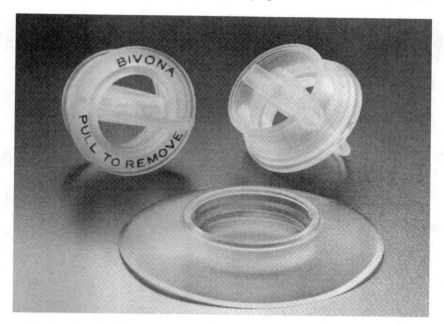

Figure 9-24. Bivona Tracheostoma Valve. (Photo courtesy of Bivona Medical Technologies.)

are available from Bivona Medical Technologies. In evaluating patient use of the valve, the speech-language pathologist focuses on the size, shape, and contour of the stoma and surrounding tissue.

Successful use of the speaking valve depends upon the ability to tape and glue the valve collar to a sufficient amount of tissue surrounding the stoma to prevent it from being dislodged by the pulmonary air pressure. Patients with sunken stomas or uneven skin tissue surrounding the stoma may not have an adequate skin surface for collar adhesion. Other factors that may influence wearing a speaking valve include phlegm production, back-pressure, age, and motivation.[29]

The first step in evaluating patient use is to attach the housing collar using a special skin adherent and double-sided tape discs or double-sided foam discs provided in the fitting kit. Once the housing collar is in place, the tracheostoma valve is fitted. The Blom-Singer Tracheostoma Valve has an internal adjustment

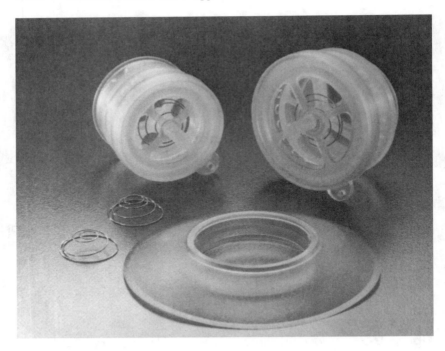

Figure 9-25. Bivona Tracheostoma Valve II. (Photo courtesy of Bivona Medical Technologies.)

sensitivity that allows the patient to adjust the valve from ultra light to medium sensitivity by rotating the faceplate. A proper valve weight must be chosen for the Bivona Tracheostoma Valve. The proper valve weight (ultra light, light, medium, or firm) is the weight that does not close during heavy respiratory effort, but will close when sufficient air pressure is exhaled to produce speech. The Bivona Tracheostoma Valve II has a set of four interchangeable springs designed to provide different degrees of sensitivity. The speech-language pathologist should help the laryngectomee select a speaking valve that requires a lower resistance during resting breathing and not too much effort to close the valve for speaking.[86]

A simple way to determine the degree of valve closure or proper valve weight (depending on the type of valve) is to have the patient walk up and down steps. Begin with the ultra-light setting or valve in place. If the valve closes when the patient is breathing heavily, turn the valve slightly or if using a valve or spring move up to the next weight. Continue this process until a valve that does not close during heavy breathing is found. Rotating the faceplate to adjust the valve sensitivity is an advantage when using the Blom-Singer Adjustable Tracheostoma Valve. The valve must be removed from the housing collar to make the proper valve or spring sensitivity adjustments for the Bivona Tracheostoma Valve or Bivona Tracheostoma Valve II, respectively.

Excessive intratracheal pressure can contribute to an adhesive seal breakdown of the housing when using the tracheostoma valve. Manometric measurements can assess intratracheal back pressure. This measurement is performed by placing the adapter from a disposable Blom-Singer Insufflation test kit into the tracheostoma valve housing and attaching a manometer to the adapter. For normal conversational intensity levels, manometric readings should range between 30 to 35 cm/H_2O. Measurements greater than 35 cm/H_2O indicates higher intratracheal airflow pressure and less time the patient may be able to wear the valve. The manometer may be used as a visual feedback tool to monitor the degree of pressure and serve to control intensity levels.[87] Contributing causes for increased intratracheal pressure may be the voice prosthesis diameter (16-Fr vs 20-Fr), the pharyngeal constrictor muscle hypertonicity, or both.

Use of the tracheostoma valve has been beneficial for many patients, especially those who are required to use both hands while working. A HumidiFiliter can be placed on the Blom-Singer Adjustable Tracheostoma Valve to moisten, warm, and filter inspired air. Some patients report a decrease in coughing with the use of the HumidiFiliter.

Coughing can present a problem for all tracheostoma valve users. The increased air pressure that is produced when coughing will close the valve requiring the valve to be completely removed. Sometimes repeated coughing will cause strain on the adhesive discs that hold the housing collar in place causing premature leaking of air around the housing. Increased mucus will also work the adhesive free from the skin. Another complication is skin irritation from the adhesive. We have found that even with a commercial skin preparation that is brushed on the skin prior to the adherent, some patients still experience skin irritation.

Summary

Although significant advances have been made in the treatment of head and neck cancer, total rehabilitation of the laryngectomized patient continues to be challenging for the patient, the patient's family, and for all professionals involved in this process. Rehabilitation involves a multidisciplinary approach in addressing the patient's physical and psychosocial needs in a comprehensive and timely manner. The speech-language pathologist's role in working with the cancer patient and family involves both counseling and management of all communication and swallowing needs. Our interactions with the cancer patient and family may, at times, be challenging and personally stressful, but most often the results of our efforts are both satisfying and rewarding. No other group of patients with communication impairments has the potential to progress from very limited communication to functional oral communication as rapidly as the laryngectomized patient.

The laryngectomized patient has several communication options from which to choose. The speech-language pathologist is encouraged to become familiar with all options and for the sake of the patient, to show no biases against any. As research continues to expand and improve these options, so, too, will the role of the speech-language pathologist also expand.

References

1. Landis SH, Murray T, Bolden S, Wingo PA. Cancer statistics, 1999. *CA Cancer J Clin.* 1999;49:8-31.
2. Carew JF, Shah JP. Advances in multimodality therapy for laryngeal cancer. *CA Cancer J Clin.* 1998;48:211-228.
3. Shah JP, Karnell LH, Hoffman HT, Ariyan S, Brown GS, Fee WZ, Glass AG, Goepfert H, Ossoff RH, Fremgen A. Patterns of care for cancer of the larynx in the United States. *Arch Otolaryngol Head Neck Surg.* 1997;123:475-483.
4. American Cancer Society. *Cancer facts and figures.* Atlanta Ga: Author; 1999.
5. Rothman KJ, Cann CI, Flanders D, Fried MP. Epidemiology of laryngeal cancer. *Epidemiol Rev.* 1980;2:195-209.
6. Casper J, Colton R. *Clinical Manual for Laryngectomy and Head/Neck Cancer Rehabilitation.* 2nd ed. San Diego, Calif: Singular Publishing Group; 1998.

7. DeWeese DD, Saunders WH, Schuller DE, Schleuning AJ. *Otolaryngology— Head and Neck Surgery.* 7th ed. St Louis, Mo: CV Mosby; 1988.

8. American Joint Committee on Cancer. *Manual for Staging of Cancer.* 5th ed. Philadelphia, Pa: Lippincott-Raven; 1997.

9. Coutard H. Roentgentherapy of epitheliomas of the tonsillar region laryngopharynx and larynx from 1920 to 1926. *Am J Roentgenol.* 1921;28:313-331.

10. Kuppersmith RB, Greco SC, Teh BS, Donovan DT, Grant W, Chiu JKC, Cain RB, Butler EB. Intensity-modulated radiotherapy: first results with this new technology on neoplasms of the head and neck. *ENT Ear Nose Throat J.* 1999;78:238-251.

11. Kian Ang K, Trotti A, Garden AS, Foote RL. Importance of overall time factor in postoperative radiotherapy. *Proceedings of the Fourth International Conference on Head and Neck Cancer.* July 28-August 1; Toronto, Canada. Arlington Va: The Society of Head and Neck Surgeons; 1996:231-235.

12. Parsons JT, Mendenhall WM, Stringer SP, Cassisi NJ, Million RR. An analysis of factores influencing the outcome of postoperative irradiation for squamous cell carcinoma of the oral cavity. *Int J Radiat Oncol Biol Phys.* 1997;39:137-148.

13. Huntley TC, Borrowdale RW. Tracheoesophageal voice restoration following laryngopharyngectomy and laryngopharyngoesophagectomy. In: Blom ED, Singer MI, Hamaker RC, eds. *Tracheoesophageal Voice Restoration Following Total Laryngectomy.* San Diego, Calif: Singular Publishing Group; 1998:41-49.

14. Ariyan S. The pectoralis major myocutaneous flap: a versatile flap for reconstruction in the head and neck. *Plast and Reconstr Surg.* 1979;63:73-81.

15. Murakami Y, Saito S, Ikari T, Haraguehi S, Okada D, Maruyama T. Esophageal reconstruction with a skin grafted pectoralis major muscle flap. *Arch Otolaryngol Head Neck Surg.* 1982;108:719.

16. Anthony JP, Singer MI, Mathes SJ. Pharyngoesophageal reconstruction using the tubed radial forearm flap. *Clin Plast Surg.* 1994;21:137-147.

17. Shangold LM, Urken ML, Lawson W. Jejunal transplantation for pharyngoesophageal reconstruction. *Otolaryngol Clin North Am.* 1991;24:1321.

18. Clayman C. *The American Medical Association Home Medical Library: Fighting Cancer.* Pleasantville, NY: The American Medical Association; 1991.

19. Raybaud-Diogen H, Fortin A, Morency R, Roy J, Monteil RA, Tetu B. Markers of radioresistance in squamous cell carcinomas of the head and neck: a clinicopathologic and immunohistochemical study. *J Clin Oncol.* 1997;15:1030-1038.

20. Iskowitz M. Historical surgery a "miracle in progress" for accident victim. *Adv Speech Lang Pathol Audiolog.* 1998;8:6-9.

21. Campinelli PA. Audiological considerations in achieving esophageal voice. *Eye Ear Nose Throat Monthly.* 1964;43:76-80.

22. Diedrich WM, Youngstrom KA. *Alaryngeal Speech.* Springfield Ill: Charles C Thomas; 1966.

23. LaBorwit L. Speech rehabilitation for laryngectomized patients. *Ear Nose Throat J.* 1980;59:82-89.

24. Clark J, Stemple J. Assessment of three modes of alaryngeal speech with a synthetic sentence identification SSI task in varying message-to-competition ratios. *J Speech Hear Res.* 1982;25:333-338.

25. Hilgers FJ, Aaronson NK, Ackerstaff AH, Schouwenburg PF, van Zandwikj N. The influence of a heat and moisture exchanger HME on the respiratory symptoms after total laryngectomy. *Clin Otolaryngol.* 1991;16:152-156.

26. Ackerstaff AH, Hilgers FJ, Aaronson HK, Balm AJ, van Zandwijk N. Improvements in respiratory and psychosocial functioning following total laryngectomy by the use of a heat and moisture exchanger. *Ann Otol Rhinol Laryngol.* 1993;102:878-883.

27. Grolman W, Schouwenburg PF. Postlaryngectomy airway humidification and air filtration. In: Blom ED, Singer MI, Hamaker RC, eds. *Tracheoesophageal Voice Restoration Following Total Laryngectomy.* San Diego, Calif: Singular Publishing Group; 1998:109-121.

28. Grolman W, Blom ED, Branson RD, Schouwenburg PF, Hamaker RC. An efficiency comparison of four heat and moisture exchangers used in the laryngectomized patient. *Laryngoscope.* 1997;107:814-820.

29. Grolman W, Schouwenburg PF, deBoer MF, Knegt PP, Spoelstra HA, Meeuwis CA. First results with the Blom-Singer adjustable tracheostoma valve. *ORL J Otorhinolaryngol Related Specialities.* 1995;57:165-170.

30. Keith R. *Looking Forward: A Guidebook for the Laryngectomy.* 2nd ed. New York, NY: Thieme Medical Publishers; 1991.

31. Gardner W. *Laryngectomee Speech Rehabilitation.* Springfield, Ill: Charles C Thomas; 1971.

32. Pressman J, Bailey B. The survey of cancer of the larynx with special reference to subtotal laryngectomy. In: Snidecor J, ed. *Speech Rehabilitation of the Laryngectomized.* Springfield, Ill: Charles C Thomas; 1968.

33. International Association of Laryngectomees. *First Aid for (Neck-Breathers) Laryngectomees* [No 4522]. New York, NY: National Office of the American Cancer Society.

34. Lauder E. *Self-Help for the Laryngectomee.* Unpublished manuscript; 1989-1990, (Available from 1115 Whisper Hollow, San Antonio, TX 78230).

35. Sindecor J. *Speech Rehabilitation of the Laryngectomized.* 2nd ed. Springfield Ill: Charles C Thomas; 1968.

36. International Association of Laryngectomees. *Laryngectomized Speaker's Source Book* [No 4521]. New York, NY: National Office of the American Cancer Society.

37. Blood G, Blood I. A tactic for facilitating social interaction with laryngectomees. *J Speech Hear Disord.* 1982;47:416-418.

38. Watterson TL, McFarlane SC. The artificial larynx. *Sem Speech and Lang: Laryngectomee Rehab.* 1995;16:205-214.

39. Keith RL, Shanks JC. Historical highlights: laryngectomy rehabilitation. In: Keith RL, Darley FL, eds. *Laryngectomee Rehabilitation.* 3rd ed. Austin, Tex: Pro-Ed; 1994:1-48.

40. Shanks JC. Essentials for alaryngeal speech: psychology and physiology. In: Keith RL, Darley FL, eds. *Laryngectomee Rehabilitation.* 3rd ed. Austin, Tex: Pro-Ed; 1994:191-203.

41. Doyle PC. *Foundations of Voice and Speech Rehabilitation Following Laryngeal Cancer.* San Diego, Calif: Singular Publishing Group; 1994.

42. Duguay MJ. Esophageal speech training: the initial phase. In: Solmon SJ, Mount KH, eds. *Alaryngeal Speech Rehabilitation for Clinicians by Clinicians.* Austin, Tex: Pro-Ed; 1991:47-78.

43. Salmon S. Methods of air intake for esophageal speech and their associated problems. In: Keith RL, Darley FL, eds. *Laryngectomee Rehabilitation.* 3rd ed. Austin, Tex: Pro-Ed; 1994:219-234.

44. Morrison W. The production of voice following total laryngectomy. *Arch Otolaryngol.* 1981;14:413-431.

45. Isshiki N, Snidecor J. Air intake and usage in esophageal speech. *Acta Oto-Laryngologica.* 1965;59:559-574.

46. Berlin CI. Clinical measurement of esophageal speech, I: Methodology and curves of skill acquisition. *J Speech Hear Disord.* 1963;28:42-51.

47. Berlin CI. Clinical measurement of esophageal speech, III: Performance of nonbiases groups. *J Speech Hear Disord.* 1964;30:174-183.

48. Van den Berg J, Moolenaar-Bijl AJ. Cricopharyngeal sphincter pitch intensity and fluency in oesophageal speech. *Practica Oto-Rhino-Laryngologica.* 1959;21:298-315.

49. Gates G, Ryan W, Cantu E, Hearne E. Current status of laryngectomy rehabilitation: causes of failure. *Am J Otolaryngol.* 1982;32:8-14.

50. Aronson A. *Clinical Voice Disorders: An Interdisciplinary Approach.* New York, NY: Brian C Decker; 1980.

51. Sloane P, Griffin J, O'Dwyer T. Esophageal insufflation and videofluoroscopy for evaluation of esophageal speech in laryngectomy patients: clinical implications. *Radiology.* 1991;181:433-438.

52. Gussenbauer C. Ueber die erste durch Th Billroth am Menschen ausgeführte Kehlkopf-Ecstirpation und die Anwendung eines kunstlichen Kokokopfes. *Arch F Klin Chir.* 1874;17:343-356.

53. Guttman MR, Rehabilitation of the voice in laryngectomized patients. *Arch Otolaryngol.* 1932;15:478-479.

54. Kolson H, Glasgold A. Tracheo-esophageal speech following laryngectomy. *Trans Am Acad Ophthalmol Otolaryngol.* 1967;71:421-425.

55. Blom E, Singer M. Surgical-prosthetic approaches for post-aryngectomy voice restoration. In: Keith RL, Darley FL. eds. *Laryngectomy Rehabilitation.* Austin, Tex: Pro-Ed; 1979.

56. Amatsu M, Matsui T, Maki T, Kanagawa K. Vocal reconstruction after total laryngectomy: a new on-stage surgical technique. *J Otolaryngol Japan.* 1977;80:779-785.

57. Arslan M, Serafini I. Reconstructive laryngectomy: report of the first 35 cases. *Ann Otol Rinol Laryngol.* 1972;81:479-486.

58. Asai R. Laryngoplasty after total laryngectomy. *Arch Otolaryngol.* 1972;95:114-119.

59. Conley J, DeAmesti F, Pierce M. A new surgical technique for the vocal rehabilitation of the laryngectomized patient. *Ann Otol Rhinol Laryngol.* 1958;67:655-664.

60. Shedd D, Schaaf N, Weinberg B. Technical aspects of reed-fistula speech following pharyngolaryngectomy. *J Surgical Oncol.* 1976;8:305-310.

61. Singer MI, Blom E. An endoscopic technique for restoration of voice after laryngectomy. *Ann Otol Rhinol Laryngol.* 1980;89:529-533.

62. Staffieri M. Laryngectomie totale avec reconstitution de la glotte phonatoire. *Rev Laryngolo Otol Rhinol.* 1973;95:63-68.

63. Taub D. Air by-pass voice prosthesis for vocal rehabilitation of laryngectomees. *Ann Otol Rhinol Laryngol.* 1975;84:45-48.

64. Freeman SB, Hamaker RC. Tracheoesophageal voice restoration at time of laryngectomy. In: Blom ED, Singer MI, Hamaker RC, eds. *Tracheoesophageal Voice Restoration Following Total Laryngectomy.* San Diego, Calif: Singular Publishing Group; 1998:19-25.

65. Singer MI, DeLassus Gress C. Secondary tracheoesophageal voice restoration. In: Blom ED, Singer MI, Hamaker RC, eds. *Tracheoesophageal Voice Restoration Following Total Laryngectomy.* San Diego, Calif: Singular Publishing Group; 1998:27-32.

66. Hamaker RC, Singer MI, Blom ED, Daniels HA. Primary voice restoration at laryngectomy. *Arch Otolaryngol.* 1985;111:182-186.

67. Donegan J, Gluckman J, Singh J. Limitations of the Blom-Singer technique for voice restoration. *Ann Otol Rhinol Laryngol.* 1981;90:495-497.

68. Andrews JC, Mickel RA, Hanson DG, Monahan GP, Ward PH. Major complications following tracheo-esophageal puncture for voice rehabilitation. *Laryngoscope.* 1987;97:562-567.

69. American Speech-Language Hearing Association. Position statement and guidelines: evaluation and treatment for tracheoesophageal fistulization/puncture. *Asha,* 1992;34(suppl7):17-21.

70. Johns ME, Cantrell RW. Voice restoration of the total laryngectomy patient: the Singer-Blom technique. *Otolaryngol Head and Neck Surg.* 1981;89:82-86.

71. Schuller DE, Jarrow JE, Kelly DR, Miglets AW. Prognostic factors affecting the success of duckbill vocal restoration. *Otolaryngol Head Neck Surg.* 1983;91:396-398.

72. Isdebski K, Reed CG, Ross JC, Hilsinger RL. Problems with tracheo-esophageal fistula voice restoration in totally laryngectomized patients. *Arch Otolaryngol Head Neck Surg.* 1994;120:840-845.

73. Simpson CB, Postma GN, Stone RE, Ossoff RH. Speech outcomes after laryngeal cancer management. *Otolaryngol Clin North Am.* 1997;30:189-205.

74. Singer MI, Blom E. Selective myotomy for voice restoration after total laryngectomy. *Arch Otolaryngol.* 1981;107:670-673.

75. Blom ED, Singer MI, Hamaker RC. An improved esophageal insufflation test. *Arch Otolaryngol.* 1985;111:211-212.

76. Martinkosky SJ. Tracheoesophageal puncture: general considerations. In: Solmon SJ, Mount KH, eds. *Alaryngeal Speech Rehabilitation for Clinicians by Clinicians.* Austin, Tex: Pro-Ed; 1991:107-138.

77. Yetiser S, Serce G, Mus N. Evaluation of esophageal speech in patients with total laryngectomy: a comparison of esophageal insufflation and intra-esophageal manometric tests. *Phonoscope.* 1998;4:255-264.

78. Hamaker RC, Cheesman AD. Surgical management of pharyngeal constrictor muscle hypertonicity. In: Blom ED, Singer MI, Hamaker RC, eds. *Tracheoesophageal Voice Restoration Following Total Laryngectomy.* San Diego, Calif: Singular Publishing Group; 1998:83-87.

79. Crary MA, Glowasky AL. Using Botulinum Toxin A to improve speech and swallowing function following total laryngectomy. *Arch Otolaryngol Head Neck Surg.* 1996;122:760-763.

80. Hoffman HT, Fisher H, VanDemark D, Peterson KL, McCulloch TM, Karnell LH, Funk GF. Botulinum neurotoxin injection after total laryngectomy. *Head and Neck.* 1997;19:92-97.

81. Hoffman HT, McCulloch TM. Botulinum neurotoxin for tracheoesophageal voice failure. In: Blom ED, Singer MI, Hamaker RC, eds. *Tracheoesophageal Voice Restoration Following Total Laryngectomy.* San Diego, Calif: Singular Publishing Group; 1998:83-87.

82. Centers for Disease Control. *Perspectives in Disease Prevention and Health Promotion.* 1988;37:377-388.

83. American Speech-Language-Hearing Association. AIDS/HIV: implications for speech-language pathologists and audiologist. *Asha.* 1990;32:46-48.

84. Leder SB, Blom ED. Tracheoesophageal voice prosthesis fitting and training. In: Blom ED, Singer MI, Hamaker RC, eds. *Tracheoesophageal Voice Restoration Following Total Laryngectomy.* San Diego, Calif: Singular Publishing Group; 1998:57-65.

85. Blom ED, Hamaker RC. Tracheoesophageal voice restoration following total laryngectomy. In: Myers EN, Suen J, eds. *Cancer of the Head and Neck.* Philadelphia, Pa: WB Saunders; 1996:839-852.

86. Grolman W, VanSteenwijk RP, Grolman E, Schouwenburg PF. Airflow and pressure characteristics of three different tracheostoma valves. *Ann Otol Rhinol Laryngol.* 1998;107:312-318.

87. Blom ED. Tracheostoma valve fitting and instruction. In: Blom ED, Singer MI, Hamaker RC, eds. *Tracheoesophageal Voice Restoration Following Total Laryngectomy.* San Diego, Calif: Singular Publishing Group; 1998:103-108.

Index